CHILD PSYCHIATRIC NURSING

Editor

Patricia Clunn, EdD, ARNP, CS

**Professor,
Department of Nursing,
University of Florida,
Miami, Florida**

With 16 illustrations

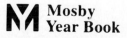

**Mosby
Year Book**

St. Louis   Baltimore   Boston   Chicago   London   Philadelphia   Sydney   Toronto

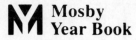
Mosby
Year Book

Dedicated to Publishing Excellence

Editor: Linda L. Duncan
Developmental Editor: Linda Stagg
Project Manager: Carol Sullivan Wiseman
Production Editor: Linda McKinley
Design: Laura Steube

Printed in the United States of America

Mosby–Year Book, Inc.
11830 Westline Industrial Drive, St. Louis, Missouri 63146

Library of Congress Cataloging in Publication Data

Child psychiatric nursing / editor, Patricia Clunn.
   p. cm.
   Includes bibliographical references.
   Includes index.
   ISBN 0-8016-0363-3
   1. Child psychiatric nursing.   I. Clunn, Patricia A.
   [DNLM: 1. Mental Disorders—in infancy & childhood.
2. Psychiatric Nursing—in infancy & childhood.   WY 160 C5361]
RJ502.3.C49 1991
610.73′68—dc20
DNLM/DLC
for Library of Congress

90–13310
CIP

GW/D/D 9 8 7 6 5 4 3 2 1

CHILD PSYCHIATRIC NURSING

Contributors

Donna C. Aguilera, PhD, FAAN, FIAEP
Consultant and Private Practice,
Sherman Oaks, California

Catherine Ayoub, EdM, RN, CS
Clinical Fellow in Psychology,
Department of Psychology,
Harvard University School of Medicine;
Judge Baker Children's Center;
Children's Hospital Medical Center,
Boston, Massachusetts

Patricia Whisonant Brown, MSN, ARNP, CS
Clinical Specialist,
Center of Excellence,
Adolescent Psychiatric Humana Hospital,
Palm Beach, Florida

Deborah Kay Brantly, MS, RNCS
Director of Nursing,
Shadow Mountain Institute,
Tulsa, Oklahoma

Margaret Burkhardt, MSN, MA
PhD Candidate,
University of Miami,
Miami, Florida;
Assistant Professor,
West Virginia University,
School of Nursing,
Charleston Division,
Charleston, West Virginia

Vanya Crabbe, MS, RN
Assistant Nursing Care Coordinator,
Four Winds Hospital,
Lemont, Illinois

Jean Heideman, MS, RN
Unit Leader, Rush Day School,
Rush Medical Center;
Instructor,
Rush College of Nursing,
Chicago, Illinois

Norman Keltner, EdD, RN
Professor,
Department of Nursing,
California State University,
Bakersfield, California

Megan McKee, MS, RN
Clinical Consultant, Mental Health Management,
McLean, Virginia

Judy A. Rollins, MS, RN
Consultant,
Washington, DC

Mary Lou Scavnicky-Mylant, PhD, RN, CPNP
Associate Professor,
University of Wyoming,
School of Nursing;
Private Practice,
Laramie, Wyoming

Donna J. Takacs, MS, RN, C
Director, Quality Attainment
Laureate Psychiatric Clinic and Hospital,
Tulsa, Oklahoma

Linda Whisonant-Haberman, MED
Program Coordinator,
Progressive Directions, Inc.,
Clarksville, Tennessee

Beatrice Crofts Yorker, JD, MS, RN
Chair,
Department of Psychiatric Mental Health Nursing,
Georgia State University,
Atlanta, Georgia

Preface

Caring for the specific mental health problems and needs of infants and children and their families has gained recognition as an important area in the field of psychiatry. This text focuses specifically on the mental health-psychiatric nursing of infants and children. The significance of child psychiatric nurse specialists and the specific body of knowledge and skills needed was highlighted with the development of a specific national certification examination and standards of practice for child psychiatric nursing and with the inclusion and expansion of the disorders usually first evident in infancy and childhood in the DSM-III and DSM-III-R.

The text provides the recent knowledge required for child psychiatric nursing in home and family environments, general and psychiatric hospitals, day care centers, schools, and community mental health centers. It is also a useful adjunct to adult psychiatric texts. The content spans the spectrum of children's mental health, emotional problems, and severe psychopathology, starting with an overview of the challenges developing children encounter in contemporary society. From this mental health framework, the text progresses to more complex psychopathology, intervention strategies, and suggestions for fostering and enhancing therapeutic treatment settings. The DSM-III-R classification and 1990 NANDA nursing diagnoses are used throughout the text and are important companions to it.

Part I focuses on the foundations of child psychiatric nursing practice. Included in this section are concepts basic to psychiatric-mental health nursing of children and their families, particularly ethical and legal considerations, the nursing process, communication with children, and the therapeutic relationship. Part II addresses prevention and early intervention. The special issues, roles, and functions of child psychiatric nurses in consultation-liaison child advocacy roles are presented in case examples. Interventions with child clients with psychologic and psychosomatic illnesses are discussed. In Part III the psychopathologic DSM-III-R disorders of childhood that may require psychiatric hospitalization and the highly coordinated efforts of the mental health interdisciplinary team are considered. Child psychiatric nurses' role as case finder, case manager, consultant, and child advocate in long-term residential treatment settings is emphasized. Some of the many assessment tools and psychologic measures for evaluation of children are also discussed. Part IV addresses specific treatment modalities designed for health promotion, maintenance, and restoration used in child psychiatric nursing. These include specialized therapies for chronically distressed children and psychosocial interventions for children with special problems, such as AIDS. Tactics for staff support that facilitate developing and maintaining children's therapeutic treatment environment and examples of treatment settings are also presented.

Child psychiatric nursing is so highly specialized that no one person holds expertise in all areas. Without the knowledge of the contributing authors, this text would not have been possible. Special appreciation to Linda Duncan, Linda Stagg, and Linda McKinley of Mosby-Year Book, Inc. for their recognition and support of the need for this text and for sharing our dedication and professional concern for children's health.

Patricia Clunn

Contents

PART IV   PSYCHOTHERAPEUTIC INTERVENTIONS

Part I

Foundations for Practice

Chapter 1

Historical Overview and Current Status of Child Psychiatric Nursing

Jean Heideman
Vanya Crabbe

All history becomes subjective; in other words there is properly no history, only biography. Every mind must know the whole lesson for itself, must go over the whole ground. What it does not see, what it does not live, it will know.

RALPH WALDO EMERSON

The history of child psychiatric nursing is brief in comparison to other clinical specialties in nursing, partly because of the only recent concern of the general public and professionals for children's health and welfare. Before the turn of the century, children lacked judicious treatment and had few rights. They were seen as an economic value and were considered the property of their parents. These past values sharply contrast current thinking, which views children as the future contributors to our world and emphasizes medical and psychiatric care for their special needs.

The evolution of the specialty area of child psychiatric nursing has been strongly influenced by the history and evolution of psychiatry, child psychiatry, and pediatrics. Psychiatry is one of the newer and least accepted specialties in medicine, and child psychiatry, with its roots in the child guidance movement, has been further isolated from the mainstream of psychiatric care (Pothier, 1984).

This chapter traces the origins and evolution of child psychiatry and child psychiatric nursing. Child psychiatric nurses have established a unique role in the multidisciplinary team, strengthening the independence of these advanced practitioners. Future role changes and research needs are also discussed.

Origins of Child Psychiatry

Before 1900, psychiatrists were almost exclusively concerned with adult behavior disorders. Although acknowledged on occasion, child behavior disorders received very little attention. Children were viewed as miniature adults, evincing similar problems and benefiting from the same reasoned advice as adults (Aries, 1962).

A more extensive view of children and a focus on the assessment and treatment of childhood disorders began in the twentieth century. Laws were passed to safeguard children's interests. The Federal Children's Bureau was established in 1912 to protect the welfare of children. In 1938, the Wages and Hour Bill prohibited employment of children under the age of 16 in hazardous occupations. The change in thinking continued with the proclamation of the International Bill of Rights for Children in 1975, the International Year of the Child.

Child Guidance Movement and Chemotherapeutic Revolution

Some of Sigmund Freud's theories of psychoanalysis led to the initial treatment of children. In 1909, Freud published his paper on the treatment of "Little Hans." Melanie Klein and Anna Freud were later pioneers in the analytic treatment of children. Shortly after the introduction of psychoanalysis in America the first child guidance clinic was founded by William Healy in 1909 in Chicago (Ollendick and Hersen, 1983). It was named the Chicago Psychopathic Institute and served the juvenile court.

The growth of child guidance clinics in the United States began slowly. These clinics provided the data base on children's mental health needs, and most were affiliated with the juvenile courts. Later, these treatment services were opened at demonstration child guidance clinics located in the community but were often isolated from medical schools or hospitals (Fagin, 1974).

In 1935, Leo Kanner published the first American textbook on the subject; it was entitled *Child Psychiatry*. The 1930s and 1940s were also marked by the beginning of the chemotherapeutic revolution. The first effective drugs used to treat children, amphetamines, were introduced. Professionals in child clinics became enthusiastic about preventing disorders in childhood, and the community was led to expect that each new child clinic made an adult mental hospital obsolete (Eisenberg, 1969). During this time, psychiatric nurses became involved in child psychiatry.

Emergence of Child Psychiatric Nursing

The child guidance movement represented an outgrowth of the social reform movement that flowered in the late nineteenth and early twentieth centuries in the United States. Previous efforts at social reform had largely focused on the care of individuals in prisons and asylums. One of the leaders in this earlier reform was Dorothea Dix, a nurse, who implored the legislature of Massachusetts in 1843 for more humane treatment conditions. She described insane persons who were locked and chained naked in cages, closets, cellars, stalls, and pens and beaten with rods (Rosen, Clark, and Kivitz, 1976). Within this group of insane persons, Dorothea Dix observed children and adolescents.

Nurses did not have an official role in the child guidance clinics. Psychiatric nursing was still largely a mixture of modified "mother's role" activities, discipline of patients, and custodial companionship care (Peplau, 1989). The psychiatrist was assigned as the therapist, the psychologist as the psychometrist, and the social worker as the history taker, family caseworker, and coordinator of necessary community resources (Fagin, 1974). When the chemotherapeutic revolution began, nurses were needed to perform the technical procedures associated with somatic treatments. When institutionalized patients became more manageable, nurses began to form therapeutic relationships, a change from their earlier custodial role. Nurses also began to recognize that additional education would further their role on the treatment team.

Federal Funding and Child Psychiatric Nursing Education

The National Mental Health Act became law in 1946. During World War II a major shift in viewing psychiatric casualties of war occurred. World War I veterans with psychiatric difficulties received little sympathy and were often viewed as cowards. The new idea that "everyone has a breaking point" generated not only sympathy but also generous funding supporting efforts addressing mental illness (Peplau, 1989). One section of the National Mental Health Act provided government funds to train much needed professionals in psychiatry, psychology, social work, and nursing. These funds stimulated the establishment of graduate programs in psychiatric nursing, ultimately leading to the development of not only psychiatric nursing but the entire field of nursing (Peplau, 1989).

In 1948 psychiatric mental health nursing was incorporated into the curriculum of nursing schools. The objectives were threefold: (1) increase the number of educated psychiatric nurses, (2) improve the quality of psychiatric nursing programs in baccalaureate schools of nursing (later known as the mental health integration projects), and (3) provide some degree of mental health education in all areas where nurses could face mental health problems (Chamberlain, 1983). Emphasis was placed on therapeutic and preventive intervention rather than on functional and custodial care.

In 1952, *Interpersonal Relations in Nursing* by Hildegard Peplau became the first published psychiatric nursing theory written by a nurse. Her classic work formed some of the groundwork for expanded roles of nurses as psychotherapists. Developed by Peplau and graduate students in psychiatric nursing at Teachers' College, Columbia University, the *tools and tasks* of infancy and childhood became guidelines in an early nursing text by Fagin and are still studied in basic psychiatric nursing programs (1972). Fagin described the role of child psychiatric nurses as intervening: (1) to assist children with new learning regarding themselves and their world, (2) to assist children and their family with relearning of roles, relationships, and expectations, and (3) to assist in restoring deprived aspects of living.

Boston University offered the first graduate program for the training of child psychiatric nurses in 1954, 8 years after the passage of the National Mental Health Act (Pothier, 1976). Six other universities soon developed programs. Also in 1954, the National Institute of Mental Health (NIMH) recognized the shortage of nurses in the specialty and the need for prevention and early intervention for disturbed children (Chamberlain, 1983). The first child psychiatric nursing project was established at NIMH to provide further funding and resources.

The professional Nurse Traineeship Program was established in 1956. Over

33,980 long-term traineeships were awarded to increase the supply of registered nurses prepared for teaching, administration, and supervision (American Nurses' Association, 1974). The strides in psychiatric nursing education were supported by NIMH funding that enabled the profession to support research training and develop doctoral programs.

In 1960, Nathan Ackerman founded The Family Institute—the first center of its kind. Psychiatric nurses became involved and gained recognition as family therapists. A summary of the events influencing child psychiatric nursing is shown in Table 1-1.

The Community Mental Health Act

In 1963, President Kennedy called for a "bold new approach" in treatment of the mentally retarded and mentally ill. That year Congress passed the Community Mental Health Act, initiating funding for community mental health centers. In the 1960s social movements that changed and challenged traditional ideologies occurred and affected nursing. The child was recognized as an individual with unique needs and problems, the family was included in the decision-making process, and child family nurses assumed their responsibility as vital contacts in the health care system (Mott, Fazekas, and James, 1985). Some nurse psychotherapists opened private practices. The American Nurses' Association (ANA) recognized the need for self-regulatory measures to protect the public and published *Standards of Psychiatric Nursing Practice* in 1966.

In 1968, members of the seven child psychiatric nursing programs met to discuss the consistency and inclusiveness of the philosophy of child psychiatric nursing. This meeting was supported by the NIMH. The conference participants discussed the philosophy, roles and images, and conceptual framework in child psychiatric nursing, and the published findings further defined the practice and functions of child psychiatric nurses. The group also publicly resolved that custodial institutions were inappropriate for the care and treatment of disturbed children (Pothier, 1984). Community centers were to provide a full range of services for children, adolescents, and adult patients. However, funding never matched the community needs, and children's services received a low priority. Only 4% of the available professional outpatient positions were filled by nurses. Access to clients was diminished because the role for nurses in large hospitals was not transferred to community settings nor was there recognition of the availability of competent, well-educated nurses (Pothier, 1984).

Changes in Child Psychiatric Nursing

During the 1970s a new political era that brought federal cuts to many mental health programs began, but private for-profit hospitals and residential care facilities for psychiatric patients expanded with the support of insurance programs (Pothier, 1984). Many of these facilities served children and adolescents and provided new opportunities for nursing. Although nursing roles were closely tied to medicine, child psychiatric nurses expanded their therapeutic role with children who were being treated in inpatient and outpatient settings and in schools (Pothier, 1984).

Table 1-1   Events Affecting Child Psychiatric Nursing

Year	Event
1909-1930	Child guidance movement began. Nurses did not have formalized role in treatment of children.
1930-1940	Chemotherapeutic revolution began. Nurses performed technical procedures. As patients became more manageable, nurses began to form therapeutic relationships.
1946	National Mental Health Act provided for training of psychiatric nurses, with funding for both graduate and undergraduate programs.
1952	Hildegard Peplau published *Interpersonal Relationships in Nursing.* First published psychiatric nursing theory and remains a classic.
1953	American Academy of Child Psychiatry formed to provide national forum for child psychiatrists.
1954	Boston University offered first graduate program for training of child psychiatric nurses. Six other universities soon developed programs.
1955	Congress approved Public Law 182, enabling Joint Commission of Mental Illness and Health to conduct survey of mental illness in United States. One recommendation included developing therapeutic roles of nurses.
1956	Professional Nurse Traineeship Program began. From fiscal year 1957 to fiscal year 1972, 33,989 long-term traineeships were awarded to increase supply of RNs prepared for teaching, administration, and supervision.
1959	Child psychiatry became official subspecialty of psychiatry.
1960	Nathan Ackerman founded Family Institute, providing a resource for nurses to receive advanced training in family therapy.
1963	*Journal of Psychiatric Nursing* and *Perspectives in Psychiatric Care* began publication.
1965	Joint Commission on Mental Health of Children was established to support child advocacy.
1967	American Nurses' Association's "Position Paper on Psychiatric Nursing" stated that psychiatric nurses functioned as clinical specialists, individual psychotherapists, as well as group, milieu, and family therapists.
1971	Advocates for Child Psychiatric Nursing, Inc. formed.
1972	Claire Fagin published the classic text *Nursing in Child Psychiatry.*
1975	International Year of the Child declared.
1980s	Child psychiatric nurses focused on theory, practice, and research.
1985	Standards of Child and Adolescent Psychiatric and Mental Health Nursing Practice approved.
1985	Claire Fagin became president of American Orthopsychiatric Association.
1988	*Journal of Child and Adolescent Psychiatric and Mental Health Nursing* began publication.

A severe nursing shortage swept the country in the mid to late 1970s, partly because of increasing career opportunities for women in other areas. In 1974, amendments to the Taft-Hartley Act allowed nurses in private hospitals the right to collective bargaining. However, nurses continued to lack a strong political base. The federal cuts of the 1970s shaped both the clinical experiences of nurses and the curriculum in graduate and undergraduate programs. Anderson (1975) states, "Child psychiatric nursing is indeed influenced by economic factors and is dependent on an outside agency for its direction in education and practice." Other problems described by Anderson included nursing's dependence on other groups to define its education and practice and the influence of federal funding on curriculum development.

CHILD PSYCHIATRY NURSING SPECIALTY ORGANIZATIONS

In 1971 the Advocates for Child Psychiatric Nursing was formed, and the first national meeting was held the next year. The name of the organization was chosen carefully (Scharer, 1985). The word *for* signified advocacy for child psychiatric nurses themselves and for psychiatric nursing. It was a clinical forum fulfilling a need for the subspecialty of child psychiatric nurses. The organization, which includes 150 to 200 individuals nationally, was incorporated in 1975.

The ANA Council on Psychiatric and Mental Health Nursing was formed in the late 1970s and developed a child and adolescent psychiatric and mental health nursing specialty group. Although the Advocates for Child Psychiatric Nursing have remained a separate organization, most child psychiatric nurses are members of both groups. The two organizations collaborated in developing *Standards of Child and Adolescent Psychiatric Nursing and Mental Health Nursing Practice* (published in 1985), and members of both groups network on other specialty issues affecting the clinical area.

STANDARDS OF PRACTICE AND ANA CERTIFICATION

The official standards of practice designate specific definitions, educational preparation, and performance expectations for both generalists and clinical specialists. Consistent with the ANA standards (ANA, 1985), they include outcome or evaluation criteria, often used in areas such as third-party payment and quality assurance.

The standards defined four distinctive, interlocking characteristics of child and adolescent psychiatric and mental health nursing practice: "A preventive approach to intervention, a consideration of developmental variables, attention to interacting social systems, and a focus on nonverbal communication and activity" (ANA, 1985). These characteristics influence every aspect of nursing practice with the child and "apply to any setting in which psychiatric and mental health nursing with children and adolescents is practiced by generalists or specialists in child and adolescent psychiatric mental health nursing" (ANA, 1985).

The roles of generalists and clinical nurse specialists practicing child and adolescent psychiatric nursing described in the ANA standards and shown in the box define the knowledge, skills, and competency required for clinicians practicing in

ANA Standards of Child and Adolescent Psychiatric and Mental Health Nursing Practice

Professional practice standards

Standard I. Theory The nurse applies appropriate, scientifically sound theory as a basis for nursing practice decisions.

Standard II. Assessment The nurse systematically collects, records, and analyzes data that are comprehensive and accurate.

Standard III. Diagnosis The nurse, in expressing conclusions supported by recorded assessment and current scientific premises, uses nursing diagnoses and/or standard classifications of mental disorders for childhood and adolescence.

Standard IV. Planning The nurse develops a nursing care plan with specific goals and interventions delineating nursing actions unique to the needs of each child or adolescent, as well as those of the family and other relevant interactive social systems.

Standard V. Intervention The nurse intervenes as guided by the nursing care plan to implement nursing actions that promote, maintain, or restore physical and mental health, prevent illness, effect rehabilitation in childhood and adolescence, and restore developmental progression.

Standard V-A. Intervention: Therapeutic Environment The nurse provides, structures, and maintains a therapeutic environment in collaboration with the child or adolescent, the family, and other health care providers.

Standard V-B. Intervention: Activities of Daily Living The nurse uses the activities of daily living in a goal-directed way to foster the physical and mental well-being of the child or adolescent and family.

Standard V-C. Intervention: Psychotherapeutic Interventions The nurse uses psychotherapeutic interventions to assist children or adolescents and families to develop, improve, or regain their adaptive functioning to promote health, prevent illness, and facilitate rehabilitation.

Standard V-D. Intervention: Psychotherapy* The child and adolescent psychiatric and mental health specialist uses advanced clinical expertise to function as a psychotherapist for the child or adolescent and family and accepts professional accountability for nursing practice.

Standard V-E. Intervention: Health Teaching and Anticipatory Guidance The nurse assists the child or adolescent and family to achieve more satisfying and productive patterns of living through health teaching and anticipatory guidance.

Standard V-F. Intervention: Somatic Therapies The nurse uses knowledge of somatic therapies with the child or adolescent and family to enhance therapeutic interventions.

Standard VI. Evaluation The nurse evaluates the response of the child or adolescent and family to nursing actions in order to revise the data base, nursing diagnoses, and nursing care plan.

Professional performance standards

Standard VII. Quality Assurance The nurse participates in peer review and other means of evaluation to ensure quality of nursing care provided for children and adolescents and their families.

From American Nurses' Association: Standards of child and adolescent psychiatric and mental health nursing practice, Kansas City, Mo, 1985, The Association.
*Standards V-D and X apply only to the clinical specialist in child and adolescent psychiatric and mental health nursing.

Continued.

ANA Standards of Child and Adolescent Psychiatric and Mental Health Nursing Practice — cont'd

Standard VIII. Continuing Education The nurse assumes responsibility for continuing education and professional development and contributes to the professional growth of others studying children's and adolescents' mental health.

Standard IX. Interdisciplinary Collaboration The nurse collaborates with other health care providers in assessing, planning, implementing, and evaluating programs and other activities related to child and adolescent psychiatric and mental health nursing.

Standard X. Use of Community Health Systems* The nurse participates with other members of the community in assessing, planning, implementing, and evaluating mental health services and community systems that attend to primary, secondary, and tertiary prevention of mental disorders in children and adolescents.

Standard XI. Research The nurse contributes to nursing and the child and adolescent psychiatric and mental health field through innovations in theory and practice and participation in research and communicates these contributions.

---

these different roles. These competencies were further clarified in the ANA's certification test for child and adolescent clinical specialists and generalists.

Current Status

Today, child psychiatric nurses are integral members of the interdisciplinary team. The 1985 ANA standards clearly state the importance of the nurse collaborating with other health care providers in assessing, planning, implementing, and evaluating programs and other activities related to child and adolescent psychiatric and mental health nursing. Collaboration occurs in teaching, supervision, research, and management.

Pothier, Norbeck, and Laliberte (1985) surveyed the members of the Advocates for Child Psychiatric Nursing and the child adolescent subgroups of ANA Council of Specialists in Psychiatric and Mental Health Nursing. They found that many prepared specialists in child and adolescent psychiatric nursing spent a larger percentage of their time working with an adult population. Children who need mental health services are not receiving them, a trend that is likely to continue because of a deficiency of both professional personnel and clinical programs. Only 5% of practicing psychiatric nurses specialize in child and adolescent treatment.

Reimbursement policies can interfere with the use of nurses in some outpatient settings and private practices. Psychiatric nurses have also been recognized as legitimate providers of third-party reimbursable services, and more than 50% of the states offer various reimbursement fees (Fagin, 1983). Given the disparity between the need for child psychiatric services and the number of qualified professionals available, interdisciplinary communication, cooperation, and collaboration needs to be strengthened (American Academy of Child Psychiatry, 1983).

Historically there has been a debate in the literature about whether nurses can be psychotherapists. The reason many nurses may experience difficulty in taking on an independent practice role may have its roots in the traditional medical setting in which nurses are often seen as adjunct staff to the therapeutic relationship between the psychiatrist and the client. Nurses must take an active role in research to show the efficacy of psychotherapy and other treatment modalities implemented by nurses. As Peplau (1989) suggests, nurses must monitor and, if necessary, examine any erosion of their identity as psychotherapists.

Both adult and child psychiatrists are moving toward a biomedical model that defines mental illness as a chemical imbalance or genetic deficiency. Some nurses will follow this trend; others will seek unique roles in private practices, schools, community settings, and employee assistance programs. Those nurses who choose to follow the trend must continue advanced therapeutic practice to prevent the return to providing adjunct and technical procedures exclusively.

Levels of Prevention

As emphasized in the standards, primary prevention in child psychiatry promotes strong relationships between child psychiatric nurses and other nurses working in child health. Current primary prevention efforts focus on many of the modern concerns in the health care system such as disease-related diagnoses. Evolving during the late 1970s, infant psychiatry has grown rapidly as reflected in its inclusion in the 1980 DSM-III. Prenatal classes for parents and consultations to parent groups are two areas in which child psychiatric nurses can offer information on normal development and the stresses of child care and parenting. Since they often have the most contact with high-risk infants in the community, child psychiatric nurses are also prepared to provide consultation to public health agencies.

Caplan (1961) described primary prevention as helping to reduce the risk of people developing mental illness. Nurses involved in primary prevention of childhood disorders also have the opportunity to participate in legislative issues related to children at a local, state, and federal level. Collaboration between child psychiatric nurses and maternal child nurses is essential to assess further needs for primary prevention projects. Common preventive activities include ongoing observation and assessment, developmental teaching, anticipating guidance, support for age-appropriate behaviors, and counseling of children and families for developmental and situational crises (ANA, 1985).

Secondary prevention activities are targeted toward individuals who have been identified with mental health problems (ANA, 1985). Case finding, early diagnosis, and effective treatment are the focuses at this level. Child psychiatric nurses may be involved in family assessments and counseling to help a family faced with a crisis, such as loss and separation by death or divorce, to progress to the next developmental stage. Once identified, children at risk for problems beyond those of normal adjustments need early intervention. Child psychiatric nurses are also involved as consultants for day care centers and schools to identify mental health needs at an early age and may provide a wealth of resources to school nurses with regular contact with school-age children. Educating children and adolescents about mental health and drug and alcoholism abuse, screening adolescents for drug use, and assessing levels of stress in children are all areas that child psychiatric nurses address.

Tertiary preventive roles include providing a daily therapeutic milieu in inpatient, residential, or day programs. Immediate therapeutic interventions dealing with behavior and emotional difficulties allow children to develop their problem-solving skills and to progress along normal developmental lines. Child psychiatric nurses conduct individual, group, and family psychotherapy at this level in both inpatient and outpatient settings. Nurses also assess the need for and help administer somatic treatments and provide education for the child and family.

INTRAPROFESSIONAL COLLABORATION

References for child psychiatric nursing indicate an overlapping of child psychiatric nursing with the theories of adult and pediatric nursing, especially in family therapy and preventive developmental mental health interventions. These areas emphasize the need for continued practice distinction by child psychiatric nurses and other nurse specialty groups.

Because of their limited number, child psychiatric clinicians need to be aware of the theoretic knowledge base and interventions performed by nurses in other areas of clinical nurse practice. The use of intradisciplinary referrals and collaboration is critical for child psychiatric clinicians to work with those children in need of their unique expertise. Possible collaborators include child psychiatric and mental retardation specialists.

Current Issues

Despite the growth of substantive knowledge in the field of child psychiatry during the past two decades as reflected in the DSM-III-R section inclusion and the ANA's recognition of the subspecialty with the published standards (1985) and certification in child psychiatric nursing (1974), most basic nursing programs do not include student learning experiences in child psychiatry and questions related to the area are not part of State Board examinations. Most nurses begin their careers without knowledge of child psychopathology and appropriate child and family nursing intervention. This limited exposure to child psychiatry may contribute to the lack of interest in graduate specialization in child psychiatric nursing. In 1989, only 11 graduate programs in the United States listed the specific offering of child and adolescent psychiatric mental health nursing master's preparation. However, other master's programs offer child psychiatric nursing as a subspecialty within the adult psychiatric nursing tract. Many graduate programs can no longer offer many clinical specialty programs because of economic constraints.

In child psychiatric care settings, the lack of prepared nurse clinicians created a service and staffing gap that was partly filled by other mental health professionals, such as social workers and psychologists, and by paraprofessional workers, such as child care workers and technicians. In nursing, this gap has been filled by other specialty areas, such as adult psychiatric, pediatric, and maternal-child health specialists.

Some nurses achieve experiences in post-master and postdoctoral internship programs, reflecting the growing trend toward adjusting academic programs and the practice requirements for certification in all clinical specialty areas. Therefore ANA credentials in child psychiatric nursing can be achieved through special petitions of nurses with masters degrees who are academically prepared in other areas, such as adult psychiatric nursing, by completing post-master internships, or by providing documentation of the child specialty content gained through continuing education and appropriate clinical practice supervision.

Because of the limited number of programs at the graduate level, few nurses are available to train other nurses in both clinical and academic settings. Of the approximately 10,000 active psychiatric mental health specialists, child psychiatric nursing specialists include less than 1000 prepared at the master or doctoral level. The nursing shortage has also contributed to fewer psychiatric nurses in practice and decreased enrollment in undergraduate and graduate nursing programs. Federal support for education has continued to decrease over the past decade. Funding by NIMH peaked in fiscal year 1969 and has continued to decline to a record low in fiscal year 1986, when only 20 projects in 16 schools received funding (Pothier, Norbeck, and Laliberte, 1985). Chamberlain (1987) also reported that only 5 projects funded by NIMH in that year were programs exclusively related to child psychiatric nursing. The majority of children and adolescents with severe emotional disorders are receiving either inadequate nursing treatment or none at all.

The number of children who need services continues to increase. To meet the demands of this growing population, more qualified child psychiatric nurses must be educated at all levels of practice. Nursing education programs need to assess the theoretic and experimental components related to severely emotionally disturbed children and their families in both undergraduate and in master and doctoral programs.

In addition to theoretic components, clinical experiences for students must also be enhanced. Clinical specialists in child and adolescent psychiatric nursing need exposure to both inpatient and outpatient settings, and collaboration with other disciplines must occur. As Peplau (1989) points out, every psychiatric nurse must become involved in encouraging schools of nursing to include adequate content and clinical experience in psychiatric nursing in all generic programs so that all nursing students are well prepared to care for psychiatric patients and interested in graduate education in psychiatric nursing.

Research and Practice Issues

Nursing research in child psychiatric nursing had been essentially nonexistent before the last decade because of the small number of doctorally prepared nurses specializing in child and adolescent psychiatric nursing. The need for research in this field is critical to further advance both the educational and clinical aspects of the specialty. Nurses need to develop outcome and treatment model studies that delineate the most effective treatment for children and adolescents. High-risk groups need to be identified and early intervention programs need to be designed and tested to prevent emotional disorders. Normal development should also be studied to determine what causes certain children to be at risk for emotional problems. Family research is needed to study both healthy interactions in high-functioning families and the effect of family treatment on families with difficulties.

Current issues affecting child psychiatric nursing include homeless children, children with AIDS, poverty, the influence of drug and alcohol use on children, adolescent suicide, and the changing structure of the family addressing single parents and blended families. Other important interests include an increase in neglect, physical and sexual child abuse and in the number of children and adolescents who abuse chemicals. Future consideration may involve children conceived through in vitro fertilization, children placed in foster care, the effect of organ transplants on emotional development, and the effect of day care treatment. Research is needed in all of these areas, and child psychiatric nurses must publish their findings.

REFERENCES

American Academy of Child Psychiatry: Child psychiatry: a plan for the coming decade, Washington, DC, 1983, American Academy of Child Psychiatry.

American Nurses' Association: Facts about nursing, 1972 and 1973, Kansas City, Mo, 1974, The Association.

American Nurses' Association Council on Psychiatric and Mental Health Nursing: Standards of child and adolescent psychiatric and mental health nursing practice, Kansas City, Mo, 1985, The Association.

American Nurses' Association Division on Certification: Knowledge, skills and abilities required for ANA certification examination in child and adolescent psychiatric mental health nursing, 1986, Kansas City, Mo, 1974, The Association.

American Psychiatric Association: Diagnostic and statistical manual of mental disorders, ed 3, Washington, DC, 1980, American Psychiatric Association.

American Psychiatric Association: Diagnostic and statistical manual of mental disorders, ed 3, rev, Washington, DC, 1987, American Psychiatric Association.

Anderson M: Forces affecting the education of child psychiatric nurses, doctoral dissertation,

Aries P: Centuries of childhood, New York, 1962, Vintage Books.

Caplan G: Prevention of mental disorders in children, New York, 1961, Basic Books, Inc.

Chamberlain J: The role of the federal government in the development of psychiatric nursing, J Psychosoc Nurs Ment Health Serv 4:21, 1983.

Chamberlain J: Update on psychiatric mental health nursing education at the federal level, Arch Psychiatr Nurs 1:132, 1987.

Eisenberg L: Child psychiatry: the past quarter century, Am J Orthopsychiatry 39:38, 1969.

Fagin C: Nursing in child psychiatry, St. Louis, 1972, The CV Mosby Co.

Fagin C: Readings in child and adolescent psychiatric nursing, St. Louis, 1974, The CV Mosby Co.

Fagin C: Concepts for the future: competition and substitution, J Psychosoc Nurs Ment Health Serv 21:36, 1983.

Kanner L: Child psychiatry: retrospect and prospect, Am J Psychiatry 117:1522, 1968.

Mott S, Fazekas N, and James S: Nursing care of children and families: a holistic approach, Menlo Park, Calif, 1985, Addison-Wesley Publishing Co, Inc.

Ollendick T and Hersen M: Handbook of child psychopathology, New York and London, 1983, Plenum Publishing Corp.

Peplau H: Future directions in psychiatric nursing from the perspective of history, J Psychosoc Nurs Ment Health Serv 27:21, 1989.

Pothier P: Mental health counseling with children, Boston, 1976, Little, Brown & Co, Inc.

Pothier P: Child psychiatric nursing, J Psychosoc Nurs Ment Health Serv 22:22, 1984.

Pothier P, Norbeck J, and Laliberte M: Child psychiatric nursing: the gap between need and utilization, J Psychosoc Nurs Ment Health Serv 23:18, 1985.

Rosen M, Clark GR, and Kivitz MS, editors: The history of mental retardation, vol 1, Collected papers, Baltimore, 1976, University Park Press.

Scharer K: An oral history of the advocates for child psychiatric nursing, Inc, interview, Nov 1985.

Chapter 2

Legal and Ethical Issues in Child Psychiatric Nursing

Beatrice Crofts Yorker

Although the past century has reflected significant progress in the law recognizing the special needs of children, many conflicting precedents still exist. This chapter addresses the major laws affecting children, children in the mental health system, the potential liability of the nurse, the advocacy role of nurses, and the ethical issues facing child psychiatric nurses.

Historical Perspective

Throughout most of recorded history, children had few rights and almost no protection under the law. Children were killed if they were the wrong sex and were used as sacrifices, cheap or free labor, and sex objects.

Ancient Hebrew law allowed parents to kill or sell their children. Roman law was dominated by the doctrine of "paterfamilias" in its approach to parents and children. Nicholas (1962) provides an explanation of this doctrine:

The family is the legal unit of society. Its head, the paterfamilias, is the only full person known to the law. His children of whatever age, though they are citizens and therefore have rights in public law, are subject to his unfettered power of life and death.

English Common Law emerged during the twelfth century. It still dominates many modern legal principles. For the first time the law dealing with persons was distinguished from the property and inheritance laws. Previously, children and wives were considered property of adult males. These new laws recognized duties of parents, for example, "to maintain, educate and protect" their children and duties of children, for example, "to honor and obey" their parents. They also recognized the power of parents over their children (Blackstone, 1765). One of these parental rights was discipline. "The English Common Law had great faith in the workings of parental affection and the thought that a parent might unnaturally brutalize his child was unthinkable" (Johnson, 1984).

By the fifteenth century the influence of Christian humanism could be seen in the law when a new concept of state intervention — provision of a guardian — emerged in the otherwise absolute domain of the father. Child advocates first took legal action to remove a child from an abusive situation in the late 1800s. The only laws then available to protect children were for the prevention of cruelty to animals (Schueller, 1984).

Research in child development had an obvious influence on the legal system when the boundaries defining children's and parents' rights were established. *Reforming the Law* (Melton, 1987) is devoted to the integration of research on child development and the social sciences into aspects of the law and the judicial process. For example, a "mature" minor may have more autonomy about using contraceptives or obtaining an abortion than a minor who does not exhibit certain decision-making capacities (*Bellotti v. Baird,* 1979). Advertising for beer and cigarettes, however, has been outlawed because minors are considered highly impressionable and unable to decide for themselves whether to use these products (Schueller, 1984).

The framework for understanding many of the issues involved in child advocacy involves the triad of parent-child-state, with considerable interdependence among the three interests. The courts must balance the right of parents to have family privacy and autonomy in raising their children and the public health and welfare interest of the state. Children have rights to be free from unnecessary interference from the state and to be protected if parents are not sufficiently providing for their welfare. Davis and Schwartz (1987) suggest that the list of interests shown in Figure 2-1 often conflict and must be balanced by the courts.

Private Law

TORTS

Much inconsistency is found in the statutory and case law regarding children's status, capacity, competence, and liabilities. Private law includes torts (private harms by one person against another) and contracts (the ability to enter into a legally binding agreement). Examples of private harms against a person include trespass, negligence, assault, and battery. The general rule is that no automatic immunity exists to protect minors from liability for their harmful acts. If a 6-year-old child tramples on the neighbors' strawberry plants, the child (not the parents) can be found liable for the damages. Children are held to the standard of care of "the reasonable child" of a similar age and experience. Minors can be held to an adult standard of care if they are engaged in an adult activity such as driving (Prosser, 1971).

Children can sue and be sued but do require an adult acting on their behalf during the proceedings. Examples of tort lawsuits brought by minors and even infants include malpractice suits for medical harm, negligence suits for injuries arising out of car accidents, and, recently, suits against parents and educators for wrongful life, inadequate parenting, excessive corporal punishment, and "educational malpractice." The child rarely wins in the latter cases (Davis and Schwartz, 1987).

CONTRACTS

In contract law the law takes almost the opposite view. Minors are protected and deemed lacking capacity, so agreements or contracts cannot be enforced against them. For example, if a minor purchases a car on credit and then defaults on the

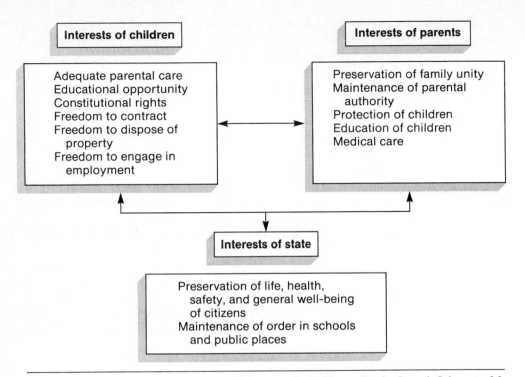

Interests of children

Adequate parental care
Educational opportunity
Constitutional rights
Freedom to contract
Freedom to dispose of
    property
Freedom to engage in
    employment

Interests of parents

Preservation of family unity
Maintenance of parental
    authority
Protection of children
Education of children
Medical care

Interests of state

Preservation of life, health,
    safety, and general well-being
    of citizens
Maintenance of order in schools
    and public places

Figure 2-1   Child advocacy: parent-child-state triad. (From Davis S and Schwartz M: Children's rights and the law, Lexington, Mass, 1987, DC Heath & Co.)

payments, "The law is of the view that the minor has the absolute power to disaffirm the contract; therefore he is entitled to return of his money and release from any further obligation" (Davis and Schwartz, 1987). However, a minor may enforce a contract against another party.

The doctrine of emancipation reduces the harshness of this law. A minor is considered emancipated or free from parental authority if married, serving in the military, living separately from the parents, or otherwise self-supporting. Emancipated minors can contract for health care services and give informed consent and may be regarded as adults in the eyes of the law.

Constitutional Law

Understanding the concept of *federalism* is essential to any discussion of constitutional law. According to the founding fathers, states were allowed to regulate most matters of day to day life. However, if the state promulgated laws that violated the Constitution or its amendments then the federal courts could intervene and strike down laws that were deemed unconstitutional.

The states have enacted a variety of laws that protect children and have mandated certain activities considered best for the child (for example, education and vaccination) in the twentieth century. Most statutes have filled a void in the legal arena of children's rights, but some laws were overly paternalistic and based on notions of antiquated morality.

When an individual believes that the law violates a constitutionally protected right, the courts apply the aforementioned balancing process between parent, child, and state. Table 2-1 illustrates the major constitutional sources used to challenge laws regulating families and children.

The Supreme Court is the final appellate tribunal where disagreements between individuals and the government are decided. Table 2-2 summarizes the landmark Supreme Court decisions affecting children.

From 1967 to 1977 a set of decisions oriented toward individual rights were handed down by the Supreme Court. The "right to privacy" became a fundamental right, flowing from certain clauses in the Constitutional amendments. The 1980s brought a change in the membership of the Court. With a new cadre of Reagan appointees, the majority vote of the 1970s dwindled to a minority vote on many issues relating to the right to privacy.

The balance between children's autonomy, parental control, and state authority ebbs and flows . . . [This] has generated some uncertainty over the Supreme Court's ability, as an institution reflecting and influencing societal values over the long term, to develop consistent, cohesive policy toward children and their position in the law (Davis and Schwartz, 1987).

Nurses must be able to conceptualize the relationship between Supreme Court decisions and the ability of states to regulate issues involving human rights.

Confidentiality

Confidentiality is a broad concept covering the areas of constitutionally based right to privacy, tortiously defined right to privacy, laws regarding confidentiality in treatment, and privilege.

RIGHT TO PRIVACY

The landmark case of *Griswold v. Connecticut* (1965) established the constitutional basis of a fundamental right to privacy. Justice Douglas explained:

Various guarantees create zones of privacy. The right of association contained in the penumbra of the First Amendment is one, as we have seen. The Third Amendment in its prohibition against the quartering of soldiers "in any house" in time of peace without the consent of the owner is another facet of that privacy. The Fourth Amendment explicitly affirms the "right of the people to be secure in their persons, houses, papers, and effects, against unreasonable searches and seizures." The Fifth Amendment in its Self-Incrimination Clause enables the citizen to create a zone of privacy which government may not force him to surrender to his detriment. The Ninth Amendment provides: "The enumeration in the Constitution, of certain rights, shall not be construed to deny or disparage others retained by the people" (*Griswold v. Connecticut,* 1965).

Although the Court recognizes this right to privacy for adults, children are rarely granted this fundamental right apart from their parents. They are permitted to search their children's rooms and possessions as they see fit. School administrators can

Table 2-1   Constitutional Sources Used to Challenge Laws Regulating Families and Children

Conditional provision	Right protected	Implications for children
First Amendment	Religious freedom; free speech; free press; right of assembly	Children may attend parochial school; Amish children may be allowed an exception to compulsory education; obscene speech *not* protected; school newspapers may be censored; manner of but *not* content of youth meetings regulated
Fourth Amendment	Protection against unreasonable searches and seizures of person, papers, houses, and effects	School lockers not protected from search and seizures; inpatient searches conducted if safety considerations balanced with reasonably conducted search
Fifth Amendment	Right against self-incrimination; protection against property or life taken without due process of law	Juvenile justice system provides safeguards of adversarial process; psychiatric hospitalizations comply with due process standards
Sixth Amendment	Right to confront witnesses; right to speedy and public trial; right to assistance of counsel	Child victims of sexual abuse may be further traumatized by court proceedings; juvenile offenders have access to speedy hearing and legal assistance
Eighth Amendment	Protection against "cruel and unusual punishment"	Hospitalized persons not involuntarily committed without rehabilitation or treatment; schools may use corporal punishment to maintain order if procedural safeguards met
Fourteenth Amendment	Right to equal protection under the law; protection against state's denial of due process	Children not discriminated against because of status (in some cases); state government may not abridge certain fundamental rights such as privacy

search student lockers to maintain order (*State v. Stein,* 1969). Students are, however, entitled to some form of due process before their constitutional freedoms are abridged.

In addition to a constitutionally based right to privacy, the common law recognized invasion of privacy as a tort. All persons are entitled to certain expectations of privacy

Table 2-2   Supreme Court Decisions Relating to Children's Rights

Individual wins	State wins
Governmental regulation is struck down as being unduly violative of rights of family autonomy, religious freedom, or privacy. Constitution protects activity from governmental intrusion.	Government has a compelling or substantial interest in regulating activity; either public health and welfare or parens patriae role of state justify governmental intrusion.

Pierce v. Society of Sisters (1925)
State may not mandate public education if parents prefer religious schooling. Family autonomy and religious freedom allow parochial education as viable alternative.

In re Gault (1967)
Supreme Court set out new guidelines for juvenile justice system to protect due process rights of minors.

Tinker v. Des Moines Independent Community School District (1969)
Schools may not force students to leave school or remove black armbands protesting Vietnam War.

Wisconsin v. Yoder (1972)
Amish parents have right to remove their children from public schools to enter farming and craft apprenticeships at age 14. Religious freedom outweighed state's public welfare interest.

Stanley v. Illinois (1972)
State cannot deprive children or parents from custody solely because of legitimacy. (This issue can be decided other way if father has shown no interest in children or their support.)

Goss v. Lopes (1975)
Students in public schools have due process rights that are violated by 10–day school suspensions.

Planned Parenthood v. Danforth (1976)
State cannot deny an abortion to minor in first 12 weeks of pregnancy, nor can it require parental consent to perform an abortion on minor. (State cannot compel a minor to have abortion if the minor does not want one but parent does.)

Carey v. Population Services International (1977)
State cannot deny contraceptive services to minors because there is no parental consent.

Jacobson v. Massachusetts (1905)
State may require mandatory vaccinations for children. Public health and welfare interests of state outweigh parent's choice.

Prince v. Massachusetts (1944)
State was not violating a family's religious freedom when it prohibited sale of religious literature on street corner by minor, even when supervised by family member. State is legitimately protecting minors.

Ginsberg v. New York (1968)
State may restrict sale of "obscenity" to minors without violating equal protection rights.

Ingraham v. Wright (1977)
Use of corporal punishment in schools is permitted if justified. Sufficient safeguards exist to protect children from "cruel and unusual punishment." State has interest in regulating education.

Parham v. J.R. (1979)
State can apply administrative procedures for committing children to state mental health facilities.

H.L. v. Matheson (1981)
State law requiring physician's to "notify if possible" parents of minors seeking abortions does not violate rights and serves an important state interest.

New York v. Ferber (1982)
State law prohibiting child sexual activity and pornography does not violate freedom of speech or privacy.

Bethel School District v. Fraser (1986)
Schools can expel students for speeches considered lewd by administrators without violating students' right to free speech or due process.

in their personal lives. Therefore, if another person deliberately publishes or makes public private information, that individual may be liable for any injury or harm that results. Nurses should be aware of the implications of negligently disclosing facts about a child or family.

CONFIDENTIALITY OF CLIENT INFORMATION

"Confidentiality is the legal and ethical responsibility to keep all information concerning patients and clients private; therefore, nurses as well as other health professionals must not divulge or release information given or available to them as part of their professional duties" (Laben and McLean, 1989). It is regulated through state laws and codes of professional ethics. Maintaining secrecy regarding psychiatric treatment is particularly important because of the stigma attached to mental illness.

Children's records are confidential, although agency administrators are sometimes required to balance the child's wishes and interests against the parents' request for such information. "Any child old enough to understand the decision not to allow the parents to view the records, should have the right to make that decision" (Schueller, 1984). Most states allow children over the age of 14 or 15 the same right that adults have to view their records, unless the viewing would have deleterious effects.

Nurses should be aware of the procedures in each agency or institution for parents to release information about their child's treatment to appropriate persons, for example, insurance carriers, school personnel, or the juvenile justice system. Even the acknowledgement of a child's presence in an inpatient facility should not be given without the parents' permission. However, detailed communications about a client may be made between treating professionals to improve patient care.

Several recognized exceptions to the principle of confidentiality in mental health treatment of children exist, including suicidal or homicidal ideations, information regarding child abuse or sex abuse, and specific information ordered by a court of law.

If the nurse must share information from an interaction, the child should be told the rationale and the limits of disclosure. In less compelling circumstances the nurse may encourage the child to share certain information with either a physician, the parents, or a teacher. Sometimes the nurse provides counseling to a child and also sees the parents during the course of treatment. Specific content revealed by the child should be protected, and the child should be told that only general information will be shared with parents. Asking the child's permission for this kind of disclosure is also useful for building a trusting relationship.

PRIVILEGE

Statutory privilege keeps the communication between specified individuals protected from disclosure. Examples of relationships with such protection include those of police and informer, physician and client, husband and wife, and attorney and client. Unfortunately, most states do not include nurses or other nondoctoral psychotherapists in their privilege statutes.

Privilege belongs to the client and can be invoked to prevent disclosure of communications requested by a court of law. An example of how privilege works as compared to confidentiality is illustrated in the following scenario. A client makes this statement to his psychiatrist during a therapy session: "I've taken steroids sometimes to try and get my stamina up for big football games. The other players pass them around." The doctor is placed on the witness stand and asked if the client told her about steroid use. The doctor must abide by the client's decision whether to reveal this information or not. However, the same statement made to a nurse may not be protected if the state law does not grant nurses privilege in a psychotherapeutic setting. A client may "waive" the privilege. For example, if a child has been molested and the therapist is on the witness stand, the child may want the therapist to reveal this information to facilitate prosecution.

Wigmore (1961) lists four tests for applying testimonial privilege:

1. In the usual circumstances of the professional relationship, does the communication originate in the confidence that it will not be disclosed?
2. Is the inviolability of that confidence essential to the achievement of the purpose of the relationship?
3. Is the relation one that should be fostered?
4. Is the expected injury to the relationship through the fear of later disclosure greater than the expected benefit to justice in obtaining the testimony?

Informed Consent

TREATMENT

Two general rules apply to children receiving medical or psychiatric treatment. The first is the basic right enumerated by Justice Cardozo in 1914: "Every human being of adult years and sound mind has the right to determine what shall be done with his own body" (*Schloendorf v. Society of New York Hospital,* 1914). The second is the general rule that a minor is not recognized as being capable of giving a valid consent to medical treatment (Wilson, 1978). Denying a minor the capacity to consent to treatment presumes that a minor cannot understand the treatment or procedure or may not appreciate the consequences of the decision. Therefore the responsibility for providing consent for treatment shifts to the legal guardian.

There are many exceptions to the latter rule, the most notable being in cases of emergency. If a child is in danger of losing life or limb and the appropriate guardian cannot provide consent in a timely manner, the law permits a health professional to proceed with lifesaving treatment without consent. Most states also allow minors to obtain medical or psychiatric treatment without parental consent if they are emancipated. Some states allow minors to consent on their own behalf if they are a "mature minor." Mississippi law states, "Any unemancipated minor of sufficient intelligence to understand and appreciate the consequences of the proposed surgical or medical treatment or procedure may consent for him or her self" (Mississippi Code Annotated, 1972).

The courts have created exceptions to the parental consent requirement for minors seeking certain treatments. These include birth control services (*Carey v. Population Services International,* 1977), obtaining an abortion in certain circumstances (*Planned Parenthood of Central Missouri v. Danforth,* 1976), and treatment for drug addiction and venereal disease (most states do not require parental consent, but some states allow the treating professional to notify the parents). Some states are considering further statutory exceptions, for example, allowing minors who have been sexually assaulted to obtain treatment without parental consent (California Civil Code 34.9).

The current status of the law in most states does not permit minors to obtain psychiatric treatment without parental consent. The problem of access to treatment can occur if minors believe that their emotional problems are related to their family or fear their parents will belittle and minimize their concerns and become angry at their desire to obtain mental health services. Nurses in mental health settings should know that parental consent must be obtained for outpatient and particularly inpatient treatment unless the state of residence has an explicit exception in the law. Verbal counseling over a crisis hot line probably does not require parental consent, particularly if the situation is an emergency. If any injury results from treatment performed without parental consent, the treating professional may be liable for assault, battery, or negligent infliction of emotional distress (Wilson, 1978).

RESEARCH

Research on children has become a highly protected activity. By today's standards the research performed on healthy children to develop rubella and poliomyelitis vaccines would not have been permitted. Some commentators believe research should never be conducted on children in institutions because of mistreatments in the past (Schueller, 1984). However, denial of research would make attaining a research base for inpatient psychiatric nursing practice almost impossible.

Parental consent must be obtained for a child to participate in research. Because children are accustomed to obeying adults, their true voluntarism is difficult to assess. Children may not have the developmental ability to appreciate the altruistic aspect of participation. Ethicists also realize that economic and social pressures may influence parents to not act in their child's best interests. For these reasons, a double-pronged approach must be used. First, the informed consent of a legal guardian must be obtained, and second, the child must "assent" to participation in the research. The child's voluntarism must be assessed, and children 7 years of age and older should sign the consent form.

Potential harm must be minimal or nonexistent. Risks are permissible only if the benefits far outweigh them, and there is no feasible alternative (Frankle, 1978). Children in the custody of the state are generally excluded from research with any potential risk unless the experimental treatment is the only available therapy for them (Beyer, 1977).

Nurses should be aware of the Institutional Review Board (IRB) requirements of their particular agency. Children and their parents should be told the purpose of the study, the possible risks, and the potential benefits and that they may discontinue their participation at any time. Research using a control group should make the experimental treatment available to that group if the treatment is found therapeutic (Keith-Spiegel, 1976).

Protecting Children from Inadequate Parenting

CHILD ABUSE

Although many of the Supreme Court decisions revolve around the right of children and parents to be free from unwarranted intrusion by the state, the area of child abuse and neglect generally evokes strong agreement that the state should exert its *parens patriae* power and protect those unable to protect themselves. All states require health care professionals to report child abuse, and child psychiatric nurses may be exposed to situations in which they suspect physical, emotional, or sexual abuse. The mere suspicion of abuse is enough to trigger the force of these laws. Health professionals are sometimes reluctant to report without hard "evidence" of child abuse. The laws are designed to encourage rather than deter child protection, so some type of immunity from suit is usually granted to the reporting professional in cases where the allegations do not result in actual findings of abuse.

Any suspected abuse should be reported to the appropriate protective services in the county or state of residence, prompting an investigation by trained protective services workers. Nurses are often concerned about the potentially adversarial nature of these interventions. Issues such as whether to notify the parents of the report of abuse must be discussed in terms of therapeutic value. The following clinical example shows the potential therapeutic effect of reporting possible abuse:

During a therapy session with a child psychiatric nurse, a father admitted to knocking dents in his truck with his fists and feared that he was "taking things out" on his 9-year-old son. During a discussion of the case in supervision the decision was made to call protective services. The nurse worried that the father might seek retribution or feel so betrayed that he would not return to therapy because of their action. The father did return to therapy the following week and appeared more relaxed. After a few months the father's live-in girlfriend told the nurse that they knew who made the referral and felt it had been the best decision in the circumstances (Chadwick, 1989).

Courts and legislators moved from an almost noninterventionist position around 1900 to a position of removing children from abusive or neglectful environments by the 1950s. This action was taken without considering the psychologic impact on the child. Social scientists have been very vocal in the legal arena regarding the devastating effect of separation from a primary caretaker (even a poor one) on a child. Bowlby's studies (1958) of attachment and hospitalism in post-World War II Germany revealed the psychologic influence of prolonged separation from a bonded relationship.

From 1950 to 1980, deplorable living conditions were included in some child abuse laws as grounds for removing a child from the home. With room in the law for subjective interpretation of conditions warranting removal, a disagreement or moral judgment about parental lifestyle by case workers or lawyers could have resulted in parents' rights being terminated. Goldstein (1973), Freud (1979), and Solnit (1986) wrote a series of books on the best interests of children, coinciding with heightened scrutiny of laws that could violate civil rights by the Supreme Court. By the mid 1970s the ability of social service agencies to make arbitrary decisions that could profoundly disrupt both parents' and children's fundamental rights curtailed these interventionist laws. A growing awareness of options available for most removed children also deterred the courts from viewing removal as a helpful intervention in many abuse situations.

The proposed "Juvenile Justice Standards Relating to Abuse and Neglect" have limited removal of a child only when one of the following conditions is met (Waddlington, Whitebread, and Davis, 1983):

1. The child has suffered or is about to suffer physical harm causing or about to cause disfigurement, impairment of a bodily function, or similar serious physical injury, and the harm is inflicted nonaccidentally by a parent.
2. The child has suffered or is about to suffer physical harm of the kind previously described because of conditions created by a parent or inadequate parental supervision.
3. The child is presently suffering serious emotional harm as evidenced by severe anxiety, depression, withdrawal, or willful aggressive behavior toward self or others, and the parents are unwilling to seek treatment.
4. The child has been sexually abused by a parent or other member of the household (or the child has been seriously harmed physically or emotionally by such an act).
5. The child is in need of medical treatment for a condition threatening loss of life, disfigurement, or impairment of bodily functions, and the parents are unwilling to seek or consent to such treatment.
6. The child is engaging in delinquent behavior fostered or encouraged by a parent.

SEXUAL ABUSE

Child sexual abuse has received much attention and has been increasingly reported over the past two decades. The balance of interests between the rights of children and rights of the accused in legal proceedings and the need for mental health practitioners well acquainted with the hearsay Rules of Evidence are two legal issues involved in this area. Only certain information from a mental health evaluation of sexual abuse is permitted as testimony, and states vary in their definitions of hearsay testimony as it applies to child victims of sex abuse (Yorker, 1988a).

Iowa and other states have enacted a protectionistic law allowing child victims to testify behind a one-way screen to avoid viewing the alleged perpetrator in open court. The Supreme Court invalidated this provision as violative of the defendant's Sixth Amendment right to "confront a witness against him." However, Justice O'Connor stated measures to protect child witnesses were permitted if the potential trauma to the child outweighed the possibility of unfair prejudice against the defendant (*Coy v. Iowa*, 1988).

Children in the Mental Health System

RIGHT TO TREATMENT

The right to treatment in mental health and psychiatric facilities has been well established for adults as well as children. A case was filed on behalf of Ricky Wyatt, an adolescent hospitalized in a state psychiatric hospital in Alabama (*Wyatt v. Stickney*, 1971). The plaintiff's case alleged that inadequate funding for the facility was impairing the standard of care and the constitutional "right to treatment" of clients in mental health facilities. The judge agreed that the clients' rights were violated by the deplorable conditions and low standards of care. The box illustrates a summary of the pertinent mandates ordered by Judge Johnson (Laben and McLean, 1989).Two controversial issues in the area of child mental health are whether the child has a right to refuse treatment and what power parents have in obtaining involuntary psychiatric committment of their children. The first issue is poorly defined in either case or statutory law. Historically the courts have deferred to parental or state administrative judgment regarding the need for psychiatric hospitalization. Any treatment provided with parental consent and deemed necessary or therapeutic by the institution cannot be refused by a minor. However, the emerging movement of client advocacy is setting guidelines regarding humane treatments and is establishing rights of clients institutionalized in psychiatric facilities.

RESTRICTIVE INTERVENTIONS

Nurses are often uncertain about the legality of certain inpatient "level" systems that may abridge fundamental rights of minor clients, for example, restricting an anorexic client's access to the bathroom or restricting mail and phone calls of a child admitted for a conduct disorder. These nursing interventions are generally sanctioned *if* the child's condition is serious enough to warrant restrictive treatment. Many of the principles regarding the rights of adult incompetent or involuntary clients can be applied to children. Nurses should be aware of institutional guidelines regarding protection of client's rights and should also obtain competent supervision when applying treatments to a minor who is vehemently refusing them.

Highly restrictive procedures, such as seclusion or restraint, should have clear protocols for initiation and monitoring by nursing staff. Invasive procedures such as ECT or forced medication cannot be given without the informed consent of a guardian. Psychosurgery is generally prohibited in the case of incompetent patients (Laben and McLean, 1989).

COMMITMENT OF MINORS

Two landmark Supreme Court decisions involving the due process rights of minors provide a confusing set of guidelines for practitioners. *In re Gault* (1967) mandated certain protective procedures before incarceration of juvenile offenders. *Parham v. J.R.* (1979) questioned the committment procedures of minors in the state of Georgia. This case was brought on behalf of over 100 youths institutionalized in state mental institutions. The Supreme Court said the existing procedure for admission requiring parental consent and a review by a "neutral factfinder" (physician or hospital administrator) provided enough review to meet the child's due process rights.

There has been intense criticism of this ruling by many legal and mental health commentators. The court based its decision on many assumptions that are not borne out by research. For example, the court assumed that parents and the state (acting *in loco parentis*) have the wisdom to ascertain appropriate need for hospitalization, when in reality the majority of children in institutions are wards of the state and not psychotic.

In short, the picture emerging from a review of the *Parham* facts was that many, perhaps most, of hospitalized children in Georgia, a state with a relatively well-developed community

---

Right to Treatment

1. Clients have right to privacy and dignity.
2. Clients have right to least restrictive conditions necessary to achieve purposes of commitment.
3. Clients shall have same rights to visitation and telephone communication as clients at other public hospitals, except to extent that the qualified mental health professional responsible for formulation of treatment plan documents special restrictions. Written order must be renewed after periodic review of treatment plan if restrictions are to continue.
4. Clients shall have unrestricted right to visitation with attorneys, private physicians, and other health professionals.
5. Clients shall have unrestricted right to send sealed mail. Clients shall have unrestricted right to receive sealed mail from their attorneys, private physicians, other mental health professionals, courts, and government officials. Clients shall have right to receive sealed mail from others, except to extent that qualified mental health professional responsible for formulation of treatment plan documents special restrictions on receipt of sealed mail. Written order must be reviewed after each periodic review of treatment plan if restrictions are to continue.
6. Clients have right to wear their clothes and to keep and use personal possessions except when such clothes or personal possessions are determined by a qualified mental health professional to be dangerous or otherwise inappropriate to treatment regimen.
7. Each client shall have comprehensive physical and mental examination and review of behavioral status within 48 hours of admission.
8. Each client shall have individualized treatment plan developed by appropriate qualified mental health professionals, including a psychiatrist, and implemented as soon as possible — no later than 5 days after admission. Each individualized treatment plan shall contain the following:
   - Statement of specific problems and needs of client
   - Statement of least restrictive treatment conditions necessary to achieve purposes of commitment
   - Description of intermediate and long-range treatment goals, with a projected timetable for attainment
   - Statement and rationale for treatment plan for intermediate and long-range goals
   - Specification of staff responsibility and description of proposed staff involvement with client to attain treatment goals
   - Criteria for release to less restrictive treatment conditions

From *Wyatt v Stickney,* 344 F Supp 373, 1971.

---

mental health system, were in the institution because their families were unable or unwilling to care for them, and the state had not developed alternative residential services (Melton, 1984).

The implications for child psychiatric nurses are effectively summarized by Mary Lou de Leon Siantz (1988) in her article "Children's Rights and Parental Rights: A

Historical Ethical/Legal Analysis." She concluded that psychiatric nurses must be aware of the due process requirements of institutionalizing of minors. "Ultimately, nurses can be a powerful influence with their 24-hour access to the child. This information should facilitate the post admission reevaluation of the child's status and need for continued commitment."

Nurses' Role

LIABILITY

The ANA standards of care for child psychiatric nurses provide professionally sanctioned standards by which a court of law can measure the performance of nurses in this subspecialty (see Chapter 1) (ANA, 1985). In addition to these standards, nurses should be acutely aware of their state's Nurse Practice Act (NPA). These acts are the actual laws defining and distinguishing nursing practice from other specialties. Many states are currently revising their NPA to recognize advanced and independent practice by nurses, and the courts have been generally supportive of nurses in expanded roles, including practice by clinical specialists in child and adolescent psychiatric nursing (*Sermchief v. Gonzales,* 1983).

Although nurses are being sued for malpractice more frequently, nurses who work in child psychiatric settings have rarely been involved in lawsuits as defendants. The few cases that exist involve nurses' failure to exercise due care with medications (*Norton v. Argonaut Insurance Co.,* 1962) or restraint (*Moore v. Halifax Hospital,* 1967) or physical injuries incurred by children while in the setting. Although suicide of a client composes a significant malpractice area in adult and adolescent psychiatric nursing, it is less common in child psychiatry. However, nurses must be aware of the legal importance of suicide precautions.

Nurses are liable for malpractice only when the following elements are present:
1. Professional duty: This duty exists if the injured plaintiff can establish that the nurse entered into a therapeutic relationship.
2. Breach: This element is most often examined by comparing the nurses actions to the "standard of care" that should be used. The standard of care is usually established through ANA standards, hospital protocols and procedures, expert witnesses, and medical records.
3. Proximate cause: A plaintiff can win the suit only if the nurse's breach actually caused the resulting injury. For example, if a nurse failed to comply with an order for 15 minute checks on a child during the night shift but the child received an injury while supervised at breakfast, no liability would be found.
4. Damages: Some type of damage must result from the negligence. Examples of damages that can be compensated monetarily include physical injuries, emotional distress, pain and suffering, loss of earning potential, and in cases of outrageously reckless or willful conduct on the part of a health professional, punitive damages.

Nurses must be concerned with the issue of restraint. Its unnecessary use can result in a lawsuit for assault, battery, or false imprisonment, but if nurses fail to restrain a child whose condition warrants intervention, the nurse can be found liable for any injuries incurred. There are far more lawsuits against nurses for failing to restrain a client than for false imprisonments or assault (Yorker, 1988b).

WITNESSES

Nurses may testify in court in several different capacities. A nurse may be asked to testify regarding knowledge gained through professional treatment of a client, for example, if a nurse has provided an assessment of a sex abuse case. Nurses may be named as a party in a lawsuit and have to testify regarding their actions, the actions of a physician, or the policies of their employing institution. Finally, nurses are becoming more visible as "expert witnesses" in malpractice suits. A nurse with advanced credentials is used to educate a jury about the standard of care that should be applied in a specified situation. Nurses should educate themselves about the process of becoming an expert witness and should charge for this consultative service. Northrop and Kelly (1987) provide an excellent guide for nurses interested in providing this service.

LEGAL ADVOCACY

Nurses should participate in the legislative process whenever possible. Writing letters to local, state, and federal lawmakers, reading proposed legislation involving children's rights and funding for programs for youth, and actively eliciting community support are all ways that nurses can participate in governmental activity.

Ethical Issues

ADVOCACY

The ANA code for nurses describes the nurse as an advocate with "primary commitment . . . to the client's care and safety" (ANA, 1976). In child psychiatric nursing, this can be very difficult.

The sensitive nurse ponders the identity of the client: Is it primarily the child, the family system, or the interests of the whole society? The nurse can muster persuasive arguments favoring the family system and still others favoring the individual child as the client in need of advocacy (Bandman and Bandman, 1985).

Nurses should be engaged in on-going clinical supervision to clarify clinical situations presenting a conflict of interest or ethical dilemma that the nurse may otherwise fail to recognize. The ANA specifies a certain number of hours of clinical supervision as eligibility requirements for certification as a clinical specialist in child and adolescent psychiatric mental health nursing.

TREATMENT

Certain treatment modalities used in psychiatric treatment of children or adolescents arouse ethical concerns. Behavioral treatment is very prevalent in child treatment. For the most part the benefits to child, parent, and milieu far outweigh any insult to the child's integrity from being "modified" by such techniques. If, however, the behavioral treatment involves aversive conditioning, nurses should be cautious. Even mild electric shocks applied to self-destructive autistic children have been questioned or entirely prohibited by hospital protocol committees. The more intrusive or invasive a procedure, the more ethical and moral scrutiny must be applied to a decision involving such treatment.

Another area of concern is the use of *therapeutic paradox*. Because paradoxical interventions often involve a certain amount of deception, these techniques are being examined in ethical terms. Mark Hirschmann (1989) is a nurse researcher investigating nursing beliefs and attitudes toward the use of paradox. He found that the majority of nurses who used therapeutic paradox believed it was an appropriate intervention. Nurses did, however, express ethical and professional concerns about the manipulative and deceptive potential in using these techniques.

REFERENCES

American Nurses' Association: Code for nurses, Kansas City, Mo, 1976, The Association.
American Nurses' Association: Standards of child and adolescent psychiatric mental health nursing practice, Kansas City, Mo, 1985, The Association.
Bandman E and Bandman B: Nursing ethics in the life span, Norfolk , Conn, 1985, Appleton-Century-Crofts.
Bellotti v Baird, 443 US 622, 1979.
Bethel School District v Fraser, 106 S Ct 3159, 1986.
Beyer H: Changes in the parent-child legal relationship: what they mean to the clinician, J Autism Child Schizophr 7:84, 1977.
Blackstone W: Commentaries on the laws of England, vol 1, London, 1765, Robert Bell Editory.
Bowlby J: Attachment and loss, vol 1, New York, 1958, Basic Books, Inc.
Chadwick F: Personal notes, Apr 25, 1989.
Carcy v Population Services International, 97 S Ct 2010, 1977.
Coy v Iowa, 108, S Ct 2798, 1988.
Davis S and Schwartz M: Children's rights and the law, Lexington, Mass, 1987, DC Heath-Lexington Books.
Frankle M: Social legal and political responses to ethical issues in the use of children as experimental subjects, J Social Issu 34:101, 1978.
In re Gault, 387 US 1, 1967.
Ginsberg v New York, 390 US 629, 1968.
Goss v Lopez, 419 US 565, 1975.
Griswold v Connecticut, 381 US 479, 1965.
Hirschmann M: Psychiatric and mental health nurses' beliefs about therapeutic paradox, J Child Adolescent Psychia Mental Health Nurs 2:7, 1989.
HL v Matheson, 450 US 398, 1981.
Ingraham v Wright, 430 US 651, 1977.
Jacobson v Massachusetts, 197 US 11, 1905.
Johnson G: Family law and culture, an overview of parental rights. In Hunter E and Hunter D, editors: Professional ethics and law in the health sciences, Malabar, Fla, 1984, RE Krieger Publishing Co, Inc.
Keith-Spiegel P: Children's rights as participants in research. In Koocher G, editor: Children's rights and the mental health professional, New York, 1976, John Wiley & Sons, Inc.
Laben J and McLean C: Legal issues and guidelines for nurses who care for the mentally ill, Owings Mills, Md, 1989, Williams & Wilkins.
Melton G: Family and mental hospital as myths: civil commitment of minors. In Repucci N and others, editors: Children's mental health and the law, 1984, Sage Publications, Inc.

Meyer v Nebraska, 262 US 390, 1923.

Mississippi Code Annotated, 41 41 3h, 1972.

Moore v Halifax Hospital, 202 So 2d 568 Fla App, 1967.

New York v Ferber, 458 US 7474, 1982.

Nicholas B: Introduction to Roman Law, Oxford, 1962, Oxford University Press, Inc.

Northrop C and Kelly M: Legal issues in nursing practice, St Louis, 1987, The CV Mosby Co.

Norton v Argonaut Insurance Co, 144 So 2d 249 La App, 1962.

Parham v JR, 442 US 584, 1979.

Pierce v Society of Sisters of the Holy Names of Jesus and Mary, 268 US 510, 1925.

Planned Parenthood of Central Missouri v Danforth, 428 US 52, 1976.

Prince v Massachusetts, 321 US 158, 1944.

Prosser W and Keeton R: Prosser and Keeton on torts, ed 5, 1984, West Publishing Co.

Schloendorf v Society of New York Hospital, 211 NY 125, 105 NE 92, 1914.

Schueller N: The rights of children. In Hunter E and Hunter D, editors: Professional ethics and law in the health sciences, Malabar, Fla, 1984, RE Krieger Publishing Co, Inc.

Sermcheif v Gonzales, 660 SW 2d 683 Mo, 1983.

Siantz ML de Leon: Children's rights and parental rights: a historical and ethical/legal analysis, J Child Adolescent Psychia Mental Health Nurs 1:14, 1988.

Stanley v Illinois, 405 US 645, 1972.

State v Stein, 456 P 2d 1 Kan, 1969.

Tinker v Des Moines Independent Community School District, 393 US 503, 1969.

Waddlington W, Whitebread C, and Davis S: Cases and materials on children in the legal system, Mineola, NY, 1983, The Foundation Press, Inc.

Wigmore J: Vol 8 Evidence section 2285, 1961, Little, Brown & Co, Inc.

Wilson J: The rights of adolescents in the mental health system, Lexington, Mass, 1978, DC Heath-Lexington Books.

Wisconsin v Yoder, 406 US 205, 1972.

Wyatt v Stickney, 344 F Supp 373, 1971.

Yorker B: The prosecution of child sexual abuse cases: legal issues related to child advocacy, J Child Adolescent Psychia Ment Health Nurs 1:50, 1988a.

Yorker B: The nurse's use of restraint with a neurologically impaired patient, J Neurosci Nurs 29:390, 1988b.

Chapter 3

Clinical Evaluation in Child Psychiatric Nursing

This chapter reviews some clinical skills required to implement child psychiatric nursing process standards II, III, and IV (ANA, 1985). The focus is on the areas to be evaluated, the skills required to assess these areas, and some of the tools available to assist the clinician. The development of a comprehensive initial data base is essential in formulating developmental and nursing diagnoses and treatment planning.

The assessment process addresses ways in which children organize the content of their experiences and a child's phase-specific uniqueness, using concepts of specific and multiple lines of development and determinants of behavior. Many of the initial assessment procedures become on-going evaluation techniques, providing benchmarks to assess treatment progress.

Assessment of Children and Families

The direction of the initial family assessment interview and clinical assessment of the child, including the mental status examination (MSE) depends on the setting, the availability of consulting professionals, and the situation of the child and family. In settings where children are referred for comprehensive diagnostic evaluation work-ups for possible hospital admission or legal dispositions (for example, child custody cases and out-of-home or correctional placement), the interdisciplinary diagnostic interview may take several hours and include neurologists, speech therapists, psychologists, nurse clinicians, child psychiatrists, and social workers. Most settings have interview protocols, specific documentation forms, and a well-designed procedure maximizing time for collaborative evaluation and diagnostic and treatment-planning formulation.

Specific evaluation forms are useful when nurse clinicians have the major responsibility for the psychodiagnostic evaluation, such as in schools and most mental health, family practice, and child health clinics. In most settings the written diagnostic evaluation and initial interview procedures provide critical measures of quality assurance.

Finances, limited professional resources, and time were not always an issue. The clinician's evaluation interviews were often more leisurely, and clients were seen several times before the psychodiagnostic formulation and treatment plan were required. However, most contemporary mental health settings require clinicians to complete full intake evaluations, formulate diagnoses, and develop initial treatment plans based on the data gathered within a short time.

The psychiatric evaluation of a child and family can be highly productive or meaningless. The success of the initial interviews depends on the appropriate methods being used, the clinician's interviewing skills, the content, and the context (ways in which the data emerge and are extended). Clinical interviewing skills include the ability to shift styles as the content regions are explored while structuring and guiding the process. Nurse clinicians need to know what questions to ask, what information is needed, and how to expand and explore areas of possible diagnostic importance as they arise, and how to structure orderly transitions between topics.

REFERRALS

Sources of referral are especially important when working with children because children seldom refer themselves for care. It is important to ascertain who requested the evaluation and if specific deposition decisions depend on the outcome. If a child is referred by a teacher, physician, or other individuals, additional clarification may be required. Clinicians must obtain permission from the child's parents or guardian before contacting any person or documented source of information (including past treatment records). The clinician should know initially what changes are expected and the perceived roles of the referring source. These aspects need to be evaluated within the cultural and social background expectations of the child and family.

Referrals result from different circumstances, including the following (Critchley, 1979):

1. A family crisis is present, with accompanying changes in the child's capacity to cope, attend school, maintain peer relationships, learn, and play.
2. An acute physical illness occurs, with concomitant depression and/or hyperactivity demonstrating denial of the illness.
3. A chronic physical illness is present, with a gradual loss of adaptive functions by the child, increased family conflicts, and a risk of family dissolution.
4. Depression in the child occurs.
5. Acute changes in the child's thinking, behavior, and expressions of feelings, such as suicidal thinking, rages, and/or withdrawal in younger children, occur often with loss of speech.

INITIAL EVALUATION PROCEDURES

The importance of conducting the initial evaluations to ensure that the child and family will complete the referral and return for treatment if necessary has been stressed in the literature. Initial evaluations need to be designed to minimize the number of "no shows" and "drop outs," that is, children and families who do not appear for the referral or do not return after the first clinic encounter. An estimated 50% of referred children and families fail to follow through or drop out after the first evaluation session (Call, 1985). Unless evaluation interviews are managed with professional skill and sensitivity, opportunities for early interventions will be lost.

Questions used to initiate a nonthreatening, inviting contact include: (1) Are evaluation and therapy separate processes? (2) How much time is needed to establish a diagnosis? (3) Should the intake worker and therapy clinician be the same individual? (4) How should the clinician initiate evaluations with the parents and child? and (5) What essential data must be identified and recorded to support initial diagnoses and planning formulations?

Answers depend on the procedures and policies of each setting, which can vary considerably. When a formal psychodiagnostic classification of the child's disorder is required, as is increasingly the case, a specific time frame in which all available information is examined and a diagnosis is determined is often set. However, intake evaluations include therapy until an evaluation conference in which clear goals are set has occurred. Without this planning phase the therapeutic process becomes obscure and complicated (Dodds, 1985).

Some clinics use intake or triage workers to conduct evaluations and assign another clinician for children's treatment. The advantages of having the same clinician perform the initial evaluation and subsequent treatment include: (1) clinicians quickly learn about the child and family by obtaining assessment information firsthand; (2) the child does not have to switch relationships, that is, terminate the relationship established with the intake worker and rebuild another with a different staff member; and (3) parents have continuity of contact with the same staff, which may be reassuring during times of crisis and emotional distress.

However, two clinicians working initially with the child and family may have different perspectives, which gives a broader viewpoint on the data, facilitates peer collaboration and review, and compensates for any "blind spots" of the intake worker or therapist. One disadvantage is that the child may experience different therapeutic responses in assessment and therapy, which may be confusing (Dodds, 1985).

Some administrators believe that using intake workers results in more efficient staff assignments and matches the child and family more effectively with the clinician's experience, style, existing case loads, and case preferences. Others claim that treatment begins with the first contact between the family and intake clinician and that the initial evaluation contributes to the child's and family's attitudes toward the process. All agree that clinicians need to monitor the therapeutic process continually to prevent the occurrence drop outs or premature termination of therapy.

The diagnostic evaluation reflects the clinician's assessment of the child's total situation, the nature of the disorder being evaluated, and the sources of information. The *four pillars of assessment* are structured interviews, observations, informal assessment, and norm-referenced tests (Sattler, 1988). The initial evaluation consists of three segments: (1) initial discussions with the guardian or parents and siblings (if available), (2) a session with the adults and siblings, and (3) beginning the child's MSE.

History of Present Illness

INITIAL CONTACT

Children usually cannot define their problem verbally and are often unaware that their parents or others perceive their behaviors as problems. When parents seek professional help for their child, they have usually tried many techniques and followed the advice of family and friends. During the initial contact the clinician must realize that parents are often suspicious and reticent to seek mental health services for their child and have come when "all else has failed." Establishing a relationship and alliance with the parents requires a helping attitude similar to a positive parent-child relationship.

History taking occurs during the first contact with the parents or guardian. The mother is usually the best historian. If possible, the comprehensive history needs to be supplemented and explored with the child during the clinical examination segment (Adams and Fras, 1988).

Many interview guides to organize the family history data exist. Although the philosophic and theoretic orientation of settings and clinicians may differ and one orientation (behavioral, cognitive, phenomenologic, or psychoanalytic) may give more emphasis or different interpretations to content area, the traditional medical model is generally used. Shown in Table 3-1, the model provides clear guidelines for the content regions to be covered. Specific content areas and assessment techniques for infants are presented in Chapter 7.

CHIEF COMPLAINTS

The first interview with the parents should be a structured process clarifying the time required and the process, roles, confidentiality, and rationale for family and individual child interviews. Identification of the chief complaint (if referred), duration of symptoms, parents' perceptions of the problem, their concerns and efforts to solve the problem, and the family history are initial topics, and clinicians record the content and process.

Some experts claim that the presenting complaints are of greater importance in child psychiatry than in adult psychiatry and that during the first stage of the evaluation, clinicians should pose the following questions (Adams and Fras, 1988):

1. What concerns you about your child?
2. When did these problems start?
3. Are they getting worse?
4. Have these problems been noticed in school as well as at home?
5. What makes them better? Worse?
6. How have these problems affected the child's life with you? With siblings, peers, teachers?
7. Has the child's school performance suffered?

PRESENT ILLNESS

Parents provide important assessment data about the child's developmental history and family structure. Records from pediatricians, information about hospitalization, baby books, and photo albums are also important. The last two items help parents cope with the stressful memories recalled during the initial interviews. Requesting parents to bring these records with them for the initial interview is helpful.

Sometimes parents deny the existence of a problem and seek professional support to prove others wrong about their child. Clinicians need to help them regain confidence in their parenting roles, and sufficient time needs to be taken to allow the

Table 3-1   Evaluation for the Child

Content region	Elements
History of present illness	Includes development and appearance of symptoms resulting in referral; description of symptoms and their progression; help sought and tried; direct quote of chief complaint by child, parents, teachers, and referral source
Family history	Includes background factors of parents, family members; educational, social, work history; psychiatric and other medical illnesses in blood-related family (for example, schizophrenia, affective disorders, mental retardation, seizure disorders, hyperactivity, alcohol and drug abuse, cancer, diabetes); interpersonal and environmental information; separations, outside help, extent of contact among family members, social groups, friends; genogram
Medical history	Includes medical review of body systems; information about medications, allergies, childhood illnesses affecting central nervous system
Developmental history	Includes pregnancy, birth, neonatal period (verbatim descriptions of child as infant); description of child's habits, play, preschool period, school, special interests, skills, friends, daily routines
MSE	Description of behavior directly observed by examiner during play/interview session (Simmons, 1969)
Neurologic examination	Includes minor signs of neurologic deficits
Psychologic tests	Diagnostic tests indicated after evaluation of data and observations

Modified from Call JD: Psychiatric evaluation of the infant and child. In Kaplan HI and Sadock BJ: Comprehensive textbook of psychiatry, ed 4, Baltimore, 1986, Williams & Wilkins, and Adams P and Fras I: Beginning child psychiatry, New York, 1988, Brunner/Mazel, Inc.

parents to identify and discuss their feelings, successes, and frustrations. Even if the problems identified by parents have little or no relationship to the child's subjective feelings of distress, it is still important to learn their concerns and resolve them concurrently if possible or suggest marital counseling.

Although in some instances (with children under the age of 4 or 5) parents and child may be treated simultaneously, the goal initially is to engage parents as collaborators. This includes directing parents to report aspects of the child's behavior occurring outside of treatment, not ask the child questions about the therapeutic relationship, support the therapeutic goals, bring the child for therapy even if unwilling, and develop tolerance of the child's behavior changes (Group for the Advancement of Psychiatry, 1982).

During the interview the clinician needs to determine what part of the problem is present illness and what part falls within the context of the child's developmental history. A chief complaint list is helpful in distinguishing between these two areas.

Family History

Many child psychiatric clinicians use genograms for the initial data organization and on-going monitoring of the child and family. Family therapists and general family practice clinicians frequently use genograms for both family therapy and medical management and preventive medicine. Therefore the family may already have an established genogram.

Genograms are based on the perspective that the family is a group of people interacting as a functional whole, with neither adults, children, nor their problems existing in a vacuum. Genograms are a schematic representation of information on the family structure, life cycle, pattern repetition across generations, life events, family functioning, relational patterns and triangles, and family balance and imbalance (Woolf, 1983).

By viewing themselves and their child within an intergenerational context, parents often feel less guilty and will discuss their relationships and participate in the therapeutic process more readily. Requiring several sessions to complete, a genogram facilitates the establishment of the therapeutic relationship with the parents and helps to alleviate initial anxiety. Clinicians will find the comprehensive text on genograms by McGoldrick and Gerson (1986) a valuable resource containing guidelines for developing genograms with the traditional, reconstituted, and single parent families. Gerson's program (1984) for computer-generated genograms is another useful tool for recording data.

Process observations made by the clinician during the interview include parental behaviors such as spontaneous seating, verbal and nonverbal patterns of communication, the dominant communicator, and the time when communication occurs. Exploration and clarification of initial presenting themes often helps the parents and is critical in developing trust in the therapeutic relationship. Parents' trust is gained and the therapeutic alliance is established if positive feedback, information, and reinforcement are provided. For example, the mother of a hyperactive child can be asked how she provides for her own well being and restoration of energies. The child's and parents' strengths are emphasized to provide the parents with hope.

ASSESSMENT OF CHILD-PARENT INTERACTIONS

Collecting data provides opportunities to asses the parent-child relationship and the parents' strengths and limitations. A child's values and conscience are developing, and children are often in a stage of intense parental identification. Thus, no matter how dysfunctional the parent-child relationship may be, children consciously and unconsciously identify with parental values and evaluations. Children seldom like, trust, or relate well to adults or professionals that their parents distrust. Clinicians should avoid being judgmental in contacts with parents and the child. The parents' child-rearing behaviors need to be carefully evaluated because they affect the child's dependence-independence needs and self-concept. The parents' potential for changing these patterns is also assessed and enhanced initially and throughout therapy.

Information about the child's peer relationships, caretakers, and school activities need to be included. When referrals are made for children in special residential schools, group or foster homes, pediatric hospitals, or inpatient child care settings, the characteristics, strengths, and limitations of the treatment environment are important considerations.

Medical History

The complete medical history of the child is usually provided by the parents and the child's pediatrician. Along with a review of the body systems, it should detail any past illnesses that may have affected the central nervous system. Additional data and tests may be required.

Developmental History

Parents are usually under stress during the initial encounters, and clinicians' requesting specific dates and information often adds to their anxiety. In addition to the assessment form, many outpatient settings use child developmental forms specifically designed to meet their philosophic perspective. In some settings, parents are sent these forms before the initial interview or are requested to take the forms home and complete them before the second interview. Having this information before the interview facilitates the diagnostic process and provides a format for the initial discussion. The composite form in the box on p. 40 is an example of the developmental data several child care centers collect from parents.

CONSTITUTIONAL-TEMPERAMENTAL ENDOWMENT

The child's temperamental disposition provides a context for the descriptions of a child's developmental milestones. The child's temperament does not relate to parental temperament, and disposition does not appear to be biologically determined. Children's temperaments do not "fit" norms of other children at the same developmental level. While not inherited or age-stage specific, temperament produces different social response styles influencing the child's developmental patterns, attachment behaviors, and development of psychopathology.

Although temperament is not a theory of development and clinicians do not confine their approach to assessment and treatment primarily on temperament, it is often prominent in the child's behavioral difficulties. The goodness of fit between the child's and parents' temperaments is an important area to be evaluated and explored as possible sources of or contributing factors to the child's problem.

Temperament refers to the child's unique style of approaching people and situations. It develops soon after birth and become a basic component of the child's personality. The nine temperamental categories identified by Chess and Thomas (1986) and their definitions and examples of parental descriptions describing the child's constitutional-temperamental endowment by age and stage are summarized in Table 3-2. This information is a useful diagnostic tracking format, identifying changes in temperamental qualities over the child's early age periods and changes during treatment.

Developmental Data From Parents

Pregnancy and delivery data

Child's early experiences in comfort and differentiation
Child's major illnesses

Physical and developmental milestones

(Age and description of problems)
Sitting
Crawling
Walking
Talking
Toilet training
Weaning
Eating
Sleeping
Current vocabulary
Behavioral problems
Self-care
Language problems

Name of pediatrician or family physician

Current medical problems and medications, if any

Psychosocial milestones

Play with peers and friends
Problems with friends
School experiences
School progress
Separation experiences and losses
Things child likes to do
Things child does not like to do
Child's stressful life events and coping mechanisms
Family history (from developing genogram)

Parental perception

How does mother describe child?
How does father describe child?
Describe child's usual day
How are limits set on child? Why? By whom?

From Beck CK, Rawlins RP, and Williams SR, editors: Mental health-psychiatric nursing: a holistic life-cycle approach, St Louis, 1987, The CV Mosby Co.

PARENTS' DEVELOPMENTAL TASKS

Evaluation of the developmental tasks provides an interactional framework of parent and child development within the family system. Therapeutic interventions with the parents are usually based on a parallel process that strengthens the parents' potential to help the child. Developmental tasks and acceptable behavioral characteristics for the child and related tasks and behaviors of the parents (Table 3-3) and minimal and extreme psychopathology related to the child and behaviors of the parents (Table 3-4) provide a record of the process initially and during later evaluations of behavioral changes in the child-parent system. Assessment data are not considered as a basis for treatment of the parent but as a way to better understand the child.

Clinical Assessment of the Child

PREPARING THE CHILD FOR EVALUATION

If parents are seen in advance or contacted by telephone following a referral, the intake worker or clinician should advise parents about ways to prepare the child for the initial clinic visit (Dodds, 1985). Explanations should facilitate honest communication between parents and their child and set the stage for a positive first encounter.

MENTAL STATUS EXAMINATION

In general psychiatry, the MSE is the diagnostic interview portion of the psychiatric evaluation. It is preceded by a complete developmental, social, and health history and physical examination in both children and adults. Its content and process are different and the results are less crucial in child psychiatry than in adult psychiatry. The MSE provides less information and fewer grossly abnormal findings because different criteria are used. Children's cognitive and affective areas have not developed enough to elicit unambiguous information, and mental status data are usually attained indirectly (Adams and Fras, 1988). Most MSE formats suggested in texts or developed in treatment settings are adaptations of the MSE presented by Simmons (1969) and Goodman and Sours (1987) (see box on p. 52).

CLINICAL OBSERVATIONS

The two approaches used to gather the data are the semistructured verbal interview and the unstructured play interview. The first approach consists of techniques that involve the child in direct conversation or that use specific games if direct conversation is inappropriate. The second approach is based on the premise that the less the intrusion, the more the child will reveal in play. Some clinicians believe it is not appropriate to use a diagnostic play interview initially and that a direct interview is the most efficient method of collecting information (see Chapter 17). During all encounters with the child, clinicians need to make continual observations of the verbal and nonverbal behaviors and evaluate the child's multiple lines of development.

VERBAL INTERVIEWS

When children are interviewed about their problem or any aspect of their lives, clinicians should use a relaxed, conversational tone of inquiry and avoid following a "structured" questionnaire. Asking about the child's home is a good starting point. Detailed descriptions of the family and relationships with siblings, parents, teachers, relatives, and peers are also important. Children usually give excellent descriptions of their chief complaints, present illness, and past medical and developmental history. As with all clients, children need to be given the chance to tell their own story in their own way (Call, 1986).

If the child's verbal communications are unclear, clinicians need to state that they do not understand and ask for additional explanations. Questions may need to be rephrased and asked several times. Clinicians should adjust communication to the child's level of thinking and talking, use third person statements, and repeat the child's words. For example, if a child responds to a question by using a series of disconnected words, the nurse may elicit elaboration by repeating the last spoken word.

Verbalizations are critical components in the diagnostic work-up. The ability to communicate verbally is the first aspect to be assessed and affects the

Text continued on p. 53.

Table 3-2   Temperamental Categories

Definition	Assessment
Activity level	
Motor component of child's functioning; diurnal proportion of active and inactive period	Data on motility during bathing, eating, playing, dressing, handling; information on sleep-wake cycle, reaching, crawling, walking
Rhythmicity	
Predictable and/or unpredictable regularity in time	Analyzed by sleep-wake cycle, hunger, feeding, eating, elimination patterns
Approach/withdrawal	
Nature of initial responses; way child responds to new stimuli, for example, toy, food, persons	Approach responses positive with smiling, reaching; withdrawal reaction negative with crying, fussing, pushing away, spitting out new food
Adaptability	
Responses to new or altered situations	Ease of modifying or altering directions

Modified from Chess S and Thomas A: Temperament in clinical practice, New York, 1986, The Guilford Press.

| Typical parental descriptions | | |
Infancy	Toddler	Middle childhood
High activity: "Moves a great deal during sleep; kicks wildly during bath; once mastered a task, keeps doing it"; low activity: "Sleeps in same position; can turn over, but doesn't do it much"	High activity: "Runs widely when friends around"; low activity: "Prefers to sit quietly drawing or looking at picture book"	High activity: "When comes home from school, outside immediately playing active games; when inside, constant acrobatics; perpetually in motion"; low activity: "Gets involved in jigsaw puzzles, sits quietly working for hours"
Regular pattern: "Nap time never changes no matter where we are"; irregular pattern: "I wouldn't know how to start toilet training since his bowel movements come anytime, one to three times a day"	High rhythmicity: "Big meal at lunch, otherwise, just picks"; low rhythmicity: "May fall asleep right after dinner, or up until midnight"	High regularity: "Wakes up like clockwork at 6 every morning"; low regularity: "Continues to do homework until finished; never gets sleepy at same time"
High approach: "Smiles at strangers; loves new food, new toys"; high withdrawal: "Ignores new toys; spits out new foods"	High approach: "Plunges right in new group, activity"; high withdrawal: "Remains outside of group and won't participate or talk to others for weeks"	High approach: "Came home from new school excited, knew everyone by name"; high withdrawal: "When starting new school subjects, gets all confused and upset"
High adaptability: "First rejects things, but in few days, enjoys them"; low adaptability: "Everytime I put on new clothes, she screams, goes on for months"	High adaptability: "When she got new tricycle, couldn't ride it, called it stupid; then practiced and mastered it, uses it all the time"; low adaptability: "Took all fall to be content going to nursery school, each time gets sick and is out few days, reluctant to go again"	High adaptability: "Attended tennis camp, adjusted to schedule and got involved first week"; low adaptability: "Started new school with different teaching style, after 3 months still gets confused and wants explanations"

Continued.

Table 3-2   Temperamental Categories — cont'd

Definition	Assessment
Threshold of responsiveness	
Intensity level of stimulation needed to evoke discernible response, irrespective of form or sensory modality affected	Reactions to sensory stimuli, environmental conditions and objects, social contacts
Intensity of reaction	
Energy of responses	Irrespective of quality or direction
Quality of mood	
	Amount of pleasant, friendly behavior contrasted with unpleasant, unfriendly behaviors

Typical parental descriptions		
Infancy	Toddler	Middle childhood
Low threshold: "If door closes, is startled; loves fruits, but add cereal, he refuses it"; high threshold: "Can get bump on head and won't cry or stop what he was doing; can't tell if soiled by actions, have to check"	Low threshold: "Will only eat eggs if fixed same way"; high threshold: "Won't complain of being cold, even though shivering and lips are blue; comfortable in any clothes"	Low threshold: "First one to notice odor or changes in room temperature"; high threshold: "Didn't notice blister on heel while playing ball; lights went out one evening, didn't notice and kept on working"
High intensity: "When hungry, screams; if hears music, laughs loudly and bounces in time"; low intensity: "Had ear infection and didn't notice; ignores loud noises"	High intensity: "Screams when can't complete task"; low intensity: "If another child takes toy, grabs it back but doesn't cry"	High intensity: "Called poor loser, yells 'opponents cheated,' throws things in anger"; low intensity: "I knew he was upset about failing test, but was 'deadpan' about it"
Negative mood: "When sees something doesn't like, whines and fusses until it's taken away; cries for 5 to 10 minutes when put to sleep"; positive mood: "If isn't smiling, is getting sick"	Negative mood: "Usually comes home from nursery school full of complaints" positive mood: "When got new shoes, ran around with joy showing everyone; he's a pleasure to take to grocery store, he's so pleasant and happy"	Negative mood: "Only back in school a week, already has list of grievances against teacher"; positive mood: "Doesn't object to helping around house; takes garbage out willingly; does whatever asked pleasantly"

Continued

Table 3-2   Temperamental Categories—cont'd

Definition	Assessment
Distractability	Effectiveness of extraneous environmental stimuli altering direction of on-going behaviors
Attention span and persistence	Length of time activity is pursued; continuation of activity in face of obstacles; maintenance of activity direction

	Typical parental descriptions	
Infancy	**Toddler**	**Middle childhood**
High distractability: "If someone passes while nursing, looks and stops sucking until person is gone"; low distractability: "Can't be sidetracked, keeps doing something until it's mastered; when hungry and has to wait, won't get involved in play, keeps crying until fed"	High distractability: "Not a nagger; if she sees something she wants, will ask then accept substitute; room is strewn with toys, scarcely begins one game when attention is caught by something else and forgets to put things away"; low distractability: "Got new blocks and wouldn't leave them to play with friend; if it's raining and she wants to go outside, will fuss and not accept substitute"	High distractability: "Homework takes so long because attention is constantly sidetracked; is constantly losing something, gets involved with something else and forgets"; low distractability: "If friends ask him to play when he's making model airplane, can't get him away; once she starts to read, we can't get her to stop until she's finished a chapter"
High persistence: "Despite efforts to distract him, he returns to task of poking in electric outlet"; long attention span: "If I give her book, will tear up paper for an hour"; lower persistence: "If bead doesn't go on string immediately, stops playing with it"; short attention span: "While loves doll, only plays with it for few minutes"	High persistence: "If pushing toy around and it gets stuck, yells until it moves or someone comes to help; doesn't give up"; long attention span: "Can be engrossed in playing for almost an hour"; low persistence and low attention span: "Asks to be taught something but loses interest after first try"	High persistence and long attention span: "Couldn't understand homework at first, but kept at it until mastered even though it took several hours"; short attention span and high persistence: "Wouldn't give up until learned part but would work about 15 minutes at a time"; short attention span and low persistence: "Decided to learn to skate, after 5 minutes, gave up"

Table 3-3   Development Tasks and Acceptable Behavioral Characteristics of the
Child and Related Tasks and Behaviors of the Parents

Tasks in process		Acceptable behavioral characteristics	
Child	Parents	Child	Parents
18 months to 5 years of age			
To reach physiologic plateaus (motor action, toilet training)	To promote training, habits, and physiologic progress	Gratification from exercise of neuromotor skills	Are moderate and flexible in training
To differentiate self and secure sense of autonomy	To aid in family and group socialization of child	Investigative, imitative imaginative play	Show pleasure and praise for child's advances
To tolerate separations from mother	To encourage speech and other learning	Actions somewhat modulated by thought, memory good; animistic and original thinking	Encourage and participate with child in learning and in play
To develop conceptual understandings and "ethical" values	To reinforce child's sense of autonomy and identity	Exercises autonomy with body (sphincter control, eating)	Set reasonable standards and controls
To master instinctual impulses (Oedipal, sexual, guilt, shame)	To set a model for "ethical" conduct	Feelings of dependence on mother and separation fears	Pace themselves to child's capacities at a given time
To assimilate and handle socialization and acculturation (aggression, relationships, activities, feelings)	To delineate male and female roles	Behavior identification with parents, siblings, peers	Consistent in own behavior, conduct, and ethics
To learn sex distinctions		Learns speech for communication	Provide emotional reassurance to child
		Awareness of own motives, beginnings of conscience	Promote peer play and guided group activity
		Intense feelings of shame, guilt, joy, love, desire to please	Reinforce child's cognition of male and female roles
		Internalized standards of "bad," "good"; beginning of reality testing	
		Broader sex curiosity and differentiation	
		Ambivalence towards dependence and independence	
		Questions birth and death	

Modified from Senn MJE and Solnit AJ: Problems in child behavior and development, Philadelphia, 1968, Lea & Febiger.

Tasks in process		Acceptable behavioral characteristics	
Child	Parents	Child	Parents
5 to 12 years of age			
To master greater physical prowess	To help child's emancipation from parents	General good health, greater body competence, acute sensory perception	Ambivalent towards child's separation but encourage independence
To further establish self-identity and sex role	To reinforce self-identification and independence	Pride and self-confidence, less dependence on parents	Mixed feelings about parent-surrogates but help child to accept them
To work towards greater independence from parents	To provide positive pattern of social and sex role behavior	Better impulse control	
To become aware of world-at-large	To facilitate learning, reasoning, communication, and experiencing	Ambivalence regarding dependency, separation and new experiences	Encourage child to participate outside the home
To develop peer and other relationships	To promote wholesome moral and ethical values	Accepts own sex role; psychosexual expression in play and fantasy	Set appropriate model of social and ethical behavior and standards
To acquire learning, new skills, and a sense of industry		Equates parents with peers and other adults	
		Aware of natural world (life, death, birth, science); subjective but realistic about world	Take pleasure in child's developing skills and abilities
		Competitive but well organized in play; enjoys peer interaction	Understand and cope with child's behavior
		Regard for collective obedience to social laws, rules, and fair play	Find other gratifications in life (activity, employment)
		Explores environment; school and neighborhood basic to social-learning experience	Are supportive toward child as required
		Cognition advancing; intuitive thinking advancing to concrete operational level; responds to learning	
		Speech becomes reasoning and expressive tool; thinking still egocentric	

Table 3-4   Minimal and Extreme Psychopathologic Conditions of the Child and Related Behaviors of the Parents

Minimal psychopathology	
Child	Parents
18 months to 5 years of age	
Poor motor coordination	Premature, coercive, or censuring training
Persistent speech problems (stammering, loss of words)	Exacting standards above child's ability to conform
Timidity towards people and experiences	Transmits anxiety and apprehension
Fears and night terrors	Unaccepting of child's efforts; intolerant towards failures
Problems with eating, sleeping, elimination, toileting, weaning	Overreacts, overprotective, overanxious
Irritability, crying, temper tantrums	Despondent, apathetic
Partial return to infantile manners	
Inability to leave mother without panic	
Fear of strangers	
Breathholding spells	
Lack of interest in other children	
5 to 12 years of age	
Anxiety and oversensitivity to new experiences (school, relationships, separation)	Disinclination to separate from child; or prematurely hastening separation
Lack of attentiveness; learning difficulties; disinterest in learning	Signs of despondency, apathy, hostility
Acting out; lying, stealing, temper outbursts, inappropriate social behavior	Foster fears, dependence, apprehension
Regressive behavior (wetting, soiling, crying, fears)	Disinterested in or rejecting of child
Appearance of compulsive mannerisms (tics, rituals)	Overly critical and censuring; undermine child's confidence
Somatic illness; eating and sleeping problems, aches, pains, digestive upsets	Inconsistent in discipline or control; erratic in behavior
Fear of illness and body injury	Offer a restrictive, overly moralistic model
Difficulties and rivalry with peers, siblings, adults; constant fighting	
Destructive tendencies; strong temper tantrums	
Inability or unwillingness to do things for self	
Moodiness and withdrawal; few friends or personal relationships.	

From Senn MJE and Solnit AJ: Problems in child behavior and development, Philadelphia, 1968, Lea & Febiger.

Extreme psychopathology	
Child	Parents

Extreme lethargy, passivity, or hypermotility

Little or no speech, noncommunicative

No response or relationship to people, symbiotic clinging to mother

Somatic ills; vomiting, constipation, diarrhea, megacolon, rash, tics

Autism, childhood psychosis

Excessive enuresis, soiling, fears

Completely infantile behavior

Play inhibited and nonconceptualized; absence or excess of autoerotic activity

Obsessive-compulsive behavior; "ritual" bound mannerisms

Impulsive destructive behavior

Severely coercive and punitive

Totally critical and rejecting

Overidentification with or overly submissive to child

Inability to accept child's sex; fosters opposite

Substitutes child for spouse; sexual expression via child

Severe repression of child's need for gratification

Deprivation of all stimulations, freedoms, and pleasures

Extreme anger and displeasure with child

Child assault and brutality

Severe depressions and withdrawal

Extreme withdrawal, apathy, depression, grief, self-destructive tendencies

Complete failure to learn

Speech difficulty, especially stuttering

Extreme and uncontrollable antisocial behavior (aggression, destruction, chronic lying, stealing, intentional cruelty to animals)

Severe obsessive-compulsive behavior (phobias, fantasies, rituals)

Inability to distinguish reality from fantasy

Excessive sexual exhibitionism, eroticism, sexual assaults on others

Extreme somatic illness: failure to thrive, anorexia, obesity, hypochondriasis, abnormal menses

Complete absence or deterioration of personal and peer relationships

Extreme depression and withdrawal; rejection of child

Intense hostility; aggression toward child

Uncontrollable fears, anxieties, guilts

Complete inability to function in family role

Severe moralistic prohibition of child's independent strivings

Child Mental Status Examination

Size and general appearance

General health and nutrition
Distinguishing physical characteristics or deformities
Habit patterns
Dress and grooming
Apparent age versus chronological age
Gender attributes
General appeal
Mannerisms and gestures

Motility

Hyperkinesis
Hypokinesis
Tics and other involuntary movements
Autoerotic movements

Coordination

Posture and gait
Balance
Gross motor movements
Fine motor movements
Writing and drawing

Speech

Receptive-expressive disorders
Auditory acuity and discrimination
Articulating defects
Disorders of intonation
Grammar
Infanfantilisms of speech
Pitch and modulation
Dysrhythmias
Pronomial reversal and gender confusion
Mutism — logorrhea
Neologisms and mannerisms of speech

Intellectual function

General information
Vocabulary
Ability to communicate
Ability to understand and respond to questions
Learning and adapting ability
Creative talent
Social awareness
Self-help functions

Modes of thinking and perception

Ego-defensive mechanisms
Hallucinations
Orientation
Self-concept and body image
Identification
Peculiar verbalizations
Preoccupations and concerns
Human references
Suspiciousness and paranoid ideation

Emotional reactions

Primary. Fearfulness, sadness, anger, anxiety, shame

Secondary. Apathy, oppositional behavior, docility, sulking, appropriateness, range of affects, regressive pull and recovery potential

Manner of relating

Capacity for separation and independent behavior
Friendliness
approach-avoidance
Agressivity
Need for approval
Age level (regressed or precocious)
Adaptability

Fantasies and dreams

Dreams
Symbolic elaboration versus undisguised concrete representation
Fantasies
Stories
Wishes
Ambitions

Character of play

Formal characteristics
Gender configurations
Transactional aspects
Characteristics versus contents

From Goodman JD and Sours J: The child mental status examination, ed 2, New York, 1987, Basic Books, Inc, Publishers.

decision to proceed with the direct interview or to use a diagnostic play session. Four aspects of the child's verbalizations should be noted (Adams and Fras, 1988):

1. Speech: Provides clues to the child's level of maturity.
2. Voice: Type, amount of inflection, an organic marker such as hoarseness or flatness should be noted. Lack of normal inflections may be due to childhood psychosis, while a monotone may suggest depression.
3. Vocabulary: Excessive baby talk or adult sophisticated vocabulary provides clues to child's social contacts.
4. Message: Content that is age, sex developmentally appropriate should be noted.

When the child's language development is age-appropriate, use of Piaget's theory of cognitive development and Chombsy's theory of language development integrates language with the assessment activities and facilitates identification of language and communication skills. The norms and age-appropriate behaviors summarized in Table 3-5 influence the assessment, and Table 3-6 provides guidelines that facilitate assessment of the language developmental level and psychologic status.

MODES OF THINKING

The relationship of speech to thought and to activities underlies the importance of evaluating children's level of speech to understand and identify their thought maturity. Clients' speech is the critical marker for formal thought disorders (FTD), one of the primary criterion for the diagnosis of schizophrenia and manic depressive illness in the DSM-III-R.

The major signs of FTD are the following:

1. Illogical utterances: Speech is characterized by the inappropriate and immature use of causal utterances or unfounded and inappropriate reasoning.
2. Incoherence: The content of speech is misunderstood due to scrambled syntax.
3. Loose associations: The topic of conversation is changed and moved to an unrelated topic.
4. Poverty of content of speech: Insufficient information is provided to the listener.

The lack of developmental guidelines for the diagnosis of FTD and the difficulties even seasoned clinicians experience in distinguishing between immature developing speech and FTD necessitates ruling out childhood schizophrenia by obtaining further psychologic evaluation. Several tools have been developed to diagnose FTD: the Thought Disorder Index (TDI) (Arbeleda and Holzman, 1985) and the Kiddie FTD scale (K-FTDS) (Caplan and others, 1989). The specific scale used to rule out or distinguish between depression and schizophrenia is the Kiddie SADS (Bierman and Schwartz, 1986; Puig-Antich and Chambers, 1978).

Neurologic and Psychologic Evaluations

NEUROLOGIC EVALUATION

Many experienced clinicians can perform a cursory neurologic examination without touching the child, and many aspects of the sensory system and neurologic development can be ascertained by carefully observing the child's posture, gait, fine

Table 3-5   Norms and Age-Appropriate Child Language Development Levels

Age	Characteristics
18 mo	Uses and understands limited number of single-word utterances rooted in action, such as "run," "walk," "give"; first verbal activity is extension of sensorimotor structure (Piaget, 1959)
2 yr	Begins putting two words together (expressing relationships)
2-3 yr	Begins using words in subject-verb-object order; adds suffix "-ing" to words; learns to use "no"
3-5 yr	Begins using "where, what, why" questions and tags ("isn't it, can't we, doesn't it?"); researchers found subjects used no tag questions at age 4, subjects used 32 tag questions per hour at age 4½ (average adult uses 2 to 3 per hour)
5-7 yr	Masters verbal intricacies; logical links grasped in manipulation of external world; thought processes include more than "surface" phenomena
11-13 yr	Separates speech from action; hypothetic and deductive thinking replace pragmatic "here and now" thinking; expresses thoughts independently of immediate experience; initiates language about past, present and future events; language becomes abstract and implements thought

Table 3-6   Guidelines for Verbal Interactions

Age	Action of clinician
≤4 yr	Limits verbalizations to words to which young child can respond; makes simple statements by "naming" feelings and objects (adds to child's language repertory and provides new option of behavior)
5 yr	Selects familiar concrete objects as play materials and uses those stimulating child to express areas of concern symbolically; engages child in dialogue during play (clarifies child's thought organization); uses verbal interactions and clarification to fill in missing data, identify and clarify child's misinterpretations, assist child in organizing experiences
9-12 yr	Expands and refines child's communication skills during dialogue; focuses on play materials to alleviate barriers stimulated by "eye-to-eye" interaction; manages perceptions of social and size differences between adults and child (can impede verbal expression); employs group therapy if indicated

and gross motor coordination, speech, and quality and tone of voice during the diagnostic interview. Initial observations may indicate the need for a comprehensive neurologic examination.

The neurologic examination delineates the distinctions between the neurologic development and the emotional/intellectual development. It also provides critical data on emotionally disturbed children.

Some games gain the child's cooperation and facilitate the neurologic examination by evaluating specific functions (Beck, Rawlins, and Williams, 1987):

1. Cerebral functions: Games such as Hide-and-seek, Simon Says, Blindman's Bluff, and naming games can be adapted to assess specific areas of cerebral functioning. Hide-and-seek can assess the child's *stereogenesis* by having the child identify objects with eyes closed. Simon Says is useful for assessing the child's temporal sequence because it requires following a series of commands.
2. Reflexes: Games such as Let's Take Turns and You Play Nurse help eliminate the child's fear of reflex hammers and other instruments used in a physical examination.
3. Cerebellar functions: Games such as Follow the Leader and Pin the Tail on the Donkey can be adapted to evaluate the child's coordination and balance. The child's ability to hop or stand on one foot, rapidly touch various body parts, and balance with eyes closed contributes to this evaluation.
4. Sensory functions: Body tapping and tickling games before the assessment of responses to touch, pain, vibration, and temperature may alleviate this sensitive aspect of assessment that involves body contact. It is suggested that this part of the neurologic examination be left to the final assessment because children often become uncooperative, affecting the other data to be gathered.
5. Cranial nerves: Following lights, whispering games, and playing dentist assist in assessing the child's visual acuity, visual fields, movement of eyeballs, jaws, sensations of taste, corneal reflexes, hearing, movement of the mouth, throat, and tongue, facial expressions, and sensations in the forehead, jaw, and cheeks.

CHILDREN'S DRAWINGS*

The child's body image is assessed as part of the physical dimension. The body schema begins at birth and unfolds through the gradual differentiation of self. The progressive inclusion of body imagery in the child's mind can be measured by children's drawings. A specific measurement, the Goodenough-Harris Draw-A-Person (DAP) test, is based on the premise relating drawings to developmental age and psychosocial perceptions. Norms for children's drawings have been established, and the child's neurologic integrity, psychomotor skills, and graphomotor and fine motor development can be assessed through the DAP test. Figure 3-1 illustrates the progressive complexity of children's drawings. The *mandala* in children's art is of interest because it is a universal religious symbol spontaneously drawn by most children.

The child's drawings of human figures is an index of the child's body image and progresses in a predictable manner. Drawings of the 3- to 4-year-old child usually depict large heads and eyes, with arms and legs as appendages of the head. Gradually the trunk appears, with arms and legs as stick appendages. The child's

---

* Modified from Beck CK, Rawlins RP, and Williams SR, editors: Mental health-psychiatric nursing: a holistic life-cycle approach, St. Louis, 1987, The CV Mosby Co.

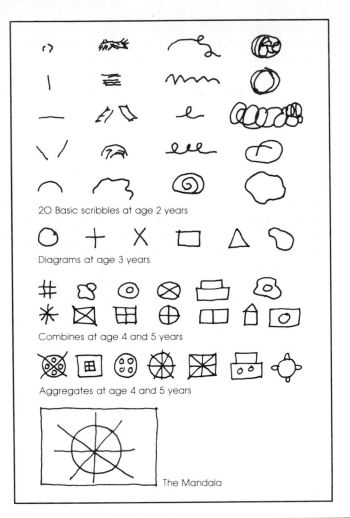

20 Basic scribbles at age 2 years

Diagrams at age 3 years

Combines at age 4 and 5 years

Aggregates at age 4 and 5 years

The Mandala

Figure 3-1   Components of children's drawing. (From Kellogg R: Stages of development of preschool art. In Lewis HP, editor: Child art: the beginning of self-affirmation, Berkeley, Calif, 1966, Diablo Press.)

overemphasis or omissions of body parts gives clues to the child's body image. Although the child's drawings are a rich source of assessment data, they are examined within the context of other assessment data for verification. For example, excessively large hands may indicate aggression, small arms and hands withdrawal and denial. Children's drawings are often used as evaluation data. For example, the child's drawings completed during assessment can be compared with drawings after the child has been in therapy to evaluate body image changes during the therapeutic process. Clearly defined body boundaries, a balance of body parts and appendages, and centering the person on the drawing paper are signs of a positive body image.

Generally, having children draw pictures of themselves and of their family provides important assessment data. When children are asked to "draw a person," they tend to concentrate on objects and details. When asked to draw a picture of themselves and their family, they project specific fears, anxieties, and concerns. In addition to viewing drawings within the child's developmental context, it is important to ask the child about the drawings because artwork can easily be misinterpreted. Winnicott (1971) suggests that the therapist draw a "squiggly" mark on a piece of paper and encourage the child to add marks to it. Once the child starts to draw, the therapist can ask the child about the marks, and the relationship can begin.

Often children draw what they cannot say. "Drawing out" the child encourages the surfacing of problem areas that otherwise may not be disclosed. Because of cultural and family taboos, children are usually unable to discuss sexual issues and anxieties. Children's drawings rarely include genitals; these omissions are normal and reflect the child's internalization of taboo topics (DiLeo JH, 1970). When the child draws genitals or stylized sexual figures, the clinician needs to realize that the child's drawing may be in response to rape trauma or sexual abuse.

PSYCHOLOGIC TEST EVALUATIONS

Most psychologic tests are *norm-referenced,* that is, psychologists have identified norms of responses for children at various developmental ages and stages. For example, the Bender Visual Motor Gestalt Test may verify a child is functioning at an immature level despite intact physical and neurologic integrity. Clinicians need to be familiar with behavior-specific tests, and in some situations, referral to a psychologist for additional testing may be appropriate (Sattler, 1988).

Diagnostic Formulations

Diagnostic formulations are developed from the composite of the information gathered and processed and are the outcome of the clinician's knowledge of normal child development and symptoms of deviations. Clinicians should not overlook important behaviors or emphasize unimportant clinical data. Kessler (1966) suggests using the following guidelines in determining if a child's behavior requires intervention:

1. Age discrepancy: Is behavior developmentally immature or precocious?
2. Frequency of occurrence: Is one symptom increasingly noted? Does a pattern exist?
3. Number of symptoms: Are the symptoms in any special area?
4. Degree of social advantage: Does the child have a support system? What is the relationship of the child's symptoms to family and peers?
5. Is the child aware of the problem? Is it causing suffering and distress?
6. Is the behavior acute or chronic?
7. What are the normal aspects of the child's behavior?
8. How does the child deal with threatening, frustrating, and challenging situations?

DEVELOPMENTAL DIAGNOSES

The developmental viewpoint believes that a child's behaviors are a product of interactions between the child's inherent tendencies, maturation patterns, and environmental influences. This perspective is a marked change from the past belief focusing on the parents' concerns and desire for change in the child. Clinicians need to distinguish the parental (or referring persons) concerns and normal maturation crises, transient growth crises, temporary reactions to interpersonal or environmental stress, regression in psychologic functions with physical injury, and normal plateaus and quit periods in development (Call, 1986).

Many experts, including Greenspan (1981), claim that the diagnostic approach in child psychiatry ideally should be developmental. Greenspan suggests using an age/stage developmental observational framework. Greenspan's method for collecting and organizing data produces information on ways in which children organize experiences and on their phase-specific uniqueness. It consists of DSM-III diagnostic labels from Axes I and II, DSM-III diagnoses based on etiologic factors, and developmental diagnoses and can be used without subscribing to a particular psychologic or psychodynamic theory. It includes the following categories, which apply to children from infancy to the age of 10:

1. Physical functioning: neurologic, sensory motor, integrative
2. Patterns of relationships
3. Overall mood or emotional tone
4. Affects
   a. Range and variety of affect
   b. Depth of affect expression
   c. Appropriateness of affect
   d. Discriminative capacity of affects
   e. Relationship of intensity of affect to stimulation or capacity for regulation of affect
5. Anxieties and fears
6. Thematic expressions
   a. Organization of thematic expression
   b. Depth and richness of thematic development
   c. Relevance in age-appropriate context
   d. Thematic sequence

The lack of a cohesive developmental focus that encompasses children's multiple developmental lines in the DSM-III and DSM-III-R has resulted in considerable dialogue in the literature (Greenspan, 1981). Critics claim the DSM-III-R diagnoses focus on syndromes and personality types that do not address adaptation or maladaptation of the child at each development level along clinically relevant lines.

MODIFIED MSE AND DEVELOPMENTAL DIAGNOSES

Critchley's outline (1979) for an MSE is practical when time, finances, and travel are an issue for the child and family. The six-step developmental framework focuses on the child's principle ego (reality-oriented) functions and capacities and is an alternative format. After the clinician collects the history and developmental data from the parents, a free play session yields the mental status data. Unstructured then structured activities follow and measure the child's sensorimotor and cognitive development. Projective techniques and questions elicit the child's understanding of the reasons for the encounter and the difficulties perceived by the child. An example of this method follows:

1. Appearance: Physical size, handicaps, mannerisms, and tics are observed. The child's dress gives clues to ego functions such as sex role identification and conformity.

2. Mood or affect: Predominant feelings (including fluctuations or changes during interview), apparent relationship of changes to interview content, and ease in venting emotions are observed.

3. Manner of relating to the clinician: Understanding of reasons for the evaluation; degree of avoidance or relatedness to the examiner, activity, verbalizations; age-appropriate conversational and social abilities, and responsiveness to suggestions and questions are evaluated.

4. Modes of thinking and intellectual functioning: Behavioral descriptions narrating the child's developmental level, predominant mode of thinking, and conceptualization of time, space, causality, and body image are observed, including inferences of thought disorders, memory, and problem-solving abilities.

5. Capacity for play and fantasy: Observations include qualitative and quantitative aspects of the child's play and fantasy materials, use of play materials, predominant themes, theme development, use of nurse by the child in play activities, quality of integration of play or fantasy, and degree of creativity or stereotype.

6. Sensorimotor development: Age-appropriate fine and gross motor activities, symmetry of movements, eye-hand coordination, right-left discrimination evaluated. Tasks presented as games such as hopping on one foot, skipping, Simon Says, drawings, and writing tasks are observed. Activities are designed to determine need for additional neurologic examination (Critchley, 1979).

Treatment Planning

Most clinicians agree that treatment planning is the acid test of clinicians' skills (Adams and Fras, 1988; Greenspan, 1981; Shea, 1988). In child psychiatry, treatment plans include activities that are supportive, healing, comforting, educating, and advocacy measures and are based on the child's and parents' developmental age and stage. For example, during the resolution of the developmental task, a period of stress and increased vulnerability — a maturations crisis — is created. Treatment plans need to include parental education about normal child development so that they are able not only to overcome the current problem but also to have a clearer concept of future developmental changes in their maturing child. Treatment plans are directed toward achieving the following goals:

1. Relieving symptoms
2. Preventing recurrence of the disorder

3. Reorienting the behavior, feelings, and thinking of the child toward healthier functioning
4. Restoring or building a more wholesome interpersonal network to support the child's welfare

The therapeutic plan guides nurse-client actions and involves setting short- and long-term goals. Most treatment plans define goals in terms of behavior. The process of planning is often therapeutic for parents and children and makes them aware of their current mental health needs.

Treatment plans depend on clinicians' awareness of treatment modalities available and their mastery of these interventions. The major types of therapies for children include pharmacotherapeutics and psychotherapies, which involve individual, family, behavioral, cognitive, and expressive therapies.

PRIMARY, SECONDARY, AND TERTIARY PREVENTION

While treatment focuses on solving problems, treatment planning should also include preventive aspects so that more serious disorders can be averted. The developmental approach to prevention is based on the assumption that the child and family have times of increased susceptibility to illness, and treatment plans should be designed to enhance resistance.

Secondary intervention plans shorten the course of illness through early identification. They include family crisis interventions and strengthening the child's and the family's support systems and involve teachers and other significant adults and children. Tertiary prevention plans stress aggressive rehabilitative activities that reduce chronicity by avoiding complications.

REFERENCES

Adams P and Fras I: Beginning child psychiatry, New York, 1988, Brunner/Mazel, Inc.

American Academy of Child Psychiatry: Child psychiatry: a plan for the coming decades, Washington, DC, 1983, American Academy of Child Psychiatry.

American Nurses' Association, Council on Psychiatric and Mental Health Nursing: Standards of child and adolescent psychiatric and mental health nursing practice, Kansas City, Mo, 1985, The Association.

Arboleda C and Holtzman PS: Thought disorders in children at risk for psychoses, Arch Gen Psychiatry 42:1004, 1985.

Beck CK, Rawlins RP, and Williams SR, editors: Mental health-psychiatric nursing: a holistic life-cycle approach, St Louis, 1987, The CV Mosby Co.

Bierman KL and Schwartz LA: Clinical child interviews: approaches in developmental considerations, J Child Adolesc Psychotherapy 3:267, 1986.

Call JD: Psychiatric evaluation of the infant and child. In Kaplan, HI and Sadock BJ, editors: Comprehensive textbook of psychiatry, ed 4, Baltimore, 1986, Williams & Wilkins.

Caplan R and others: The Kiddie formal thought disorder rating scale: clinical assessment reliability and validity, J Am Acad Child Adolesc Psychiatry 3:408, 1989.

Chess S and Thomas A: Temperament in clinical practice, New York, 1986, The Guilford Press.

Christ AE: Cognitive assessment of the psychotic child: a Piageian framework. In Chess S, and Thomas A, editors: Annual progress in child psychiatry and child development, New York, 1976, Brunner/Mazel, Inc.

Clunn P: The child. In Beck CK, Rawlins RP, and Williams SR, editors: Mental health-psychiatric nursing: a holistic life-cycle approach, St. Louis, 1987, The CV Mosby Co.

Critchley DS: Mental status examination with children and adolescents: a developmental approach, Nurs Clin North Am 14:429, Sept 1979.

DiLeo JH: Young children and their drawings, New York, 1970, Brunner/Mazel, Inc.

Dodds JB: A child psychotherapy primer, New York, 1985, Human Sciences Press, Inc.

Elkind D: Piagetian psychology and the practice of child psychiatry, J Am Acad Child Psychiatry 21:435, 1982.

Gerson R and McGoldrick M: Genograms gathered and displayed by the computer. In Zimmer J, editor: Clinics of primary care: computers in family medicine, Philadelphia, 1986, WB Saunders Co.

Goodman JD and Sours J: The child mental status examination, ed 2, New York, 1987, Basic Books, Inc, Publishers.

Greenspan S: Intelligence and adaptation: an integration of psychoanalytic and Piagetian developmental psychology, Psychol Issues Monograph, No. 47/48, 1979.

Greenspan S: Clinical interview of the child, New York, 1981, McGraw-Hill, Inc.

Group for the Advancement of Psychiatry, Committee on Child Psychiatry: The process of child therapy, New York, 1982, Brunner/Mazel, Inc.

Kessler J: Psychopathology of childhood, New Jersey, 1966, Prentice Hall.

McGoldrick M and Gerson R: Genograms in family assessment, New York, 1985, WW Norton & Co, Inc.

Menninger Foundation, Children's Division: Disturbed children, San Francisco, 1969, Josey-Bass, Inc, Publishers.

Puig-Antich J and Chambers W: The schedule for reactive disorders and schizophrenia for school-aged children (Kiddie SADS), New York, 1978, New York State Psychiatric Institute.

Sattler JM: Assessment of children, ed 3, San Diego, 1988, JM Sattler, Publisher.

Senn MJE and Solnit AJ: Problems in child behavior and development, Philadelphia, 1968, Lea & Febiger.

Shea SC: Psychiatric interviewing: the art of understanding, Philadelphia, 1988, WB Saunders Co.

Simmons JE: Psychiatric examination of children, Philadelphia, 1969, Lea & Febiger.

Starkey PJ: Genograms: a guide to understanding one's own family system, Perspect Psychiatr Care 19:164, 1981.

Williams JB and Wilson HS: A psychiatric nursing perspective on DSM-III, J Psychiosoc Nurs Ment Health Serv 20:14, 1982.

Winnicott DW: Playing and reality, New York, 1971, Basic Books, Inc, Publishers.

Woolf VV: Family network systems in transgenerational psychotherapy: the theory, advantages and expanded application of the genogram, Fam Ther 10:219, 1983.

Chapter 4

Theoretic Bases for Child Psychiatric Nursing

Child psychiatric nursing interventions support normal growth and development and are based on developmental theories from physiologic, psychologic, cognitive, social, sensorimotor, moral, and philosophic sources. This knowledge base includes the concepts of temperament, coping styles, individual traits, interacting systems, and nonverbal communication such as body movements, play, and other symbolic expressive activities (ANA, 1985).

All clinicians in psychiatric mental health nursing base their practice on theories from the psychosocial and biophysical sciences and use both medical and behavioral models of mental health and illness. Child psychiatric nurses also draw on theories such as systems, symbolic interactions, communication, interpersonal, learning, psychoanalysis, stress, and crisis (Beck, Rawlins, and Williams, 1988). The focus of this chapter is on classical and contemporary theories of child development, child psychopathology, psychology, and child psychiatry.

Theoretic Foundations

Biologic and social sciences provide the theoretic underpinning of the multiple lines of child growth and development emphasized in the child standards (ANA, 1985). These sciences have also contributed to the epidemiologic knowledge base needed for prevention interventions of childhood psychopathology such as complications, familial patterns, prevalence, sex ratio, course, associated etiologic features, relationship of child to adult disorders, gender ratio, and geographic and social class incidence.

Psychiatry includes the disciplines of psychology, sociology, anthropology, political science, social work, family studies, medical sociology, social history, general systems, and women's studies. Without a basic knowledge in these areas, child psychiatric nurses are hampered in practice. The current status and contributions of these sciences are summarized in the box. Most disciplines are more concerned with different aspects of child development and psychiatry than with different explanations of the same behavior.

The inclusion of legal and ethical areas of child mental health reflects the trend toward closer scrutiny of the field by the federal government, hospital administrators,

Theoretic Foundations for Psychiatric Nursing

Basic biologic sciences

Neurosciences: Biophysics is based on the assumption that determinants of psychopathology are deficiencies in anatomy, physiology, or biochemistry. Biophysical data are the basis of psychopathology, and biophysical methods are the primary therapeutic measures. The biophysical disease model focuses on the development of the structure and functioning of the brain. Neuroscience subspecialties (for example, neuroanatomy, neurochemistry, neurophysiology, neuropathology, neuroendocrinology, and brain chemistry) have contributed to neuroendocrinology. Diagnosis is more complex, with efforts toward supplementing symptomatic criteria with laboratory tests and biologic markers. Advances include blood studies, CAT scans, and dexamethasone suppression tests (DST). Understanding of child psychopharmacology (see Chapter 16), including sites and mechanisms of drug actions, brain chemicals, and mind altering drugs, has been a revolution in child psychiatry care.

Genetics: Early identification of DSM-III-R Axis II conditions (autism, mental retardation, developmental disorders) is now possible through genetic research. Genegenic type identification has evolved to identifying disorders that are not genetically transmitted but demonstrate a high family incidence, for example, conduct, obsessive, reading disorders, alcohol and drug abuse, depression, and functional enuresis.

Ethnology: Science of behavior biology compares species close to humans by using animal research, for example, Harlow's attachment behavior with monkeys, Lorenz's study of aggression, and Tinbergers' work with birds. The initial scientific focus was on genetically determined behavior typical of a species, theorized to be fixed, with releasing mechanisms, sign stimuli, and a hydraulic model of motivation to explain displacement activities (Lorenz, 1956). It expanded to learning and environmental stimulation to become the field of human ethnology, influencing psychoanalysts such as Bowlby (1958, 1969). While making generalizations from animal studies to humans is precarious and crossing species lines is risky (Adams and Fras, 1988), the research approach, methods, concepts, theories, and techniques are easily applied to child study; most research in human ethnology is done on children.

Behavioral and biosocial sciences

Social cultural: The focus is on the public health model, including preventive programs, therapeutic communities, crisis intervention therapies, and social-action research. Concepts of social, community, individual casework, group work, collaboration with schools and other community organizations, and an advocacy model within the community are involved.

Clinical child psychology: This behavioral science has its origins in psychology. Developmental psychology includes the study of normal development related to aspects of perception, sensory, motor, and cognitive performance and empirical approaches to emotions and social cognition. The theories and research of experts, such as Binet, Simon, and Rutter, are known for their significant contributions to psychologic testing. The contributions of Piaget and Werner have advanced understanding of the symbolic functioning in children. The psychoanalytic approach

Continued

Theoretic Foundations for Child Psychiatric Nursing — cont'd

Behavioral and biosocial sciences — cont'd

views normal child development from the perspective that adult psychopathology is the direct product of continued operations of childhood events, processes, anxieties, and unconscious defensive maneuvers. These theories seek to explain unconscious phenomena. Phenomenologic theorists hold that the characteristics of each individual's conscious experience is the primary focus of clinical science. The ideas of existential theorists, such as May and Kelly, and the self theory of Roger are included. Behavioral theorists view subjective introspection as unscientific and define environmental influences on behavior objectively. They believe that patho-logic behavior is learned and develops according to the same laws governing the development of normal behavior and that disturbed behavior differs from normal behavior only in magnitude, frequency, and social adaptiveness. Interpersonal theorists, such as Meyer, Sullivan, Fromm-Reichmann, Fromm, and Horney, broadened psychotherapy to include family and group therapies. They focus on small groups involving face-to-face relationships.

Psychology epidemiology: This science includes the study of incidence, morbidity, mortality, natural history, and the prevalence of mental illness. Social psychiatry is based on the work of Adolf Meyer. It is the theoretic basis for both social psychiatry and community mental health. It involves risk factors and psychosocial etiology of children's mental illness and includes the theories and research of Rutter, Shaffer, Pasamanick, and Offer.

Systems science: This branch of the behavioral biosocial sciences includes inte-grated theories of crisis intervention and living systems. Integrative theorists be-lieve that psychologic processes are multidetermined and multidimensional and that single-level approaches are narrow. The bio-psycho-social model includes all aspects of the individual holistic approach. It involves the mechanistic para-digm of input, output, and subsystems; the theoretic rationale for family and group psychotherapy, verbal, nonverbal, syntactic, and symbolic communication theories. It includes the theories of Bateson, Lymann, Winn, Jackson, and Satir.

Ecology: This science studies the mutual interactions between people and their environment. Ecology focuses on social groups rather than unconnected individuals (Bronfrenbrenner, 1974). Theorists believe that groups have a life and force of their own, which is more than and different from the sum of the separate effects of individuals on them. Ecologic interventions influence the interaction of groups within environmental settings. The theories apply to schools, milieu settings, and social organizations with recognizable boundary and purpose affecting children's growth and attainment.

Ethical-legal: Because of its origins in juvenile courts and child guidance clinics, child psychiatry has strong advocacy perspectives. It works closely with the legal system and influences political action in national, judicial, and legislative issues. It addresses school truancy, delinquency, adoption, foster home placement, child custody, abuse, rights of children to treatment, rights of handicapped children, children's due process, and their capacity for participation in treatment decisions.

and third-party payers, resulting in an increased emphasis on self-regulation, monitoring, and peer review. Many experts emphasize the need for basic and continuing education course requirements in legal and ethical issues for all clinicians practicing in psychiatry (Schetaky and Benedek, 1985).

CONTEMPORARY SCHOOLS OF CHILD PSYCHOPATHOLOGY

Psychopathology, the study of abnormal behavior, has not developed as a separate academic discipline or scientific field in adult or child psychiatry. The need to develop a science of psychopathology was recognized over 80 years ago when the American Psychopathological Association was founded; however, the association has not developed into the multidisciplinary scientific society envisioned (Klerman, 1986). There is no "single journal devoted to this topic, although important aspects of psychopathology appear in many journals of psychiatry, clinical and consulting psychology, anthropology, social work and medicine" (Klerman, 1986).

Some experts cite the divisions and rivalries that persist in the field as a contributing factor to the absence of a dominant paradigm (Fagin, 1983; Klerman, 1986). For over 50 years the competing four core mental health professions (psychiatry, psychology, social work, and nursing) have been rivals for public attention, quality students, government and foundation funds, and individual and third-party fees for treatment. Others claim that the lack of interest in psychopathology from 1940 to 1970 reflects a skepticism about and disinterest in diagnosis and classification of mental disorders. This view is attributed to the lack of pervasive, generally accepted models of psychopathology. Another contributing factor is that when adult mental disorders were treated by dynamic psychotherapy, the need for diagnosis for differential treatment assignments was usually immaterial (Klerman, 1986). Even without a unified framework, remarkable scientific advances were made during the last few decades resulting in a phenomenal paradigm shift and a reformulation of psychiatric disorders, as seen in the DSM-III (1980) and DSM-III-R (1987). With the use of the DSM-III and DSM-III-R, treatment decisions can be grounded on a nosologic base with specific treatments designated for categoric disorders.

The DSM-III-R is increasingly being used as a framework for teaching and research in the mental health fields, and psychopathology has permeated clinical practice and reduced some of the traditional controversies and competition (Klerman, 1986). Theories relevant to child psychopathology are shown in Table 4-1.

The DSM-III multiaxial psychiatric evaluation system yields psychologic and physiologic data that will contribute future clarification of possible etiologic factors in mental diseases and facilitates planning treatments and formulating prognoses. The DSM-III-R has been compared to the child's functional dimension (Table 4–2) and has a fourfold increase in categories as compared to similar sections in the DSM-III, reflecting the "great increase in knowledge in this area" (Webb and others, 1981).

The V multiaxial codes are used for problems not attributable to a mental disorder by assessing the severity of psychosocial stressors. The V codes introduced social and culturally mediated stress factors into the DSM-III-R diagnostic system (see Chapter 5). The case example on pp. 67 and 68 illustrates a diagnostic formulation using the DSM-III-R Axes.

Table 4-1   Contemporary Schools of Psychopathology

School	Major U.S. proponents	Theoretic sources	Research emphases	Therapeutic emphases
Biologic	Kety Winokur E. Robins Snyder	Nineteenth-century Continental schools of biology and medicine	Genetic studies, CNS research	Pharmaco-therapy
Psycho-analytic	Erikson Mahler Kohut Kernberg	Freudian psychoanalytic concepts and American modifications, particularly ego psychology and self psychology	Personality disorders	Intensive, insight-oriented dynamic psychotherapy and psychoanalysis
Interpersonal	Sullivan Fromm-Reichmann Fromm Horney Arieti	G. H. Mead, C. H. Colley, and the Chicago school of symbolic interactionists	Adult relations on marriage, work, and community	Broadened psychotherapeutic framework to include family and group therapies Psychotherapy with ambulatory patients with schizophrenia, depression, and other severe conditions
Social	Meyer Leighton Lindemann Caplan	Conceptual and empirical frameworks derived from sociology, anthropology, and other social sciences	Epidemiologic studies and large-scale social analyses	Community mental health services
Behavioral-cognitive	Wolpe Eysenck Beck	Pavlovian and Skinnerian theory Cognitive psychology	Behavioral analysis of symptoms Learning theory	Behavior therapies Cognitive therapy

From Klerman, GL: Historical perspectives on contemporary schools of psychopathology. In Millon T and Klerman GL, editors: Contemporary directions in psychopathology: toward the DSM-IV, New York, 1986, The Guilford Press.

Table 4-2   Functional Classification of DSM-III-R Disorders of Childhood

Function	Classification
Intellectual	Mental retardation (IQ below 70) with possible causes including biologic deficits such as fetal trauma, chromosome deficits, inadequate fetal oxygenation due to maternal toxins (for example, alcohol, tobacco); mild: IQ of 50-70 (educable); moderate: IQ of 35-49 (trainable); severe: IQ of 20-34; profound: IQ below 20
Physical	Includes eating disorders (anorexia, bulimia; pica; rumination in infancy), atypical stereotyped movement disorders (transient, chronic motor tic, Tourette's disorder); other disorders with physical manifestations (stuttering, functional enuresis, functional encopresis, sleepwalking, sleep terror disorder)
Developmental	Involves psychologic functions required to develop social skills, language, attention, perception, reality testing, movement; includes infantile autism, pervasive developmental disorders, atypical pervasive developmental disorder
Emotional	Includes anxiety disorders (separation, avoidance, overanxiety) and others (reactive, attachment, schizoid, mutism, oppositional, identity)
Behavioral	Includes attention deficit (inattention, impulsion, hyperkinesis), conduct disorder (patterns violate rights of others and social norms); undersocialized individual shows reduced or absent bonding or loyalties; socialized individual shows some social attachment, aggressive-nonaggressive atypical individual demonstrates socially age-inappropriate behaviors

Modified from Webb LJ and others: DSM-III training guide, New York, 1981, Brunner/Mazel, Inc. and American Psychiatric Association: Diagnostic and statistical manual of mental disorders, ed 3, Washington, DC, 1987, American Psychiatric Association.

Case Example

Eight-year-old Stuart was referred to the local child guidance clinic by his physician because of a history of overactivity, school problems, onset of illness within the family, and poor social relations.

The mother reported that Stuart was overly active as an infant and toddler. His teachers found him difficult to control once he started school. He is described as extremely impulsive and distractible, moving about tirelessly from one activity to the next. At present he knows his alphabet and a few words on sight, but he cannot read a full sentence. His math skills are also minimal. Because of these learning difficulties, Stuart is in a small, self-contained class for learning-disabled children. His teacher reports that he is immature and restless, responds best in a structured, one-on-one situation, but is considered the class pest because he is continually annoying the other children and is disobedient.

Since the start of the school year, he has soiled his pants on numerous occasions, does not seem to have any special friends, and has been reported on different occasions by the school bus driver for hitting other children and throwing things on the bus.

His mother reports that Stuart responds to some disciplining, but lately he has started sassing back and swearing at her. He frequently throws temper tantrums, especially if she asks him to do something or denies his requests. His constant badgering and whining are irritating for her, especially since her husband has been in and out of the hospital for the past six months with a terminal illness. Because of his illness, the father has been minimally involved with Stuart's discipline for the last 2 years.

DIAGNOSIS

Axis I: 314.01 Attention deficit disorder with hyperactivity
         318.81 Oppositional disorder
         307.70 Functional encopresis
Axis II: 315.00 Developmental reading disorder
         315.10 Developmental arithmetic disorder
Axis IV: Severe — 5
Axis V: Poor — 5

DISCUSSION

Stuart has symptoms typical of ADD with hyperactivity, as well as the additional burden of learning problems. His oppositional behavior (disobedience, throwing, hitting, tantrums) and soiling seem to coincide with the worsening of his father's illness. Because these behaviors have persisted for so long, diagnosis of Oppositional disorder and encopresis is made, and a stressor is recorded on Axis IV rather than using the diagnosis of adjustment disorder.

From Rapaport JL and Ismond DR: DSM-III training guide for diagnosis of childhood disorders, New York, 1984, Brunner/Mazel, Inc.

Changing Paradigms of Child Development

Before the sixteenth century, children were considered miniature adults (performinism) in Western cultures. Few distinctions were made between the emotional and mental maturity and immaturity of children and adults. Some historical accounts describe children at 5 or 6 years of age reading and writing — reports that seem exaggerated and beyond the biologic capacities and stage-age concepts of contemporary theories. Some historians suggest that concepts of child development are created by society and scientists and that science has essentially created today's children and the stages of development (Aries, 1962; Plotz, 1988; van den Berg, 1961).

Until the sixteenth and seventeenth centuries, inheritance was viewed as the primary factor in human development (Havighurst, 1973; Murray and Zentner, 1985). When social values changed, the task of scientists was to study and explain child development. They focused on identifying and documenting aspects of child development based on assumptions and definitions that remained relatively unchallenged until the 1960s.

Most child historians also claim that the cult of childhood — childhood as a cultural and social category — began in the sixteenth century, peaked in the twentieth century, and is now drawing to an end. Many of the social institutions (such as the family) formed to protect children are disappearing (Plotz, 1988).

The classical developmental theorists used a framework of ordered changes over time that arose in systematic ways and passed through predetermined, epigenic stages; developmental events were dispersed in time and meaningfully and lawfully related to one another. They assumed that children organized more of what they were to progressively and predictably achieved higher levels of complexity or abstraction. For example, through increasing symbolization abilities, children cognitively develop time-binding capacities and can grasp past as well as future events. The theories of Freud, Piaget, Erikson, and Kohlberg were based on traditional premises about human development and emphasized continuity, predictability, and critical periods. The study of transformation from one stage to another and the variables that affect these transformations constituted the study of human development (McNeill, 1966). Most concepts were biologic and stressed the organization of life processes, openness, and the capacity to change. Selection, a vital concept of development, held that human development was a response to choices and that humans responded to routines by developing habits while the increased complexity of the developmental processes reached a final, stable state.

Epigenetic concepts theorized that human dimensions evolved over time, and the timing of development was internally controlled by the biologic nature of the species. New phenomena and properties did not exist in miniature before they emerged; teleology, development, and change had purpose and meaning and enabled children to seek a predestined state, as if an invisible organizational force existed that directed them to a developmental end point.

Children's behavior was viewed as appropriate or inappropriate compared to characteristic norms set for children of the same age and stage. Therefore a behavior had different meaning during infancy than during later childhood, and no behavior had only one meaning.

Growth was defined as the physical or physiologic change with passage of time, learning, behavior modification from experience, and maturation (the process of moving and unfolding human potential).

Some classical theorists stressed the internal determination of development and the importance of successfully completing one stage before progressing; others stressed external influences on development and the importance of interpersonal relationships in modifying behaviors from an unsuccessfully completed stage.

Psychoanalytic theorists used the concepts of id, ego, and superego as components of development. Although differing in many other respects, classical child developmental theories concurred on four components of developmental stages:

1. Each stage is qualitatively different from the preceding stage.
2. Each stage occurs in an invariant sequence.
3. Each stage is age-related within general age groupings.
4. Each stage demonstrates a newer, more complex system of organization.

Through the mid-1960s, many theories were proposed, spanning a spectrum of explanations for progressive development. Some theories claimed that infants were born with and thus had no need to learn from experience (Jung's racial consciousness concept) or that humans were born with characteristics making them human (Freud's instinct theory). In contrast, the theories of humanism, behaviorism, and cultural relativism focused on environment rather than genetic endowment. These humanistic positions emphasized the development of normative patterns.

Nagal (1957) was one of the first scientists to observe that development was both a process and the product of a process. He theorized that development involved two components—a system possessing a definite structure and a definite set of preexisting capacities: "a sequential set of changes in the system, yielding relatively permanent but novel increments not only in its structure but in its modes of operation as well." Nagel's premises were expanded in the 1960s and a definition of human development according to two models of change was generally accepted. These models differentiated between universal sequences and individual differences. The organismic (structural) model viewed life events as components of the organized complexity. The mechanistic (behavioral) model viewed life events as distinct causes of particular outcomes. The definition of an organismic model was the first time that life events were viewed as important.

During the 1970s, research in human development reflected a paradigm change to the life-span context (Schaie, 1984). This perspective is based on different premises than classical developmental theories and a comparison of the two concepts is shown in the box. It proposes that people continue to develop and change throughout life. Life-span theorists considered change and stress major causes of mental illness, occurring at any time during the life cycle. This theory was initially accompanied by an intensified rejection of traditional psychologic theories and practices and led to gradual synthesis and acceptance of the contributions of the classical schools.

For the first time in centuries, change, self-actualization, and growth were considered possible in adults. Many healthy, normal people began seeking help through human potential therapies with the goal of improving their adult lives. This perspective changed the social concept of therapy from applying only to severe pathology to enriching and improving the lives of normal people. Childhood traumas were no longer seen as permeate and irreversible.

The view that development is a lifelong process is not new; it can be traced back to second century Hindu scriptures, which state that a person's true education does not begin until after the birth of the first grandchild. Grandparents were encouraged to abandon worldly possessions and go on pilgrimages to fulfill their only responsibility—the search for the eternal self. When Freud and his followers gathered in Vienna to develop psychoanalysis, Jung made a major contribution to the understanding of life-span development with his descriptions of the individuation-separation process (Campbell, 1987). However, the initial scientific focus on life-span development was ignored by society, whose major fascination was Freudian theories of the unconscious and childhood psychosexual development.

Medical historian Aries (1962), compares the rediscovery of life-span philosophy to a pendulum that has swung too far, with adults overzealously preoccupied with

---

Contrasting Premises of Child and Life-Cycle Developmental Theorists

Child developmentalist

Infancy and early childhood are the major life periods for the origin and occurrence of developmental change.

Change as development is similar to the concept of growth in biology, that is, unilinear, end state-oriented, irreversible, and qualitative.

Development is based on the age-related principles of ontogeny. Age graded mechanisms such as biologic maturation and socialization are predictable age-graded phases, and the successful completion of each is critical to the successive task or stage-phase accomplishment.

Mechanistic and organismic paradigms result in end states.

Life-cycle developmentalist

Human development is a lifelong process, and no one period of the life cycle has primacy in the origin and occurrence of developmental changes.

Growth and differentiation concepts of child development are but one of a number of developmental phenomena.

There are many origins of development that may occur at any time in the life cycle that are critical factors in shaping human development. These nonnormative events include career change, accidents, migration, divorce, and illness.

The individual acts on the environment, and selection occurs through this active and selective behavior. The contextual and dialectical conception of human development holds that there are not always the same end states.

Modified from Baltes P: On the potential and limits of child development: life span developmental perspective, Newsletter of the Society for Research in Child Development, Summer 1979.

---

self-development and neglecting and abusing dependent children and the elderly. He optimistically predicts that after a social philosophic reorientation a new period will emerge, one that equally respects and values the potential and contributions of all members at all stages of life.

Biologic Theories of Child Development

TRAITS, TEMPERAMENT, AND PERSONALITY

Personality is defined as the elements that constitute and characterize children's total reaction to their environment. Temperament is their behavior style of reacting to the environment (Chess and Thomas, 1986) and is related to the trait theory—the oldest explanatory model for individual personality attributes. In addition to the types shown in Table 3-2, temperament has also been classified according to a perceptual construct, that is, a mother's view (easy, slow-to-warm-up, difficult, and intermediate). Although not genetic, these inborn traits produce different social response styles that influence attachment patterns and the development of psychopathology.

Life-span researchers have used longitudinal studies to study the stability and changes in personality traits over time. The age at which personality stabilizes is not known, but there is little evidence that major changes occur. The question is not when or ways in which personality changes, but how stability is maintained.

BODY IMAGE AND BODY BOUNDARIES

Body image is a biophysical concept that also spans biologic and social dimensions of child development. It is dynamic and fluid, unfolding through interpersonal, environmental, and body-ideal imagery and adjusting in response to physical growth and life experiences. Maturing children gradually differentiate themselves as separate objects from their mother, and their body schema becomes relatively fixed and stable by the end of adolescence.

According to Schilder (1970), everything that individuals know or feel about their body is learned, except for neurologic functioning. The perceptions of body parts are on the reality, conscious fantasy, and unconscious symbolic levels. This three-dimensional interpretation of body image is generally viewed as a central component of personality. Schilder noted that body image occurs through continuous interaction with the environment. This social dimension includes interpersonal awareness that children use to perceive ways in which they affect others, resulting in adjustments. Emotions function as social and not psychologic components; the stronger the perceived emotional bond, the more intense the effect of the significant other on children's body image.

Failure of adults to perceive the body parts is dramatically observed in the phantom limb phenomenon, a psychologic and/or neurologic form of denial in which memory traces at subconscious levels respond as if the receptor still exists. Body-image distortions also contribute to anorexia and bulimia in young children.

Observations of the variations in surgical clients' response to body-image altering procedures illustrate the unique, unconscious, symbolic meaning given to body parts. Amputations, mastectomies, hysterectomies, vasotomies, colostomies, rhinoplasties, and cosmetic surgery may evoke severe body-image disturbances. Children may show a lack of interest; adults may display frigidity or impotence.

Body boundaries are an important aspect of the body-image concept in children. They usually coincide with the physical border of the body, and when there are discrepancies between the actual body and the idealized mental image of the body, ego defenses may form.

Small children have weak body boundaries, as observed in their terrified reactions to someone cutting their hair or nails, body parts that are within their body boundaries. Children with severe mental disorders, such as schizophrenia, are often deficient in their body boundaries and images. They lack the ability to localize, discriminate, and give meaning to mental body images.

Before adolescence, girls usually have higher body barriers than boys, partly because of the anatomic location of the genitals. Female genitalia are internal and protected, but male genitalia are outside the body, making boys more vulnerable to body boundary problems (Erikson, 1968). During adolescence, boys have higher body barriers than girls because they can visually perceive genital maturation and change and can tie many body sensations to observations. The prepubital female experiencing growing pains has no external signs for body-imagery adjustments and may therefore have greater difficulty accepting puberty and menstruation as a normal process.

NURSING APPLICATIONS

The progressive inclusion of body parts and organs in children's body imagery can be easily assessed through drawings. These drawings, the projective "Draw A Person" tests, determine if body imagery is developing normally (see Chapter 3). Questions that elicit verbal children's body image include the following:
1. How would you describe yourself physically?
2. How do you feel about your body?
3. What do you value most and least about your body?
4. If you could, how would you change your body?

Often the nurse can detect the beginning of body image problems by observing whether children are having strange body sensations or are more aware of one body part than another. The nurse may inadvertently hamper the therapeutic relationship if children's body image, body buffer zone, and personal space are not considered.

Children relate touching to parenting and attachment bonding. Nuances of transference in which children express feelings toward the nurse that they feel for their parents may occur without careful monitoring of these issues. For example, children fearful of their parents may be fearful of the nurse. The nurse may also knowingly take on more of the parental role than appropriate, and children's dependency needs and tendency to overidentify may stimulate countertransference. A nurse's negative parental attitudes become competitive to the parents, and the children frequently become depressed after termination of the nurse-client relationship.

Children's high or low body-barrier assessment also demonstrates distinctions useful in planning interventions when body-image discrepancies are suspected. High body-barrier children perceive definite boundaries between their body and other objects and are independent with low field dependency. Low body-barrier children are more field dependent, rely more on peers for support, and attach or extend their body images to objects and possessions (for example, cars, adornments, and attire). Extreme low body-barrier children *depersonalize* — attribute parts of their body and/or thoughts to others. These children cannot discriminate between external and internal body stimuli. They may exhibit *catatonic withdrawal*, a severe affirmation of body boundaries and a lack of sensation in body parts because of constricted posture and denial of external sensory input.

Psychologic Theories of Child Development

PSYCHOANALYSIS

Psychoanalysis is a broad field covering almost every domain of human activity. Freud developed psychoanalytic theory from the clinical treatment and observations of adult clients. Free associations concerning present problems, past experiences, and relationships to important others were disclosed through transference, which uncovered the early developmental process and unconscious influences. Reconstruction focused on past developmental points of arrest and unintegrated conflicts in developmental transitions.

Using Maxwell's theory of a fixed reservoir of energy that was transformed yet conserved and Darwin's emphasis on the central role of sexuality, Freud formulated the first comprehensive theory of childhood personality development for the psychoanalytic treatment of adults. Anna Freud, his daughter, applied and expanded these theories to child treatment, making a major contribution to the psychoanalytic study of the child.

Freud's concept of infantile sexuality and his emphasis on mother-child attachment were other theoretic legacies. He was one of the first theorists to stress the stages of development and the influence of early childhood experiences on adult behavior. He stated that the first 5 years of life were the most important and that by the age of 5 a child's basic character was formed and unchangeable. Of the five developmental stages, his theory delineates three being completed before the age of 5. In Freudian theory, no stage is ever completely replaced by the subsequent stage, and psychologic residues from all psychosexual developmental stages are found in adults.

Although Freud considered his Oedipal complex theory a major contribution, contemporary critics view it as one of his most controversial concepts. It did, however, relate the biologic nature of humans with their dependency on their parents, from which the psychoanalytic theories of object relations and attachment emerged.

Generalizing from reconstructions of the past and an adult's view to a model of child treatment was difficult for early child psychoanalysts eager to test Sigmund Freud's theories with children. Because the transference process differed, applying the classical psychoanalytic process was an obstacle. Early efforts in child psychoanalysis failed, and it was not until the field of clinical child psychology grew and contributed observations of well-adjusted children in their natural environment that a different, more appropriate method of child psychotherapy and child analysis emerged. Therefore, child psychiatry did not develop until after adult psychoanalysis was well established, and sources for theory development were child psychotherapy, clinical observations of children, and Freud's clinical adult reconstructions.

Freud's concepts of splinting of ego, the executive, autonomous ego, and the ego's dual task of dealing with external and internal object relations, adaptive functions, and coping styles was the theoretical basis from which Melanie Kline developed the concept of the adaptive functions of the ego. Later, the field of ego psychology and the British school of object relations emerged and departed from Freud's original theories to become one of the major areas of contemporary theories of child psychiatry.

The neo-Freudian theorists emphasized biosocial and cultural interactions and followed the premises of human development used by the classical analytic group. These theorists include Karen Horney, Alfred Adler, Eric Fromm, Abraham Kardiner, and Harry Stack Sullivan.

INTERPERSONAL THEORIES

Harry Stack Sullivan, the founder of interpersonal psychiatry, developed a theory of child development focusing on relationships between and among people. The central theme of Sullivan's theories (1953) revolved around anxiety and emphasized society as the creator of personality. The concepts that people can change and that environment is important in forming personality profoundly influenced the development of contemporary anthropology (Kluckhohn, 1944).

Sullivan's concept of the conscious and unconscious mind was described using the terms *witting* and *unwittingly*. He stressed that individuals learned to behave in certain ways because of interpersonal relations and called behavior patterns *dynamism,* a concept similar to Freudian defense mechanisms. The dynamism arising from anxiety was termed the *self-system.* It protects the individual and is the product of the irrational aspects of environment and culture. This system interferes with constructive changes in the personality by preventing objective self-assessment of behavior. It is continually reinforced throughout life and colors all experiences.

Theories of affective development describe the simultaneous internal and external processes in development of the self-concept: (1) the active, individual child's role and (2) the appraisals of the child from significant others. When the latter is negative, such as in child abuse and neglect, children will often internalize the negative feelings into their developing self-concept and act on them.

Sullivan's theories bridged psychiatry, psychology, and sociology, an alliance from which the field of social psychology grew, and moved dynamic psychiatry from the Freudian focus on the treatment of neurotics to original and valuable clinical work with hospitalized schizophrenic patients. The use of his interpersonal concepts in practice have been expanded with the interpersonal theory of Hildegard Peplau (1951).

Cognitive Theories in Child Development and Child Disorders

Cognition plays a critical role in both child development and child psychiatric disorders, and the study of thought processes is a central feature in child psychiatry. Abnormalities in thinking, such as delusions and hallucinations, concern all psychiatric disciplines, and cognitive deficits account for many childhood psychopathologic conditions, including mental retardation, developmental delay, and related biologic organic disorders.

Piaget's theory of children's growth of intellect revolutionized earlier views. His theory established that children think differently than adults and that they often spontaneously learn without input from adults. Piaget refined his theory through empirical research challenging many long-standing psychoanalytic premises, including the Freudian concepts of the unconscious, intrapsychic defense mechanisms, and the relationship of the unconscious to dream analysis. Piagetian theory expressed the view that children learn through imitation and play, activities demonstrating the dual process of assimilation and accommodation (Nars, 1966; Singer and Revenson, 1978). It described stages and ages of cognitive maturation.

The preoperational period begins with reflective intelligence and requires symbolic representations. Once children understand the permanent existence of objects (internal representations), they begin to symbolize, that is, mentally manipulate represented objects in their absence. Initially, infants rely on narcissistic, motivational models (for example, the stars go to bed because children do). Children cannot keep two interdependent dimensions in mind at the same time (conservation), put themselves in another's place (decentralization), or see things from another point of view. These cognitive operations are available once children reach the concrete operational stage.

Piaget developed a six stage developmental sequence showing ways in which children progress from believing dreams are real-life occurrences to believing dreams exist outside themselves and are visible to others. His theory of cognitive development refuted the Freudian notion of memory during early childhood and demonstrated that their understanding of internal representations did not occur until the age of 6. It also posited that normal children progress to the next stage once there are signs of mental operations from the higher stage, even though earlier forms of thinking persist.

Piaget claimed that cognitive developmental stages are not caused by genetic predisposition but by children's intrinsic growth. His definition of intelligence included intellectual activities, such as reasoning, remembering, and perceptions, which contrasted with the traditional, specific IQ-measurement concepts. His research also verified that the first three stages of cognitive development applied to children of all cultures. Changes at adolescence occurred when the intellectual processes of formal operations matured and thinking became less individualized and more influenced by environmental factors (Pulaski, 1971).

Piaget did not view the external environment as influencing intellectual development but as a source of interesting, conflicting information, stimulating children's thinking and growth. Piaget posited stimulation came from children's peers during play and conversations, and his theories of children's growth of social thinking paralleled his theory of cognitive development.

Schemata are patterns of actions or thoughts that form a structural framework for processing incoming data. This structure is altered by the continuous action of assimilation and accommodation. During assimilation, external stimuli are altered to fit the schema, and in accommodation the schema adjusts to the stimuli. Although usually balanced, accommodation is more apparent during imitation (role-modeling), and assimilation is dominant during play. (Piaget, 1962).

Cognitive development integrates the previous structure into new and more complex behavior patterns. The speed of progress through the stages is affected by individual differences and social influences. After children have developed abstract thinking fully, they are capable of the mental operations needed by adults. No new structures occur after adolescence. Unlike other theorists, Piaget did not suggest that adults rework or adapt previous stages and problems.

COGNITIVE PROCESSING AND DEFICITS

The research of many disciplines has contributed to changes in the understanding of children's developing cognition. The reciprocity between the cognitive and affective domains and the interaction of cognitive processing and cognitive deficits are emphasized. Although these areas are not easily separated, they have significant theoretic and practice implications.

Scientists studying the aging process in 1950s discovered that cognitive deficits in the aged were reversible and that learning was a continuous life process. These findings contradicted the long-held assumption that adults, the aged, and cognitively impaired children were biologically limited in their learning potential. As a result the discipline of adult education emerged, and behavioral and social-learning theories were adapted to psychiatric care of adults and the aged. Parent self-help groups were developed, designed to teach parents management of their normal as well as difficult children. Adults are now taught how to parent through methods such as parent effectiveness programs (PET).

Advances in the understanding of cognitive processing resulted in the following trends:

1. There is a renewed interest in the self-system, and the mediating roles of personal qualities, such as self-esteem, self-efficacy, and locus of control, are more clinically and theoretically important.

2. The extent to which children's cognitive capacities regulate their susceptibility to different life experiences is emphasized. Rutter (1972) found that very young infants are not as seriously debilitated by separations from their parents as previously believed because they are not capable of forming enduring, selective attachment cognitions. Older children are less vulnerable to the ill effects of separation because they are capable of maintaining relationships through memory, even when separated.

3. There is increased attention to individuals' interpretation of experiences. Kagan (1984) claims that infants' limited abilities to process experiences is the reason for experiences during infancy rarely leading to lasting psychologic damage. In contrast, Bowlby (1984) suggests that the loss of a parent during infancy or childhood causes a negative set creating a tendency to respond with depression to a later loss because of lasting impairment to children's sense of self-esteem or self-efficacy.

4. Cognitions are viewed as important causal factors in the genesis and prolongation of psychiatric disorders, especially depression. Beck and others (1967) theorized that depression is not only a profoundly depressed mood but also a cognitive state characterized by a negative view of the self, the life situation, and the future. The belief that individuals are powerless to influence negative experiences prevents coping actions.

Some cognitive deficits may cause mental diseases that indirectly underlie social deviance and social impairment. For example, autistic children fail to engage in normal, reciprocal exchanges and to make and maintain love relationships. Attention deficits may constitute the core of both hyperkinetic disorders and schizophrenia. Researcher's suggest an association between language retardation and psychiatric disorders and between reading disabilities and conduct disorders. Christ (1976) found that most deviant school-age children characteristically function at either the sensorimotor or the preoperational level. The sensorimotor period begins at birth and ends when children actively manipulate their environment. Sensorimotor-period children are usually fixated at the secondary circular reaction stage, set at between 4 and 8 months of age. Deviant children engage in repetitive actions, and although they may accommodate, the process is not the same as in normal children. They avoid change and have a defensive need for sameness, usually making no efforts to generalize.

NURSING APPLICATIONS

To encourage developmental strides, clinicians should introduce new materials that motivate initiation of generalization, any sign of which is positive movement and growth. Children functioning in the sensorimotor stage are limited to stimulus-response, trial-and-error learning. Management should be based on what they can cognitively understand, and punishment, praise, and management using behavior modification are indicated. Specific visual demonstrations with verbal reinforcements (showing and telling) are also therapeutic. Children's cognitive status can be tested using tests such as the Piaget's Conservation Test (Tolpin, 1978).

Several notable articles in nursing literature clarify the developmental concepts of Piaget and their application to child nursing. Pothier (1970) provides an assessment tool and interventions (Table 4-3). McRae's study (1977) includes two case studies illustrating the use of Piaget's theory in educating single parents.

Language Development

Mastery of language is a major developmental task of childhood. Linguistic and cognitive structures have parallel development, exemplifying progression along multiple lines. Speech (ideation), thoughts (cognition), and locomotion (walking) foster children's development in the emotional and social dimensions and in the evolution of a separate self-concept. Balance among these developmental lines is essential for mental health.

Before 1975, explanations of the development of language were generally based on the behavioral-learning theories of Skinner. These storage-bin or babble-luck theories hypothesized that children learned language by storing sentences they had heard and then pulled sentences from the bin when they needed them. Skinner's theory was based on his observations that all babies babbled, regardless of the cultural language learned and that, by luck, children would babble a sound parents reinforced.

Extending Piaget's concepts, Chomsky (1975) proposed a theory of language development that has contributed to the subspecialty of psycholinguistics, and subsequent research and theories have profoundly altered communication interventions with normal and emotionally disturbed children (Gardner, 1985). Chomsky's theory provided a cognitive developmental perspective suggesting that children establish internal rules of grammar to convey intended meanings. Children use and interpret new sentences through internal cognitive operations called *transformations* — the reordering of words into sentences.

Language growth is characterized by a fixed gross motor developmental schedule following universal sequences. Children initially use noun-phrases, such as "I want," and then develop structure-dependent grammar spontaneously because of an innate maturation process — the language acquisition device (LAD). It helps children establish rules and regularities and is similar to the innate schematic tendencies of birds as shown in their species-specific songs.

Although rudimentary at birth, the LAD matures with the central nervous system, and activities and play foster the use of words. Mastery proceeds from one word to two, and syntactical rules of inflections, phrases, structures, and negatives are also learned progressively. Children initially verbalize perceptions by naming them and then proceed to verbalizing emotions. The naming of objects and feelings reinforces children's sense of control of feelings and helps them to distinguish what is real.

The development of language facilitates reality testing and is basic to self-identity and differentiation spanning all dimensions of the developing child. Clinicians should use age-appropriate verbal interactions, play, symbolic expressive activities, and games (ANA, 1985). Norms and ways of talking to children at different ages are shown in Tables 3-5 and 3-6.

Moral Development

Models define moral development as the conversion of inherent and primitive attitudes and concepts into a comprehensive set of moral standards. This transformation process is part of and depends on the aggregate cognitive growth of children, emerging as they reorder their social world. Their progression through a series of stages or patterns of thought is constructed through active experience and is invariant in order for all persons and cultures. Other explanatory models of moral development are found in psychoanalytic and social-learning theories (see boxes on pp. 84 and 85).

Theories of moral development began with Freud's theory relating superego formation to castration anxiety. Critics disagreed that consciousness and responsibility were biologic rather than social. Piaget's view was that justice was the core of morality. To identify the moral cognitive developmental process, Kohlberg (1964) developed a series of moral dilemma examples suitable for boys 10 to 16 years of age. They had to choose between alternative actions either in conformity with rules and authority or in accordance with the needs of others. Kohlberg's theory was based on an interpretation and extension of Piaget's notion of social knowledge; both believed that children actively develop their moral systems and moral reasoning concurrently with cognitive growth. Kohlberg's stages began with an obedience and punishment orientation and progressed to self-accepted moral principles that were developmentally fixed, invariant, and universal. Kohlberg's research confirmed Piaget's findings that the level of boys' moral reasoning depends on their age and maturity. He further refined the theory by defining different types of moral reasoning and classifying these types into levels (Omery, 1983).

Current research and theorists studying moral and cognitive development dispute Kohlberg's theory, claiming it to be gender based. Others believe that emerging that concepts of morality can be observed much earlier and are interrelated with the emergence of a sense of self. This development is attributed to biologic maturation in the developing child, with the specificity of some neurons intensified by environmental exposure and reinforcement while the specificity of others fade from disuse. Gilligan defined moral development as "the expanding conception of the social world reflected in the understanding and resolution of the inevitable conflicts that arise between self and others."

Table 4-3   Assessment Tool Based on Piaget Developmental Stages

Stages		Age (weeks)	Behavior	Imitation	Play
1. Reflexes		0-4	Sucking Vision Hearing Prehension	Assimilates crying of others into own	None Autistic
2. Primary	2a	5-7	Hand to mouth coordination	Habitually observes others	Pleasure of activity
Adaptive Circular	2b	8-11	Head moves in coordination with vision, hearing		
	2c		Directs object in hand to mouth Sucking		
3. Secondary	3a	18-20	Reaches for objects	Imitates sounds and movement in repertory	Pleasure of activity
Adaptive Circular	3b	21-25	Grasps objects Transfers hand to hand		
	3c	26-29	Changes body position to reach objects Uses hand independently, makes interesting sights last longer		
4. Coordination Secondary Adaptation		30-33	Manipulates objects with both hands Combines two objects in one activity	Imitates new models, sound patterns	Ritual activity (bedtime)
5. Tertiary Adaptive Circular	5a	42-47	Searches for objects out of sight Predicts outcomes	Active Deliberate	Turns activity ritual into play
	5b	48-51	Repeats actions to original stimulus Solicits help		
	5c	52-55	Uses gestures and responds to them		

From Pothier P: The developmental concepts of Piaget applied to nursing assessment and interventions with atypical children, JPN and Mental Health Services, p 30, Jan/Feb 1970.

Object	Space	Causality	Play material-activity
Undifferen-tiated	Collection of spaces	Action Tension Need rhythm	Pacifier Red balloon over head Soft tone bell Cradle gym Rattle Cuddle toys
Undifferen-tiated	Collection of spaces	Begins to see difference in action and result Self-acting on things	Mobile Manipulate shape, size, texture, weight
Attempts to recapture Sensorimo-tor rela-tions and objects	Depth near and far Coordinates vi-sion and pre-ension	Sees self acting on things	Soft colored nested boxes Mirror Squeak toys Plastic tube-marbles Turning handles Turning dials, wheels Develop repertoire of put in, take out, shake, rattle, squeeze
Object Performance	Masters rela-tions of self to objects	Causality recog-nized only when he acts	Squeeze box Horn, harmonica, castinets Jack-in-box, xylophone Bead stringing Large straws, bubble pipe Prepare for eating Roll ball, peek-a-boo Wave bye-bye
Looks where objects last seen	Understands ob-ject as seper-ate, indepen-dent of child's action	Sees self as cause of and recipient of causes	Pat-a-cake Works for toys covered, in a bag, in boxes

Continued

Table 4-3   Assessment Tool Based on Piaget Developmental Stages—cont'd

Stages		Age (weeks)	Behavior	Imitation	Play
6. Invention of new means through mental combinations	6a	56-59	Responds to single commands	Imitates new and complex models	True make-believe fantasy
	6b	60-64	Uses objects and people to gain goals Follows sequences of displacement Identifies objects on request	Imitates domestic activity	
	6c	65-70	Delayed imitation Identifies objects in pictures Identifies body parts		

Freud and other early psychosexual developmental theorists strongly influenced Kohlberg's theory, and these early theorists believed that emotions were the basis for cognitive and moral development. Freud said the id (the emotions) came first, and the ego (the basis for thought and logic) followed after the resolution of conflict. Nineteenth century theorists placed emotions primary in their theories and felt thought was the necessary coping device to deal with conflict. The theory of Kagan and contemporary scientists is directly opposite, alleging brain maturation is accompanied by the emergence of cognitive competency. Thus, children cannot show stranger anxiety or fear of their mother leaving until they are cognitively mature enough to remember the past; children cannot experience guilt until they are mature enough to recognize alternate actions. These new findings affirm that most of the profound emotions and conflicts children experience must wait for cognitive maturation and advances. The environment (including parenting) mesh with genes and the maturation of biologic programming to sculpt the mind (Kagan, 1990).

According to Kagan's research (1990), between the ages of 18 and 24 months normal children become aware that they have intentions and feelings and that they can act. This is a remarkable insight, resulting from the maturing brain and living in a world of interactions. Thus, no matter how many interactions children have had before the middle of the second year, the sense of self cannot be derived from experiences.

According to this research, the developing sense of self can be tested using a simple *rouge test.* A dab of rouge is applied to the end of a child's nose, and the child is placed in front of a mirror. Children less than 18 months of age will not reach up and touch their nose because they do not recognize the face in the mirror as their face. By 18 to 20 months of age, children will touch the rouge on their nose because the sense of self has matured.

Object	Space	Causality	Play material-activity
Mastery of existence as things apart	Keeps account of movement in space	Foresees an effect given its cause	Puzzles □ ○ Puts in pieces on request Strings bead colors on request Play peg people in pull toy Placement of shapes, colors on flannel board Buttoning Zippering Latches and locks Garden tools Playhouse set up—dolls Nested eggs to unfold Books—stories Music—action songs Games—identifies body parts

Another behavioral sign of the emergence of a sense of self and moral maturation is children's use of words such as "I," "me," and "mine." Deaf children of deaf parents who are learning sign language make the sign for "I" and touch themselves at the same age as children with normal hearing. This profound finding suggests a biologically unfolding time table in the development of a sense of self and moral principles.

The developmental milestone of the moral sense can also be clinically observed. When playing, children show concern and distress when they find a flawed toy. They cry and reject the toy or object, saying it is "broken," "dirty," or "bad." They become disturbed and take the toy to their mother or therapist, implying that something is wrong and needs to be fixed. This perception is maturational, and no child younger than 12 to 18 months responds in this way.

The flawed toy response indicates that a child has a primitive understanding of the integrity of objects, and if this integrity is violated, someone has done something wrong. Kagan claims that this emergence of a moral sense is one of the most profound developmental accomplishments and is as important as physical milestones and that it should be observed and assessed.

Thus, the sense of self and the moral sense are two qualities programmed by biology and emerge during development, and from this perspective, other qualities shown by the developing child emerge and fall in place. For example, the terrible twos are not characterized as a period of stubbornness but as a time when children are trying to establish the difference between right and wrong and when the relationship between thought or cognition and emotions becomes clear. Most nursing practice, educational programs, and published research are based on Kohlberg's model, and nurses have just begun to explore how to develop more principled thinking in themselves and their clients (Omery, 1983).

Moral Development: Freudian Psychoanalytic Concepts

Castration anxiety: Fear of castration, which induces a repression of sexual desire for the mother and hostility toward the father.

Identification: Method by which a person takes over the features of another person and makes them a corporate part of the personality.

Introjection: Mechanism by which the superego is incorporated into the personality.

Oedipus complex: Sexual attraction for the parent of the opposite sex and hostility toward the parent of the same sex.

Penis envy: Discovery by the female of the absence of the penis and the subsequent desire to possess the penis she lacks.

Phallic stage: Third stage of personality development during which the sexual and aggressive feelings associated with the function of the genitals comes into focus.

Superego: Part of the personality that represents the moral standards of society as conveyed to a person by the parents.

From Omery A: Moral development: a differential evaluation of dominant models, ANS 10:5, 1983.

Moral Development: Kohlberg's Cognitive-Development Model

Level I: Preconventional morality

Level of morality in which the perspective is egocentric.

Stage 1: Heteronomous morality. Right is might, the reason for doing right is to avoid punishment by those with superior power.

Stage 2: Instrumental morality. Right is following rules when it is to someone's immediate interest; acting to meet one's own interest and needs and letting others do the same. Right is also what is fair, what is an equal exchange, a deal, or an agreement.

Level II: Conventional morality

Level of morality in which the perspective is societal.

Stage 3: Mutual morality. Right is living up to what is expected or what people generally expect of people in a certain role. Being good is important and means having good motives, showing concern for and about others, and keeping mutual relationships.

Stage 4: Social system morality. Right is fulfilling the actual duties agreed on. Laws are to be upheld except in extreme cases where they conflict with other fixed social duties. Right is also contributing to society, the group, or the institution.

Level III: Postconventional morality

Level of morality in which the perspective is universal.

Stage 5: Social contract morality. Right is being aware that people hold a variety of values and opinions, and that most values and rules are relative to the groups'. These relative rules would usually be upheld, however, in the interest of impartiality and because they are the social contract. Some nonrelative values and rights such as life and liberty, however, must be upheld in any society and regardless of majority opinion.

Stage 6: Universal ethical (principled) morality. Right is following self-chosen ethical principles. Particular laws or social agreements are usually valid because they rest on such principles. When laws violate these principles, one acts in accordance with the principle. Principles are universal principles of justice, the equality of human rights, and respect for the dignity of human beings as individuals.

From Omery A: Moral development: a differential evaluation of dominant models, ANS 10:5, 1983.

Moral Development: Gilligan's Cognitive-Developmental Model

Level I: Orientation to individual survival

Morality is sanctions imposed by society. Being moral is surviving by being submissive to authority. The perspective is egocentric. Transition from selfishness to responsibility. Responsibility for and to others is more important than surviving through submission.

Level II: Goodness as self-sacrifice

Goodness is viewed as relying on shared norms or expectations. Being moral is first of all and above all not hurting others, with no thought of the hurt that might be done to self.

Transition from goodness to truth. Responsibility for not hurting others shifts to include not only others, but self.

Level III: Morality of nonviolence

The injunction against hurting becomes the moral principle governing all moral judgments. This injunction includes an equality of self and others. Care, instead of individual rights, becomes the universal obligation.

From Omery A: Moral development: a differential evaluation of dominant models, ANS 10:6, 1983.

Ego Psychology

Theories of emotional development used in child psychiatry have generally evolved from ego psychology, which bridges psychoanalysis and developmental psychology. It uses a structural approach to understand children by focusing on the ego or self as an independent agent. Theorists supporting this viewpoint believe that the ego is a rational agent responsible for intellectual and social achievement and consists of an energy source, motives, and interests. Ego psychologists include Heinz Hartmann, Ernst Kris, Harry Lowenstein, and David Rapaport.

Two dominant approaches to theory development have been used by ego psychologists. The approach used by theorists, such as Piaget, Chomsky, and Kohlberg focused on children's conflict-free ego functions. In contrast, Anna Freud, Margaret Mahler, and Eric Erikson studied the ego as it defends, synthesizes, and assists the developing personality in response to conflict.

DEVELOPMENTAL LINES: ANNA FREUD

The basic tenets of Ann Freud's seminal theory of developmental lines (1964) followed Sigmund Freud's analytic theory, stressing that ego defenses available to children depend on their maturation level. For example, the mental mechanism of repression emerges from the superego, which does not develop until children reach the Oedipal stage. Her theory was unique, however, in conceptualizing the role of defense mechanisms.

Propositions Regarding Developmental Lines

1. . . . the concept of developmental lines, contributed to both from the side of the id and of ego development; these developmental lines lead from the child's state of immaturity to the gradual setting up of a mature personality and are, in fact, the result of interaction between maturation, adaptation, and structuralization.
2. Under the influences of internal and external factors, . . . lines of development may proceed at a fairly equal rate, i.e., harmoniously, or with high divergences in speed, leading to the many existent imbalances, variations, and incongruities in personality development (e.g. excessive speech and thought development combined with infantilism of needs, fantasies, and wishes).
3. The more mature levels of development replace the earlier ones. In short, growth proceeds in a straight progressive line until maturity is reached, invalidated only by intervening severe illness or injuries, and at the end by the destructive involuntary processes of old age.
4. The status of these developmental lines is revealed clearly whenever a child is confronted with one of the many situations in life which pose for him a difficult problem of mastery. . . . Examples of such situations as they occur in the life of every child are the following: separation from the mother; birth of a sibling; illness and surgical intervention; hospitalization; entry into nursery school; school entry; the step from the triangular oedipal situation into a community of peers, the step from play to work, tolerance for the new genital strivings in preadolescence and adolescence, the steps from the infantile objects within the family to new love objects outside the family.

From The writings of Anna Freud, 7 vols, New York, 1965–1974, International Universities Press, Inc.

According to Anna Freud, children are not capable of free association or self-reflective introspection, and to evolve communication of their intense experiences, clinicians must offer them opportunities for role playing and other activities with toys and games according to their developmental interests and tolerance. In early adolescence, introspection and free-association processes become dependable (A. Freud, 1965).

She described her theory of developmental lines as the "unfolding maturational progress through time of the changes which occur in the evolving psychic structure and function as part of the child's normal growth process" (A. Freud, 1964). Both biologic and environmental factors contributed to the developmental process of the psychic structure. The metaphysiologic profile of children consists of dynamic, genetic, economic, structural, and adaptive data. Anna Freud's propositions regarding the theory of developmental lines are shown in the box, and phases of the theory of developmental lines are summarized in the box on pp. 88–92.

Text continued on p. 93.

Propositions Regarding Developmental Lines — cont'd

5. It is not true that children become abnormal for any one reason, whether this is not being loved enough by the parents; or rejected; or not being given a feeling of security; or being overprotected; or separated; or clung to, etc. The truth is that the growth and development of the human individual, body and mind, is a complex matter. Human individuals are born with varying endowments into environments of infinite variety. Their development will in each case depend on the interaction between the inner and outer forces which come into play. A favorable environment will help those whose endowment is poor; on the other hand, children with a good endowment will show more resilience under the pressure of adverse outside influences. Every child is born different, has a different rate of growth, and experiences different growing pains and conflicts.

6. The disharmony and disequilibrium between the lines of development . . . serve to highlight precocity or retardation of specific ego functions as well as the relative preponderence of certain ego functions over others."

7. . . . progression is not the only force in operation and that equal attention needs to be paid to the regressive moves which are its inevitable accompaniment and counterpart.

8. Once we accept regression as a normal process, we also accept that movement along these lines is in the nature of a two-way traffic. During the whole period of growth, then, it has to be considered legitimate for children to revert periodically, to lose controls again after they have been established, to reinstate early sleeping and eating patterns (for example, in illness) to seek shelter and safety (especially in anxiety and distress) by returning to early forms of being protected and comforted in the symbiotic and preoedipal mother relationship (especially at bedtime). Far from interfering with forward development, it will be beneficial for its freedom if the way back is not blocked altogether by environmental disapproval and by internal repressions and restrictions.

    To the disequilibrium in the child's personality which is caused by development on the various lines progressing toward maturity at different speeds, we have to add now the unevennesses which are due to regressions of the different elements of the structure and of their combinations. On this basis it becomes easier to understand why there is so much deviation from straight-forward growth and from the average picture of a hypothetically "normal" child. With the interactions between progression and regression being as complex as they are, the disharmonics, imbalances, intricacies of development, in short the *variations of normality,* become innumerable.

9. All workers in education, and quite especially teachers, suffer from the fact that their training applies only to specific age-groups — toddlers, under-fives, school children, adolescents — and that they are deprived of the opportunity to see human growth in progress in an unbroken line, with the events of each successive phase being understood as influenced by previous experience and as pre-determining the later stages.

Developmental Lines

Libidinal phases—from dependency to emotional self-reliance and adult object relationships

Phase 1.
1. Subphase A (2–3 months): Mutual mother infant narcissism/autistic phase in which babies do not perceive themselves as separate entities and do not perceive outer reality. Ego boundries are indistinct, and infants and mothers are as one.
2. Subphase B (3–6 months): Phase of symbiotic unity/mother-child dual unity.
   a. Rudimentary ego emerges from the id.
   b. Early formation of visually dominated engrams and visual distancing in relationship to the mother occurs.
3. Phase of separation-individuation.
   a. First subphase (5-10 months): Differentiation occurs. Infants move out of the symbiotic orbit and develop distance perception, recognize mother as specific object, exhibit stranger-anxiety phenomenon, and are relatively impervious to hurts and falls.
   b. Second subphase (10-15 months): Infants' practicing phase occurs. They explore objects and areas distant from their mother and frequently return for emotional refueling.
   c. Third subphase (15-25 months): Rapprochement stage occurs. Toddlers remain close to their mother by using language and are more sensitive to hurts and falls.

Phase 2.
1. The part-object or need-fulfilling, anaclitic relationship, which is based on the urgency of the child's body needs and drives derives and is intermittent and fluctuating, since object cathexis is sent out under the impact of imperative desires and withdrawn again when satisfaction has been reached.
2. Manifested introjection of the parental objects and of guilt in very young children occurs.
3. Proper failure of the mother to play her part as a reliable need-fulfilling and comfort-giving agency will cause breakdown in individuation, or anaclitic depression, or other manifestations of deprivations, or precocious ego development, or what has been called a "false self."

Phase 3: Object constancy. Children maintain a positive inner image of the object in the external absence of the object, permitting lengthening temporary separation from their mother.

Phase 4: Anal-sadistic stage. The ambivalent attitude of pre-Oedipal children is characterized by the clinging attitude of toddlers, resulting from pre-Oedipal ambivalence and not maternal spoiling.

Phase 5: Object-centered phallic-oedipal stage. Possessiveness of the parent of the opposite sex, jealousy and rivalry with the same-sexed parent, protectiveness, curiosity, and bids for admiration and exhibitionistic attitudes are displayed. In girls a phallic-Oedipal (masculine) relationship to the mother is seen preceding the Oedipal relationship to the father. Mutuality of object relations is also demonstrated.

From Firestone J and Clunn P: The theory of Anna Freud. Unpublished paper presented at the University of Florida, Gainesville, 1977.

Developmental Lines — cont'd

Phase 6: Latency period.

1. Post-Oedipal lessening of drive urgency and transfer of libido from parental figures to peers, community groups, teachers, leaders, and impersonal ideals occurs.
2. Fantasy is characterized by disillusionment of parents, family romance, twin fantasy, and adoption fantasy.
3. Period of integration into group life and community occurs.

Phase 7: Preadolescent prelude to the adolescent revolt. A return to early attitudes and behaviors, especially of the part object, need-fulfilling, and ambivalent type occurs.

Phase 8: Adolescent struggle. Denying, loosening, and shedding of ties to infantile objects, defending against pregenitality, and establishing genital supremacy with libidinal cathexis transferred to objects of the opposite sex outside the family are displayed.

Toward bodily independence — from suckling to rational eating

. The food-mother equation persists through phases 1-4 and provides the rationale for the mother's subjective conviction of the child's refusal of food as a personal affront. This can be circumvented by the substitution of another person at meal times.

Phase 1. Being nursed at the breast or bottle, by the clock or on demand, with the common difficulties about intake caused partly by the infant's normal fluctuations of appetite and intestinal upsets, partly by the mother's attitudes and anxieties regarding feeding; interference with need satisfaction caused by hunger periods, undue waiting for meals, rationing or forced feeding set up the first — and often lasting — disturbances in the positive relationship to food. Pleasure sucking appears as a forerunner, byproduct of, substitute for, or interference with feeding (The writings of Anna Freud, 1965).

Phase 2. Weaning from breast or bottle, initiated either by the infant or according to the mother's wishes. In the latter instance, and especially if carried out abruptly, the infant's protest against oral deprivation has adverse results for the normal pleasure in food. Difficulties may occur over the introduction of solids, new tastes and consistencies being either welcomed or rejected.

Phase 3. ... the transition from being fed to self-feeding with or without implements, "food" and "mother" still being identified with each other.

Phase 4. ... self-feeding with the use of spoon, fork, etc., the disagreements with the mother about the quantity of intake being shifted often to the form of intake, i.e., table manners; meals as a general battleground on which the difficulties of the mother-child relationship can be fought out; craving for sweets as a phase-adequate substitute for oral sucking pleasures; food fads as a result of anal training, i.e., of the newly acquired reaction formation of disgust.

Phase 5. ... gradual fading out of the equation food-mother in the Oedipal period. Irrational attitudes toward eating are now determined by infantile sexual theories, i.e., fantasies of impregnation through the mouth (fear of poison), pregnancy (fear of getting fat), anal birth (fear of intake and output), as well as by reaction formation against cannibalism and sadism.

Continued

Developmental Lines — cont'd

Phase 6. . . . gradual fading out of the sexualization of eating in the latency period, with pleasure in eating retained or even increased. Increase in the rational attitudes to food and self-determination in eating, the earlier experiences on this line being decisive in shaping the individual's food habits in adult life, tastes, preferences, as well as eventual addictions or aversions with regard to food and drink (The writings of Anna Freud, 1965).

From wetting and soiling to bladder and bowel control

Conflicts between id, ego, superego, and environmental forces become obvious in the control, modification, and transformation of the urethral and anal trends as opposed to the intact survival of drive derivatives.

Phase 1. Infants have complete freedom to wet and soil, which is determined environmentally, not maturationally. The mother's methods, timing, and quality of interference are based on her needs and not the infant's needs. This phase may last from a few days (training from birth based on reflex action) to 2 or 3 years (training based on object relatedness and ego control).

Phase 2. The dominant role passes from the oral to the anal zone.
1. Bodily products are highly cathected with libido and are precious to children. They can be treated as gifts to be surrendered to their mother with love.
2. Bodily products are also cathected with aggression and can be used as weapons discharging rage, anger, and disappointment within the object relationship.
3. Toddler's attitude toward the object world is dominated by ambivalence.
4. Children's training will strongly reflect the toilet training received by the mother.

Phase 3.
1. Children introject the mother's and the environment's attitudes toward cleanliness, bodily wastes, and their own self-worth.
2. Strict training results in children holding back and becoming constipated, negative, stubborn, and stingy.
3. Permissive training results in children considering bodily wastes as important and precious. These children may be perceived as outgoing, generous, and active in trying to please others.
4. Toilet training with a specific toilet or potty chair may not generalize to other places. Children may withold urination or defecation or display enuresis and encopresis.

Phase 4.
1. Bladder and bowel control become wholly secure. The concern for cleanliness is disconnected from object ties and attains the status of an autonomous ego and superego concern.

From irresponsibility to responsibility in body management

Well-mothered children show relative indifference and unconcern in the care of their body and in protection from harm. Badly mothered or motherless children may adopt the mother's role (The writings of Anna Freud, 1965).

Phase 1. Infants alter the direction of aggression from on their body to the external world. Pain barriers are established.

Developmental Lines — cont'd

Phase 2. Orientation to the external world, understanding of cause and effect, and control of dangerous wishes serving the reality principle occur.

Phase 3. Children voluntarily endorse the rules of hygiene and medical necessities.
1. This developmental line is closely entwined with the oral and anal instinct, the libidinous phases, and other developmental lines.
2. Obstructive and uncompromising difficulties often last until the end of adolescence and may represent the last symbiosis between mother and child.

From egocentricity to companionship

Phase 1. . . . a selfish, narcissistically oriented outlook on the object world, in which other children either do not figure at all or are perceived only in their role as disturbers of the mother-child relationship and rivals for the parents' love (The writings of Anna Freud, 1965).

Phase 2. . . . other children related to as lifeless objects, i.e., toys which can be handled, pushed around, sought out, and discarded as the mood demands, with no positive or negative response expected from them

Phase 3. . . . other children related to as helpmates in carrying out a desired task such as playing, building, destroying, causing mischief of some kind, etc., the duration of the partnership being determined by the task, and secondary to it.

Phase 4. . . . other children as partners and objects in their own right, whom the child can admire, fear, or compete with, whom he loves or hates, with whose feelings he identifies, whose wishes he acknowledges and often respects, and with whom he can share possessions on a basis of equality (The writings of Anna Freud, 1965). Children in the third phase can successfully become integrated into a nursery group of peers or can contribute to a family constellation containing older siblings. The fourth stage equips children for companionship, enmities, and friendships.

From the body to the toy and from play to work

Phase 1. The first evidence of infants' play involves autoerotic pleasure involving the mouth, fingers, toes, vision, the entire surface of the skin, and similar play on their mother's body (usually during feeding), with no clear distinction between infants and their mother.

Phase 2. Properties first cathected in infants' and their mother's body are now transferred to a soft substance such as a teddy bear, blanket, or similar object, cathecting with narcissistic and object libido.

Phase 3.
1. Infants generalize a specific object to a more indiscriminate liking for soft toys.
2. Symbolic objects are alternately cuddled and mistreated (cathected with libido and aggression).
3. Toddlers project and express a range of ambivalence toward inanimate objects.

Continued

Developmental Lines — cont'd

Phase 4. Cuddly objects are gradually discarded except when assisting children in transition into narcissistic withdrawal needed for sleep. They are replaced by the following sequential play materials:

1. Toys offering opportunities for ego activities such as filling-emptying, opening-shutting, fitting in and messing are first used. This represents interest being displaced from body openings and their functions.
2. Movable toys providing pleasure in motility are then used.
3. Building materials for construction and destruction are employed.
4. Toys serving the expression of masculine and feminine trends and attitudes are used:
   a. In solitary play
   b. To display the Oedipal object (serving phallic exhibitionism)
   c. To stage situations of the Oedipus complex in group play (stage 3 on the developmental line toward companionship must be reached)

Phase 5.

1. Transition period in which children displace satisfaction with the play activity to the end result occurs.
2. The Montessori teaching method uses objects serving the dual role of play and work (for example, cuisinere rods, counting beads, and blocks).

Phase 6.

1. The ability to play changes into the ability to work.
   a. Materials formerly used in an aggressive and destructive way are used to build, create, and learn.
   b. Immediate pleasure in the play activity is postponed, and maximum pleasure is invested in the final outcome.
   c. Period of transition from the pleasure principle to the reality principle occurs. This is developmentally essential for success in work during latency and adolescence and in maturity.
4. Allied activities significant for personality development occur.
   a. Daydreaming is demonstrated.
   b. Games derived from the imaginative group activities of the Oedipal period (Phase 4) develop from symbolic and highly formed expressive trends toward aggressive attack, defense, and competition. They are governed by inflexible rules, adaptation to reality and tolerance for frustration are necessary.
   c. Hobbies are undertaken for pleasure with comparitive disregard for external pressures and necessities. They may pursue sublimated aims to gratify erotic or aggressive drives and appear at the beginning of the latency period.

SOCIAL AND CULTURAL CONTEXT OF DEVELOPMENT: ERIKSON

Erikson's theory of development combines the biologic elements of Freud and the social influences of Sullivan. Erikson was the first theorist to include adulthood as a stage of growth, and his theory is the framework for the formulation of many life-span developmental theories.

Erikson was strongly influenced by Anna Freud's theory of developmental lines and expanded her theory to a social and cultural context. His developmental stages paralleled the psychosexual stages developed by Sigmund Freud and included play constructions, which he viewed as stages of ritualism of life. Erikson emphasized that culture was the interplay of customs and that children's play helps resolve conflicts or developmental crises.

For each developmental stage there are problems to be solved and attitudes and abilities to be developed. Conflicts are not completely resolved, and residues are carried forward to be addressed later. The outcomes of each stage can be positive or negative and will affect the identify or the self throughout life.

Erikson's thoughts on the father's role changed after World War II when he theorized that men could admit to feminine interests without having their masculinity threatened. Older parents could no longer serve as role models to new generations of mothers and fathers because their own parental behaviors no longer sufficed. Families depended more on mutual regulations than on traditions of the elders and became little Congresses in which no single pressure group (parents, older children, or younger children) could be eliminated by coalitions. While Erikson's original formulation of development remains the same as initially conceived, his theories on the process through the stages and on families' impact and role on the stages have changed.

OBJECT RELATIONS: MELANIE KLEIN

Melanie Klein was one of the first theorists to describe attachment disorders in young children. She called the painful anxiety children experience when first separated from their reassuring mother a *depressive position,* a normal developmental stage during which children learn to modify ambivalence and sustain periodic loss. Klein's theories expanded and refined Spitz's descriptions (1965) of *anaclitic depressions.* Spitz observed failure to thrive and marasmus among infants and young children in orphanages who were prematurely separated from parents during World War II. Symbiotic reactions, the opposite behavioral manifestations of anaclitic depressions, occurred when children and their parents failed to negotiate the separation-individuation process. Symbiosis is a close association necessary for survival that does not harm either participant. Since school attendance is the first enforced separation of mother and child, symbiotic reactions often are initially manifested in school phobias.

It was generally believed that the emotions of depression and grief were not possible for young children because of developmental unreadiness. Mourning includes the grieving process, which requires a mature psychic structure and the passage of time for psychologic pain to be gradually experienced and resolved. The process of introjection and identification with a lost love object does not become dominant until adolescence.

Melanie Klein's therapeutic approach was to relate directly to the unconscious processes, even in the youngest child. She assumed that interpretation should be directed toward the deep origins of disorder and constructed a model that applied to the earliest stages of infancy. Klein took the ideas of Freud and Abraham and elaborated them into the object relationship theory of personality structure.

SEPARATION-INDIVIDUATION: MARGARET MAHLER

Psychoanalytic explanations contributed greatly to the early understanding of the deviant child. Most theories included concepts of early mother-child bonding and symbiotic attachments of the separation-individuation process. Only through their mother can children identify ego boundaries, their body, and their identity, a process that Mahler (1975) theorized occurred in the four age-related subphases. Failure to successfully negotiate these phases may be the precursor of mental disorders including borderline pathologic conditions.

As Table 4-4 indicates, while the ego is being established, children learn to walk and move away from their symbiotic mother. This physical distancing may cause panic: children feel their ego is threatened with total destruction. If they cannot return to the supportive relationship and restore it, they cannot maintain ego development and may regress to the time of total dependence (symbiotic period).

The relationship during the practice phase is close to parasitism in which close association is harmful to one or both of the members. Children are afraid of losing themselves or their mother (identical entities to children) by developing and of being completely smothered by regression. To control the degree of symbiosis, children direct most of their energy in magic rituals keeping their mother at the right distance.

Failure to negotiate the separation process successfully at any step has been associated with specific personality disorder behaviors presenting in early childhood. For example, individuals with a dependent personality allow others to assume responsibility for their life and avoid being self-reliant. They experience acute discomfort when alone, even briefly. Individuals with a borderline personality react with infantile rage and vacillate between intense hunger for love and affection and intense rejection of love objects.

Despite early deficits, many individuals have stable ego deficits and maintain reality except under extreme stress in which they manifest transient psychotic episodes.

The four defense mechanisms usually encountered with persons who have failed to negotiate the stages of the separation-individuation process successfully are the following:

1. Splitting (primitive dissociation): The opposing affective states of love and hate are kept separate. Splitting occurs during the infantile period and is similar to the splitting underlying the development of psychoses (Kernberg, 1980). Split feelings are a response to a series of psychic traumas rather than to a specific event. The ego is weak and unable to achieve adequate integration of good and bad object images, leaving children vulnerable to regression. Split feelings are absorbed by the ego and become character traits. In psychoses, split feelings are repressed and become precursors to anxiety and guilt. In neurotics, repression provides the central defense mechanism.

Table 4-4   Separation-Individuation

Phase	Developmental tasks	Possible pathologic outcomes
Autistic (0-3 mo)	Attachment to mother and/or caretaker; develops pleasurable associations with appearance of mother's person (face) and pleasurable sensations with relief from body tensions	No attachment with caretaker may result in infantile autism
Symbiotic (3 mo)	Attachment develops during symbiosis and differentiates; moves from inner-directed organization to external world, initiated by social smile; perceptual gestalt of mother and infant's emerging body image and self-representation; increased eye contact, curiosity, exploring actions, cooing; infant and mother share common boundary; infant has illusion of self as source of nurture	Ego regresses to primitive delusional state (symbiotic child psychosis)
Differentiation (4–6 mo)	Begins to hatch from symbiotic orbit; differentiation begins; infant cries, reaches out for mother when she moves away	Clings/rejects transitional objects; ambivalence, behavioral problems may result from long separation; repeated separations during first 3 mo of life may result in anaclitic depression; if mothering inadequate or inconsistant, infant cannot synthesize discordant elements of good and bad, begins endowing objects (toys, blankets) with mother's soothing qualities

Continued

2. Protective identification: Feelings are projected onto another person to justify expressions of anger and self-protection.
3. Devaluation: To defend against their own feelings of inadequacy, individuals criticize others.
4. Omnipotence: Individuals have fantasies of greatness and exaggerated importance.

Table 4-4   Separation-Individuation—cont'd

Phase	Developmental tasks	Possible pathologic outcomes
Practice (7–12 mo)	Autonomous functions emerge; practices with curiosity, joy of mastery; increased independent sense of self, autonomy; relations with mother move from primary need satisfaction to attachment; slowly learns to tolerate separations, trust transitional objects; stranger anxiety develops (8 mo)	Self-love and enchantment related to narcissism; magical omnipotence occurs
Rapprochement	Masters cognitively intensified separation anxiety; affirms sense of basic trust and sense of omnipotence in symbiotic dual unity with mother; compensates for diminished sense of omnipotence through growth of ego capacity and sense of autonomy; firms core sense of self; establishes ego controls, modulates strong libidinal-aggressive urges (infantile rage); heals tendency to intrapsychic splitting of good and bad; supplants splitting mechanism with repression to curb unacceptable feelings and actions toward love objects (Settlege, 1964)	Narcissistic enchantment moves to vulnerability; borderlines experience conflict between need for security and fear of engulfment

ATTACHMENT AND BONDING: JOHN BOWLBY

Bowlby's theory of attachment (1969) suggested that the most important emotional deprivation is any interference with the child/parent relationship. According to his theory, attachment is a hypothetic construct reflecting the quality of the affectional ties between infant and parents that develops over time. Bowlby defined deprivation as the removal of something one has had and privation as an absence from the beginning. Bowlby's theories involved concepts concerning the father and children's extended family; concepts of multiple mothering; professionalized mothering (for example, a kibbutz); and supplementary mothering. Bowlby's theory held that the physical presence of the mother was essential for infant nurturing, and he stressed the harmful effects of separation. His theories influenced public policies such as the rights of mothers to keep contact with children admitted to the hospital. Bowlby emphasized the role of the family as a promoter of children's mental health.

MILESTONES OF EMOTIONAL DEVELOPMENT: GREENSPAN

Current concepts of human behavior that provide a clinical approach to normal child development include Greenspan's milestone model which involves multiple lines of development and multiple determinants of development, an integration of classical developmental and contemporary theories. It includes Anna Freud's concepts of developmental lines, Erikson's psychosocial stages of development, Mahler's theories of attachment, and Piaget's cognitive theories.

This developmental approach is the framework for the assessment and on-going evaluation of children's developmental progress (see Table 7–1) at each stage and their response to therapeutic interventions. Greenspan's theory includes the following:
1. Children's overall physical and neurologic integrity as it pertains to their ability to function
2. Children's overall emotional tone
3. Children's capacity for human relationships with family, peers, and other adults
4. Children's emotions or affects in terms of range, depth, and stability
5. Children's anxieties and fears involving the decoding of special, deeply felt concerns that are readily expressed or that require depth psychology

The Atheoretic DSM-III-R

The recognition, modification, and expansion of child psychiatry and the theories of child development have created a redefinition of the state of the art in the field as marked by the inclusion of child psychiatry in the DSM-III and DSM-III-R (see Appendix A). Parallel to these advances, certification in child and adolescent psychiatric mental health nursing and child specialty practice standards were developed in nursing.

Some child psychiatric clinicians oppose the lack of a developmental framework in the DSM-III-R and claim that using a system developed for adults not only is impractical but also leads to inaccuracies. Some of the contributions and advantages and criticisms and disadvantages of the child psychiatric diagnostic groups are presented in the box.

Child psychiatric nurses can draw on other psychologically oriented developmental models for practice. Numerous efforts to synthesize and reconcile competing paradigms (Stiles, 1982) have had little success, which weakens the influence of the mental health profession (Fagin, 1983; Pardes and Pincus, 1983). The different theories create another therapeutic issue—diagnostic formulations. Concerns and dilemmas about which diagnostic system to follow are even more complex for child than adult psychiatric nurses because of the need for developmental diagnostic statements.

Contributions of the DSM-III-R

1. It provides a new language and paradigm; DSM-III classification reaffirms the concept of multiple, separate disorders.
2. Operational criteria for all disorders described throughout the nosology both include and exclude.
3. Diagnostic criteria are based on manifest descriptive psychopathology and not on causation, inferences, or criteria from presumed causation or etiology, with the exception of organic disorders.
4. First official nomenclature tested for reliability in field tests involving clinical practitioners, it generated statistical evidence and fostered acceptance, reliability, feasibility, and utility of diagnostic schemes; continued field studies yielded refinements published in DSM-III-R (1987); DSM-IV will be published in 1992 and will be compatible with revised ICD-10.
5. Multiaxial system accommodates the multiplicity of clients' lives and experiences (Klerman, 1986).
6. It includes separate child psychiatric section, suggesting official acceptance and recognition of this area.
7. Pediatric disorders section defines disorders studied and treated for years but not described in earlier DSM editions, including infantile autism, pervasive developmental disorders, learning disorders, anorexia, bulimia, pica, sleep, and sleepwalking disorders; redefinition of mental retardation based on research advances in that area is also included (Levy, 1982).
8. It specifies adult diagnoses that can be made for children and gives special instructions for using adult disorder diagnoses with children.
9. Axis II emphasizes specific childhood developmental delays.
10. Diagnoses section facilitates clinical research and scientific communication, expands the number of diagnoses for children, and provides a specific definition of a mental disorder; multiaxial system gives more complete description.

REFERENCES

Adams P and Fras I: Beginning child psychiatry, New York, 1988, Brunner/Mazel, Inc.

American Nurses' Association: Standards of mental health nursing practice, Kansas City, Mo, 1985, The Association.

American Psychiatric Association: Diagnostic and statistical manual of mental disorders, ed 3, rev, Washington, DC, 1987, American Psychiatric Association.

Aries P: Centuries of childhood: a social history of family life, New York, 1962, Alfred A Knopf, Inc (Translated by R Baldick).

Beck CK, Rawlins RP, and Williams SR, editors: Mental health-psychiatric nursing: a holistic life-cycle approach, St Louis, 1987, The CV Mosby Co.

Belenky MS and others: Women's ways of knowing the development of self, voice, and mind, New York, 1986, Basic Books, Inc, Publishers.

Bowlby J: Attachment and loss, London, 1969, The Hogarth Press, Ltd.

Bowlby J: Attachment and loss: retrospect and prospect. In Chess S and Thomas A, editors: Annual progress in child psychiatry and child development, New York, 1984, Brunner/Mazel, Inc.

Bronfenbrenner U: Freudian theories of identification and their derivatives, Child Dev 31:15, 1960.

Bronfenbrenner U: Developmental research, public policy and the ecology of childhood, Child Dev 45:1, 1974.

Campbell J, editor: The portable Jung, New York, 1971, Viking Press (Translated by RFC Hull).

Chess S and Thomas A: Temperament in clinical practice, New York, 1986, The Guilford Press.

Christ AE: Cognitive assessment of the psychotic child: a Piageian framework. In Chess S and Thomas A, editors: Annual progress in child psychiatry and child development, New York, 1976, Brunner/Mazel, Inc.

Coler MS: Diagnoses for child and adolescent psychiatric nursing, J Child Adolesc Psychia Ment Health Nurs 2:117, 1989.

Erikson E: Identity, youth and crisis, New York, 1968, WW Norton & Co, Inc.

Fagin C: Concepts for the future: competition and substitution, J Psychiatric Nurs Ment Health Serv 21:36, 1983.

Greenspan S: Clinical interview of the child, New York, 1981, McGraw-Hill Book Co.

Havighurst R: History of developmental psychology: personality development through the life span. In Baltes P and Schaie K, editors: Life span developmental psychology: personality and socialization, New York, 1973, Academic Press, Inc.

Kagan J: The emergence of self. In Chess S and Thomas A, editors: Annual progress in child psychiatry and child development, New York, 1984, Brunner/Mazel, Inc.

Kagan J: In Restak R: The mind, New York, 1990, Bantom Books.

Kernberg O: Internal world and external reality: object relations theory applied, New York, 1980, Jason Aronson, Inc.

Klerman GL: Historical perspectives on contemporary schools of psychopathology. In Millon T and Klerman GL, editors: Contemporary directions in psychopathology: toward the DSM-IV, New York, 1986, The Guilford Press.

Kluckhohn C: The influence of psychiatry on anthropology in America during the past one hundred years. In Hall JK, editor: One hundred years of American psychiatry, New York, 1944, Columbia University Press.

Kohlberg L: Development of moral character and moral ideology. In Hoffman ML and Hoffman LW, editors: Review of child development research, New York, 1964, Russell Sage Foundation.

Lorenz K: Evolution and the modification of behavior, Chicago, 1956, University of Chicago Press.

McNeil EB: The concept of human development, Belmont, Calif, 1966, Wadsworth, Inc.

McRae M: An approach to the single parent dilemma, MCNP p 164, May/June 1977.

Murray R and Zentner J: Nursing assessment and health promotion through the life span, ed 3, Englewood Cliffs, NJ, 1985, Prentice-Hall, Inc.

Nagel E: Determinism and development. In Harris DB, editor: The concept of development, Minneapolis, 1957, University of Minnesota Press.

Nars ML: The superego and moral development in the theories of Freud and Piaget, Psychoanal Study Child 21:187, 1966.

Omery A: Moral development: a differential evaluation of dominant models, ANS 6:1, 1983.

Pardes H and Pincus HA: Challenges to academic psychiatry, Am J Psychiatry 140:1117, 1983.

Peplau HE: A shift in thinking: instrument and manual for understanding behavior. Unpublished manuscript, 1951.

Piaget J; Play, dreams and imagination in childhood, New York, 1962, WW Norton & Co, Inc (Translated by C Gattegno and FM Hodgson).

Plotz : The disappearance of childhood: parent-child role reversals in after the first death and a solitary blue, Children's Literature in Education 19:67, 1988.

Pothier P: The developmental concepts of Piaget applied to nursing assessment and interventions with atypical children, JPN and Mental Health Services p 30, Jan/Feb 1970.

Pulaski MAS: Understanding Piaget: an introduction to children's cognitive development, New York, 1971, Harper & Row, Publishers, Inc.

Rutter M: Maternal deprivation reassessed, New York, 1972, Penguin Books.

Schaie K: Historical time and cohort effects. In McClusky K and Reese H, editors: Life-span developmental psychology: historical and generational effects, New York, 1984, Academic Press, Inc.

Schetaky DH and Benedek EP: Emerging issues in child psychiatry and the law, New York, 1985, Brunner/Mazel, Inc.

Schilder P: The image and appearance of the human body, New York, 1970, International Universities Press, Inc.

Settlege C: Psychoanalytic theory in relation to the nosology of childhood disorders, J Am Psychoanal Assoc 12:776, 1964.

Singer DG and Revenson TA: A Piaget primer: how children think, New York, 1978, American Library Publishing Co, Inc.

Spitz RA: The first year of life, New York, 1965, International Universities Press, Inc.

Stiles WB: Psychotherapeutic process: is there a common care? In Aby LE and Stuart IR, editors: The new therapies: a sourcebook, New York, 1982, Van Nostrand Reinhold Co, Inc.

Sullivan HS: The interpersonal theory of psychiatry, New York, 1953, WW Norton & Co, Inc.

Tolpin M: Self-objects and Oedipal objects: a critical developmental review, Psychoanal Study Child 33:167, 1978.

van den Berg JH: The changing nature of man, New York, 1961, WW Norton & Co, Inc.

Webb LJ and others: DSM-III training guide, New York, 1981, Brunner/Mazel, Inc.

The writings of Anna Freud, 7 vols, New York, 1965–1974, International Universities Press, Inc.

Zilbergeld B: The shrinking of America: myths of psychological change, Boston, 1983, Little, Brown & Co, Inc.

Chapter 5

Sociology and Psychosocial Theories of Child Development

Psychiatry has been dominated by psychologic theories and treatment approaches for many decades, and it was not until the late 1960s that community psychiatry, grounded in sociology, became a dominant force. In contrast to traditional psychiatry, community psychiatry focuses on the interplay of an individual's environment, life experiences, and biological endowment; interventions focus on prevention. The DSM-III included aspects of the sociologic perspective by adding Axes IV and V, and psychosocial concepts are also emphasized in the standards V-A, V-B, and V-E of the Child and Adolescent Mental Health Nursing Practice (ANA, 1985).

The term *sociocultural* generally refers to combined concepts from the social and cultural sciences. Although some concepts are interrelated, the need to "unpackage" and separate concepts from these two disciplines has been stressed increasingly in the literature (Whiting and Whiting, 1975).

Culture is viewed as the matrix within which psychologic and sociologic forces operate and become meaningful to humans. Traditionally, the discipline of anthropology focuses on the study of culture, and the discipline of sociology is concerned with the social context of mental illness.

Mental disorders are a major social problem in the United States as shown by the many sociologic studies identifying a significant relationship between social factors and psychiatric conditions. The major sociologic theorists are Meyer, Leighton, Lindemann, and Caplan, whose theories emphasize community mental health services and prevention (see Table 4-1).

Definitions and Distinctions

Historically, a social definition of mental disorders was the significant deviation from standards of behavior that were generally regarded as normal by the majority of people in the group or society (Cockerham, 1985). Although the locus of a pathologic mental condition exists within an individual, the basis for determining illness depends on social criteria in most cases. When a disruption of or disregard for social norms occurs, a person's state of mind is questioned.

Social definitions of normality are especially important in child psychiatry because the family or significant other makes the initial diagnosis leading to referral. Children are usually unaware that their behaviors are a problem because of their immature and limited social perceptions and their limited verbal abilities. The psychiatric examination for generalized impairments in social functioning and adaptation in the DSM-III-R Axes IV and V is based on clinicians' understanding of norms, roles, and social expectations.

EPIDEMIOLOGIC APPROACHES

Sociology has two dominant theoretic perspectives: the macro approach, which studies society as a whole, and the micro approach. Many theories and interventions in family violence are based on the micro perspective and are of importance to child clinicians working with children of dysfunctional families (Gelles, 1987). Examples of sociologic macro concerns are conflict-resolution theories concentrating on disputes between social classes or interest groups.

Collaboration between sociology and psychiatry is best known by the landmark research of Hollingshead, a sociologist, and Redlich, a psychiatrist (1958), who developed the Hollingshead Index of Social Position scale (SES). Their findings played a central role in the debates before the passage of the 1962 Community Mental Health Act, and some experts claim that the SES is the best known social psychologic scale in the world (Cockerham, 1985; Rigier and Burke, 1985).

According to social epidemiologic research findings, social class, socioeconomic position, and incidence of mental disorder are strongly associated. The highest rates of mental disorders (especially schizophrenia and personality disorders) are found among the lowest socioeconomic groups. Affective and anxiety disorders more frequently occur in the upper socioeconomic groups. Members of the lower class are more susceptible to mental disorder, but genetics, social stress, social selection, and social drift are also contributing sociologic factors. People with mental disorders often "drift downward" in social class status.

Sociologic theories and research address risk factors, the social experience of being a mental client, the relationship of social group membership to mental illness, the impact of informal sources of support (notably family and friends), and dominant social modes of coping with severe life situations. Current sociologic clinical research includes studies of compliance (Mechanic, 1980), stigma (Cockerham, 1985), social support, and social networks (Sarason and Sarason, 1985).

SOCIAL INTERACTION APPROACHES

The micro approach studies subsystems and social structures that are components of the larger social system. Theories and clinical research in this area are of special interest to child psychiatric nurses because the focus is on interpersonal interactions of individuals while participating in a collective life. Scientists in this area focus on theories of social learning, behavior modification techniques that use social reinforcements, and labeling and symbolic interaction theories.

Mead's symbolic interaction theory (1964) was strongly influenced by Harry Stack Sullivan's interpersonal theory of psychiatry (1953) and the assumption that humans were self-directed on the basis of shared, symbolic meanings. Mead's theory was based on the assumption that self-concept was a result of interactions with others. Consistent and sufficiently bizarre failure in this area is the reason for being defined as mentally ill.

Expanding the concept that deviant acts become symbolically attached to people labeled as socially offensive, Scheff (1975) proposed the widely accepted sociologic notion that different social groups create deviance and mental illness by making rules and labeling infractions of them as deviant. Deviance is therefore not a quality of the act a person commits but a consequence of the definition. Once labeled, people are given deviant roles and status and treated accordingly.

This labeling theory does not explain the factors that cause mental disorders or the reasons for certain people becoming mentally ill while others in the same social situation do not. It does explain ways in which labeling places people in circumstances leading to behavior signified by the label.

Labeling theories also address the effects of psychiatric factors such as social class, family influence, marital status, the attainment of a lawyer, and the implementation of legal challenges to psychiatric decisions. The more affluent the family, the more control they have over relatives admitted to or released from psychiatric facilities. Another psychiatric factor is the social mechanisms of stigma, a powerfully rejecting force in society. Although stigmatizing labels may be discarded, many child clinicians are reticent to label developing children with the more severe DSM-III-R diagnoses because development and maturation change personality. Thus, "adjustment reactions" have historically been the preferred psychiatric diagnoses for children.

Families label children brought for psychiatric care, and these children are referred to as the "identified client" by professionals, inferring that the family or society has identified the child as "sick." Social group systems theory holds that systems send out their weakest member, and the immature, vulnerable child is often the system's messenger. Families and peer groups also label members by using nicknames, which often reinforce the labeled person's self-concept. Family scripting often becomes a child's "self-fulfilling prophesy." When a nurse responds to a client differently, a change in the client's language, thoughts, and behaviors will occur (Peplau, 1952).

FUNCTIONAL APPROACHES

Functional theories hold that individual human behavior is shaped by society and its norms and values. The functional perspective was the organizing framework for Durkheim's seminal epidemiologic study of suicide (1951) in which he based cues for lethality assessment on statistically verified population characteristics. Durkheim developed a nosology of self-destructive behavior and used social interaction descriptive terms: *egoistic* referred to individuals not integrated into any social group, family, community, or religion; *altruistic* referred to individuals integrated into a social group but who had committed suicide to support an altruistic belief (for example, members of the Jim Jones' Guiana community); and *anomie* referred to individuals who were left without the ordinary norms of social behavior, held values no longer relevant, and had lost their ties to society or their social group.

Sociologic concepts, such as anomie and learned helplessness, are frequently used to explain children's deviant behaviors. Carter's classical study of learned helplessness found that anomie among staff members in a psychiatric residency training program promoted suicide among patients, illustrating ways in which poor relations are transmitted within a social system and create despair (Cockerham, 1985). Other sociologic studies have found that large-scale social changes over which children and their family have no control correlate with increased rates of mental disorders and hospitalization (Benner, 1973).

Wellness, Prevention, and Community Mental Health Concepts

During the past 20 years, a gradual and fundamental paradigm shift toward the promotion of wellness in the health-care field has occurred. This paradigm shift has had the strongest impact on community mental health and is viewed by some experts as the logical evolution and continuation of the preventive approaches formulated by Caplan (1974) and other advocates of the community mental health movement.

The "wellness" era follows a postmedical or health era that extended from 1920 to the 1960s in which allopathic medicine was the dominant system. The shift was described by Capra (1982) in *The Turning Point* as follows:

For the past 300 years, our culture has been dominated by the view of the human body as a machine, to be analyzed in terms of its parts. The mind is separated from the body, disease is seen as a malfunctioning of biological mechanisms, and health is defined as the absence of disease. This view is now slowly being eclipsed by a holistic and ecological conception of the world that sees the universe not as a machine but rather as a living system, a view that emphasizes the essential interrelatedness and interdependence of all phenomena and tries to understand nature not only in terms of fundamental structures but in terms of underlying dynamic processes. It would seem that the system's view of living organisms can provide the ideal bases for a new approach to health and health care that is fully consistent with the new paradigm and is rooted in our cultural heritage. The system's view of health is profoundly ecological and thus in harmony with the Hippocratic tradition that lies at the roots of Western medicine. It is a view based on scientific notions and expressed in terms of concepts and symbols that are part of our everyday language. At the same time the new framework naturally takes into account the spiritual dimensions of health and is thus in harmony with the views of many spiritual traditions. Systems thinking is process thinking, and hence the system's view sees health in terms of an on-going process.

The wellness paradigm has four dominant determinants:
1. Individual behavior (use of drugs, lack of exercise)
2. Social organization (stress, social support, burn out)
3. Physical environment (pollution, school setting)
4. Economic status (poverty, overconsumption)

This emerging era requires different tools, actors, interests, and understandings of society and life. The wellness model's definition of health differs from the earlier sociologic definition:

Health is really a multidimensional phenomenon involving interdependent physical, psychological, and social aspects. The common representation of health and illness as opposite ends of a one-dimensional continuum is quite misleading. Physical disease may be balanced by a positive mental attitude and social support, so that the overall state is one of well-being. On the other hand, emotional problems of social isolation can make a person feel sick in spite of physical fitness (Capra, 1982).

Advocates of the health model claim that the traditional pattern of covering up social problems needs to be avoided. For example, older approaches diagnosed and treated children's hyperactivity and learning disabilities rather than examine the inadequacy of diets and schools. (Capra, 1982).

Health is thought to be outside the scope of most clinical work, and no wellness taxonomies exist. Clinicians have "clinical eyes trained to detect the most minuscule aspects of disease, however, they have paid little attention to health and well-being" (Anthony and Cohler, 1987). Nursing is the exception—health is a concept found in all nursing theoretic frameworks and is prominent in all clinical areas. Nursing has been cited as one of the potential leaders and contributors in the wellness paradigm:

> Professional nurses, and those with public health training particularly, may develop an entirely new low technology system of holistic primary care. Such a system is badly needed, and no other professional group is as well-equipped to develop it (Hanlon and Pickett, 1984).

Although prevention is emphasized in current psychosocial literature, two competing viewpoints are emerging. One is an analytic position focusing on theoretic hypothesis testing and diagnostic formulations. The other is an "applied" perspective consisting of descriptions of interventions that facilitate program and clinical intervention evaluations (Rook and Dooley, 1985). Prevention is geared toward intervention before or independent of the development of emotional disorders in high-risk populations, and the applied approach requires clinicians to move from abstract theoretic and definitional levels to practical and concrete levels for evaluation.

PRIMARY PREVENTION

An instrument developed by Perlmutter, Vayda, and Woodburn (1982) to evaluate prevention programs is an example of the applied approach. The need for the instrument grew from the evaluation requirements of federally funded, socially oriented mental health prevention programs. Evaluations of interventions were a major problem because prevention levels overlapped, resulting in definitional difficulties for practicing clinicians, clinical researchers, and funding sources.

Caplan's definition (1974) was used to distinguish among the three levels of prevention:

> Primary prevention aims at reducing the incidence of new cases of mental disorder in the population by combating harmful forces that operate in the community and by strengthening the capacity of people to withstand stress. Secondary prevention aims at reducing the duration of cases of mental disorder that occur in spite of the programs of primary prevention. By shortening the duration of existing cases, the prevalence of mental disorder in the community is reduced. . . .Tertiary prevention aims at reducing the community rate of residual defect that is sequel to mental disorders. It seeks to ensure that people who have recovered from a mental disorder will be hampered as little as possible by their past difficulties in returning to full participation in the occupational and social life of the community.

As the box illustrates, groups are identified by occupational affiliations and are not associated with a therapeutic function (such as schools and the PTA) in primary-level programs. Secondary-level programs reach target populations in occupational or

Programs in Prevention

Programs in primary prevention

1. A program of group sessions for parents of newborn mentally retarded children working around the area of parental anxiety and guilt
2. Providing consultation to a marriage counseling service based in a local church
3. A program training former gang members to become gang workers
4. A crisis-oriented intervention program for rape victims based in emergency rooms of local hospitals
5. Organizing a tenants' rights group at a catchment area housing project
6. Working with local school PTAs to develop drug abuse prevention programs
7. Developing and staffing a prenatal care program for unwed adolescents
8. A program to sensitize local primary school teachers to the problems of single-parent families
9. Offering discussion groups for men and women to cope with issues raised by the women's liberation movement
10. A program offering consultation to private nursing homes on ways of enriching the social experience of patients

Programs in secondary prevention

1. A follow-up on all callers to the center who failed to keep an initial appointment for treatment
2. A twenty-four-hour emergency home-visiting team.
3. A program at a school for blind children to offer first aid to children who appear emotionally upset
4. A round-the-clock consultation service for general practitioners in the catchment area who have individual cases with emotional problems
5. A training program for local police in handling persons with symptoms of emotional disorder
6. An open house at the center with tours and presentations that inform catchment area residents about treatment services
7. A program for management level personnel of local industries about symptom recognition and referral techniques
8. A training program for nurses at a local general hospital about methods of identifying symptoms of emotional disorder among patients
9. A teenage "Pal" program for elementary school children who receive treatment from the center
10. Counseling services for mothers who experience postpartum depression

From Perlmutter FD, Vayda AM, and Woodburn PK: An instrument for differentiating programs in prevention: primary, secondary, and tertiary. In Perlmutter FD, editor: New directions for mental health services: mental health promotion and primary prevention, New York, 1982, Jossey-Bass, Inc, Publishers.

Continued

Programs in Prevention — cont'd

Programs in tertiary prevention

1. A program to acquaint center staff with resocialization services
2. A Saturday night social program for adult mentally retarded clients of the center
3. A program of vocational and aptitude testing for all newly released outpatients with referrals to training and jobs
4. A program to escort patients discharged from an inpatient unit to their first appointment for after-care
5. A training program to enable paraprofessional staff of mental hospitals to teach patients self-care, homemaking, and budgeting
6. A program working with boarding homes proprietors on the problems of after-care patients housed in these homes
7. A short-term homemaker service to assist mothers discharged from an inpatient unit
8. A program to familiarize halfway house residents with local transportation systems and shopping facilities
9. A clerical service for universities and businesses that provides hospitalized mental patients with income and job experience
10. A program for families of discharged patients about the need for support during the transition period

---

educational settings. In tertiary-level prevention programs, the target of the intervention may not be clients. For example, the paraprofessional child care staff members are the target populations; however, the children are the beneficiaries. Primary-prevention activities, referred to as KISS (Key Integrative Social Systems), are not found at agencies that deal with mental illness; other social institutions involved in the normal process of living are the settings of choice (Bower, 1972).

Psychosocial, Life-Span, and Child Developmental Theories

The life-span and child development principles of continuity are both based on the assumption that attitudes and behavioral responses found in behavior pathology are related to and stem from normal biosocial behavior. However, life-span theorists hold that there are no radical changes or stages, just steady accretions and higher intensities of response. Some claim that stages are artifacts of theory and reject developmental profiles as confining the child to certain response sets (Anthony, 1987). Their research methods focus on interindividual differences in long-term sequences and patterns of intraindividual (personal) change and long-term patterns of changes of interindividual (social and cultural) differences (Brim, 1980).

Although life-span theories complement rather than conflict with classical child developmental theories, some scientists question the basic assumptions. Behaviorists stress that it is difficult to extinguish behaviors learned during early childhood because of the influential conditions of parental identification and reinforcement.

Psychoanalysts note that sources of anxiety generated during infancy and childhood do not change with age, nor can they be altered. Social psychologists argue that the self-image developed in childhood becomes a self-fulfilling prophecy (Danish, Smyer, and Nowak, 1980).

LIFE EVENTS

Just as anxiety, conflict, ages, and stages are unifying concepts in child development theories, the concepts of life events unite life-span theories. They are defined as notable individual occurrences that are physical, social, and/or cultural and are characterized as the following:

1. Normative individual life events: Experiences people expect as part of the "usual" life course are included. Individual life events are not age-stage graded; however, some (such as child bearing) are influenced by biology. Childhood examples include the birth of siblings and the start of school each fall.
2. Cultural events: Experiences that do not occur in the "normative" life course (yet affect many), are major social events, have an immediate effect on the individual, and influence historical changes on a culture are included. Childhood examples include wars, catastrophes, economic depressions, and hurricanes.
3. Cohorts: Persons born at the same time whose lives are affected by the same cultural events fit this definition. As each new generation enters the "stream of history," they differ from earlier cohorts because of intervening social changes. Human development is determined by these historical changes. Childhood examples include dietary changes (prevalence of fast food), health practices (fitness programs for infants), and education (requirement for AIDS courses for elementary school children).
4. Timing of events: Experiences are influenced by social and cultural events that alter the balance of available educational, health, career, and employment contexts. For cultural events to affect development, they must be linked to the interpersonal environment, which occurs in four contexts: (1) family, (2) social and community, (3) occupation and career, and (4) friendship networks. Childhood examples include social changes (alterations in social resources), parental career changes because of economic changes creating a decrease in available jobs and career options, and changes in cohort size and composition because of migrations and geographic differences in sex ratios.
5. Sequencing of life events: Patterned changes vary individually, implying sensitivity to time of cultural events over the life span and the historical context in which they occur. Childhood examples include the birth of a sibling—an event that does not have uniform meaning. For example, this life event has a different meaning for the oldest child than for the youngest child in a family. Giving birth to a child is different for a 14-year-old unwed girl than for a 16-year-old unwed girl or a 35-year-old woman.
6. On time and off time: Life-span concepts are related to the times in life people expect life events to occur. Timing is determined by individual choices and cultural occurrences. Out-of-sequence events are more stressful than

expected life events. Childhood examples include repeating a grade and getting out of time and experiencing birth of a sibling for a child whose mother is older.

7. Clustering, accumulation, and duration of life events: These critical life-event characteristics are not integrative, partially resolved, or evolving. Childhood examples include life changes (developing a chronic illness or an acute fatal illness), family relocations, and parental unemployment.

LIFE-EVENT SCALES

Social adjustment life-event inventories measuring life events and changes have been developed for children at four different age levels by Coddington (1972), who followed Holmes and Rahe's adult format (1967). The scales are based on the assumption that life changes are cumulative and a causative factor in physical and mental diseases in adults and children.

The types of social changes children experience are assigned life change units (LCUs). Coddington used weights predetermined by teachers, mental health workers, and pediatricians to initially determine children's LCUs. He found that teachers' perceptions of the severity of the life changes and the time required for children to adjust differed significantly from the scores assigned by mental health workers and pediatricians. Adults also judged discomfort of events differently than children. These discrepancies were a major criticism of Coddington's work, and item ratings were later adjusted and norms were standardized.

Life events on the scales are fairly common occurrences that require or signify change in children's adjustment. Since different life events necessitate different lengths of time to adjust, different weights or scores are assigned to the scale item as LCUs. Life change scores increase with age: "Normal, healthy" children in elementary school average 102.8 LCUs, and children in junior high school average 195.6 LCUs (Coddington, 1972). The scale-assigned, life change values also differ for children at different ages; for example, the death of a parent has a weight of 89 LCUs for preschoolers and a weight of 109 LCUs for children ages 6 to 11.

The scales can be self-administered if the reading skills are present (usually at ages 8 to 12). A life change score (LCS) is computed that can be compared to established, national norms. Both adult and child Social Readjustment Rating Scales (SRRS) are predictive screening tools, and cumulative scores of 200 or more indicates a high potential for mental or physical illness in the following 2 years (Table 5-1 and Table 5-2).

The scales include social, physical, and economic items of both positive and negative stress comparable to situational crises. Although many psychologic experiences are significant (such as being "born again"), these changes are not classified as life events but are viewed as causes or outcomes of physical, biologic, and social experiences. Conceptual analysis of the scale demonstrates this finding :

1. Biologic events: These experiences include developmental changes in body size and structure and in the brain, hormonal, and central nervous systems (for example, physical changes resulting from physical growth during childhood and physical changes indicating the onset of puberty).

Table 5-1   Life Event Scale for Preschool Age Group

Life event	Life change units
Beginning nursery school	42
Increase in number of arguments with parents	39
Change in parents' financial status	21
Birth of brother or sister	50
Decrease in number of arguments between parents	21
Change of father's occupation requiring increased absence from home	39
Death of grandparent	30
Outstanding personal achievement	23
Serious illness requiring hospitalization of parent	51
Brother or sister leaving home	39
Serious illness requiring hospitalization for brother or sister	37
Mother beginning to work outside home	47
Change to new nursery school	33
Change in child's acceptance by peers	38
Decrease in number of arguments with parents	22
Serious illness requiring hospitalization of child	59
Loss of job by parent	23
Death of close friend	38
Having visible congenital deformity	39
Addition of third adult to family	39
Marital separation of parents	74
Discovery of being adopted child	33
Jail sentence of parent for 30 days or less	34
Death of parent	89
Divorce of parents	78
Acquiring visible deformity	52
Death of brother or sister	59
Marriage of parent to stepparent	62
Jail sentence of parent for 1 year or more	67

From Coddington RD: The significance of life events as etiological factors in the diseases of children: a study of normal populations, Psychosom Res 16:205, 1972.

2. Social events: Social roles the children play in family, work, community, and friendship situations (for example, being an only child, the oldest child, or the youngest child; starting elementary or junior high school; developing friendships; and joining boy or girl scouts) are normative changes (Havighurst, 1962). Nonnormative changes include crimes against a person.

3. Physical events: These include characteristics of the physical world. Diurnal cycles (change of seasons) and weather limit activities or create biologic problems such as colds, pneumonia, and allergies. Nonnormative physical changes include earthquakes, fire, and tornadoes.

Results of some research studies using the life change scales are summarized by the following statements (Minter and Kimball, 1980):

1. Clusters of life changes precede the onset of reported illness.

Table 5-2   Life Event Scale for Ages 6 through 11 Years*

Life event	Life change units
Death of parent	109
Death of brother or sister	86
Divorce of parents	73
Marital separation of parents	66
Death of grandparent	56
Hospitalization of parent	52
Marriage of parent to stepparent	53
Birth of brother or sister	50
Hospitalization of brother or sister	47
Loss of job by parent	37
Major increase in parents' income	28
Major decrease in parents' income	29
Start of new problem between parents	44
End of problem between parents	27
Change of father's occupation requiring increased absence from home	39
New adult moving into home	41
Mother beginning to work outside home	40
Being told you are very attractive by friend	25
Beginning first grade	20
Move to new school district	35
Failing a grade in school	45
Suspension from school	30
Start of new problem between you and your parents	43
End of a problem between you and parents	34
Recognition for excelling in sport or other activity	21
Appearance in juvenile court	33
Failing to achieve something you really wanted	28
Becoming adult member of church	21
Being invited to join social organization	15
Death of pet	40
Being hospitalized for illness or injury	53
Death of close friend	52
Becoming involved with drugs	38
Stopping use of drugs	23
Finding an adult who really respects you	20
Outstanding personal achievement (special prize)	34

Courtesy R.D. Coddington, New Orleans, La.
*The purpose of this form is to record events that occurred in the child's life during a 3-month period.

2. When LCU scores for several years are increased, a significant relationship of high LCUs and illness is found.
3. In most studies, a small number of subjects had the most illness episodes.
4. More illness episodes occurred during stressful periods.
5. High LCUs precede acute manifestations of chronic illnesses.

Life event scales using open-ended questions have been developed for specific socioeconomic groups. A life event scale identifying the relationship of disrupting life events with the occurrences of psychiatric disorders in lower socioeconomic groups was developed (Dohrenwend and others, 1978). This scale, the Psychiatric Epidemiologic Research Inventory (PERI) consists of items developed from a list of life events described as significant by members of the lower socioeconomic groups. Unlike the critical "past 2 years" predictive model used by life change researchers with normative samples, remote losses were found to be crucial and cumulative. Subjects become "losers" with "accident-prone" life patterns, research findings that stressed the importance of considering individuals' perception of an event, their cognitive style or pattern, and their optimistic or pessimistic expectations of life.

By using a combination of life change scales and the open-ended question format, Colton (1985) conducted an extensive study to identify the existence of and differences between children's life change and stress. Children were asked open-ended questions eliciting their perception of life events, and adjustments in scores were made if any life events or stress items had not occurred.

LIFE-SPAN/CHILD DEVELOPMENT THEORY

The most pertinent life-span theories for child psychiatric nursing are Selye's General Adaptation Syndrome (GAS) (1956) and Erikson's psychosocial developmental theory (1955). Erickson developed one of the few classical developmental theories spanning human development from the cradle to the grave.

Several psychoanalytically oriented life-span theorists have extended and tested Erikson's theory using longitudinal and cross-sectional life-span research methods. These scientists (Brim, 1980; Levinson, 1978; Neugarten, 1976; Vaillant and Milofsky, 1980) combined the basic assumptions and definitions of life events with Erikson's epigenic stages of the life cycle and definition of conflicts, that is, a normative life crisis or times when adults or children are confronted by conflicting psychosocial tasks affecting ego development. As each task is mastered, a gain is made that adds a new ego quality and another dimension of personality strength.

Neugarten (1976) found three major age-related differences between adults and children:

1. There is a shift in time perspective, with chronologic ages and stages being relatively unimportant.
2. Adult life-span development is a "psychology of timing" and not of ages and stages. Although stress and conflict are not inherent in adult developmental transitions, stress occurs as a result of the "asynchronousness" or poor timing of life events.
3. Human development is not paced by crises but by average, expected events in the life cycle. Unanticipated events are traumatic.

Levinson's life-span theories were widely known by the lay public through his popular paperback *The Seasons of a Man's Life* (1978) and Sheehy's *Passages* (1976), America's number one bestseller during the 1970s. At that time the general public and professionals were concerned about the high incidence of coronary heart disease in young and middle-aged men. Levinson's research identified "normal" develop-

Stage 8 Integrity

Stage 7a Keepers of the Meaning

Stage 7 Generativity

Stage 6a Career Consolidation

------------------------------------ Intimacy ----------------------------------
Stage 6

Stage 5 Identity

Stage 4 Industry

Stage 3 Initiative

Stage 2 Autonomy

Stage 1 Basic Trust

Figure 5-1   Schematic diagram of the stages in the modified Erikson model. (From Vaillant GL and Milofsky E: Natural history of male psychological health: empirical evidence for Erikson's model of the life cycle, Am J Psychiatry 137:1349, 1980.)

mental tasks for the midlife male, as well as popularizing concepts concerning patterns of behaviors, life styles, and prevention. The public was educated to recognize Type A behaviors, and *risk factors* and *lifestyles* became part of everyday language.

Levinson found that transitional periods, such as adolescent turmoil and other role changes poorly mediated with culture, result from individual psychopathology rather than from development. The application of Levinson's research to child coping and vulnerability studies has resulted in the identification of Type A behaviors in elementary school children (Anthony and Cohler, 1987), with suggestions for life-style changes designed to alter children's lifestyle being developed and tested.

STUDY OF ADULT DEVELOPMENT

The Harvard Medical School's longitudinal study of adult development, conducted by George Vaillant and others (1977, 1980), has also become well known for its con-tributions to the understanding of male life-span development. Descriptions of male coping, resilience, and invulnerability provided data on male development over a 40-year time span (Felsman and Vaillant, 1987). Based on his longitudinal study results, Vaillant suggested that Erikson's hierarchy of developmental tasks—a "step" model with an ascending order of complexity—be replaced by a spiral model. This model separated less stable life periods, during which adults focus on the "reworking of identity" and values, from more stable periods, during which adults are more pre-occupied with preservation of sameness and autonomy. The compatibility of Vail-lant's spiral model and Martha Rogers' "slinky" model is noteworthy (Figure 5-1).

Using ego psychology and life-span concepts, researchers placed defenses used by the study participants on a developmental hierarchy and classified behaviors as adaptive if they minimized regression and led to conflict resolution and maladaptive if they led to avoidance of conflict, unnecessary regression, and impeded realistic gratification. Four maturity levels of defenses were identified from this research data:

1. Narcissistic defenses (onset: <5 years of age): Include projection, denial, and distortion
2. Immature defenses (onset: Between 3 and 16 years of age): Include projection, schizoid fantasy, passive-aggressive behavior, hypochondria, and acting-out behavior
3. Neurotic defenses (onset: 3 years of age and continues throughout adult life): Include intellectualization, repression, displacement, reaction formation, and dissociation
4. Mature defenses (onset: 12 years of age and continues throughout adult life): Include altruism, humor, suppression, anticipation, and sublimation

Dependent behaviors were defined as the reliance on another person, object, or substance for support. Five factors are involved: physical contact, attention, proximity, physical help, and approval and praise. Dependent behavior is adaptive during infancy and illness. When people are inappropriately or excessively dependent on substances or others, their behavior is maladaptive. Independent behavior comes from within, is free from external support, and includes taking initiative, overcoming obstacles, persisting, wanting to do something, and wanting to do things alone.

Vaillant also added two levels of male development, extending Erikson's seven life stages to nine:

6a. Career consolidation versus self-absorption: Research participants rarely achieved career consolidation until they completed the task of intimacy. The implications of this developmental level are contrary to social expectations that males establish careers before marrying and beginning family responsibilities and affect currently held concepts of father-infant parental involvement.
7a. Keepers of the meaning versus rigidity: Distinctions were found among older men Erikson identified as experiencing tensions of generativity versus rigidity. Male respondents were more preoccupied with transmission and preservation of culture than with caring for others. Involving "grandfathers" in children's life would provide for this developmental task.

STRESS THEORIES

The second group of life-span theories relevant for child psychiatric clinicians focus on the role of events as precursors to response outcomes. These nondevelopment views are based on Selye's general adaptation theory (1956) and include the theories of Lazarus and Launier (1978), Dohrenwend and Dohrenwend (1981), and scientists from disciplines currently studying the developing concepts of coping, vulnerability, and risk during childhood.

There are many definitions of stress, which is a construct that has touched almost every aspect of life and is a central concern in health care. The first official recognition of stress as a legitimate health factor was given by the surgeon general in 1979 in the publication *Healthy People.* Referring to sociologic survey data, the surgeon general stated that when stress reached excessive proportions, psychologic changes could be so dramatic that they could have serious implications for physical and mental health. Estimates were that as many as 25%

of all Americans suffered from the ill effects of excessive stress and that the majority of Americans die from illnesses that are stress related. It was also estimated that approximately 50% of all clients seen in general medical practice suffered from stress-related problems (Everly and Sobelman, 1987). As a result of the surgeon general's emphasis, stress became a major scientific concern during the 1980s, and concerted efforts to study stress reduction and prevention were established.

Stress theorists are from many disciplines and theoretic backgrounds and focus their interest on stress-induced illness and resilience. Some researchers are concerned with particular amounts of stress, such as life-threatening stresses leading to posttraumatic stress disorders, while others study life events and changes as stressors that result in psychosomatic illness.

The variety of stress theories and multiplicity of interpretations of stress responses emphasize that the concept of stress covers a spectrum of individual responses. Therefore life-span theories based on stress concepts are more ambiguous and diverse than the ego-psychologic life-span theories based on Erikson's theory, partly due to the development of concepts of stress and the GAS during the past 30 years.

Definitions of stress have changed considerably since Selye first introduced a biochemical model viewing stress at the physiologic and biochemical levels of functioning. At that time, stress referred to a body's physiologic patterns preparing the person for "flight or fight." Stress was initially seen as being identical to anxiety and was attributed to intrapsychic and conflict-laden (endogenous) factors. With scientific advances in the understanding of cognition and perception and the shift from an emphasis on drives, tensions, and intrapsychic energy, stress was differentiated from anxiety and presently relates to the external, psychosocial, environmentally related factors.

The social systems model of human stress response has six interrelated aspects: (1) environmental events, (2) the cognitive affective domain, (3) the neurologic triggering mechanism, (4) physiologic stress response axes, (5) coping, and (6) target organs effects. Although stress is activated by stressors (environmental stimuli), their existence cannot lead to action unless they are actively appraised for their effects on the perceiver (Arnold, 1984). The anatomic locus of the appraisals, the cingulate gyrus, interfaces with the limbic-prefrontal neocortical areas. In the first step, appraisal of information from every sense modality — sight, smells, movement, and somatic sensations — is perceived and sent to the occipital association areas. The second step is the movement from perception to cognitive appraisal. In the third phase the appraisal moves to the neurologic triggering mechanism and then on to the physiologic stress-response axis, which includes neurologic, neuroendocrine, and global stress responses.

Coping occurs in the final phase of a system's model of stress. In this model, stress is defined as action-oriented and intrapsychic efforts designed to manage (master, tolerate, or reduce) environmental and internal demands and conflicts. When coping occurs before the occurrence of a stressful confrontation, it is an *anticipatory confrontation* and consists of environmental or cognitive manipulations attenuating or controlling the stress response (Cohen and Lazarus, 1979). If anticipatory responses fail, the physiologic mechanisms are activated.

Stress is affected by the following elements:
1. A set of antecedent stressors (life events)
2. Mediating factors that include inner resources (physical health) and external resources (income, social support)
3. Social-psychologic adaptation syndrome (changes in affect, orientation, beliefs, or activities)
4. Adaptive or maladaptive response outcomes (physical or mental diseases)

COGNITIVE STRESS THEORIES

Lazarus (1981) developed a cognitive model of stress addressing the key concepts of appraisal, coping, and outcomes. He defined coping as the adaptational outcome of stress and stated that coping processes were more critical than understanding the "weight" of life events. The major functions of coping are to solve problems (better the situation by changing actions or the threatening environment) and to regulate emotions (manage the somatic and subjective components of stress-related emotions to control the degree of the response). Coping modes serve problem-solving and emotional regulatory functions:
1. Information seeking: This mode is directly related to individuals' social support system and available people to provide the needed information. To regulate emotional distress, they may ignore or deny the negative implications of the information.
2. Direct coping action: Noncognitive activities, such as expressing anger, seeking revenge, taking medications, and jogging to preserve health, are aimed at the self or environment and are anticipatory coping actions.
3. Inhibition of action: This mode involves holding back or avoiding actions that poorly fit the moment.
4. Intrapsychic mode: This mode includes cognitive elements that regulate emotions, for example, self-deceptive defenses of denial, reaction formation, projection, avoidance, detachment, and intellectualization.

Some children respond to the slightest threat from the outside and feel that they are at the mercy of external forces. These children tend to compete constantly and excessively against everyone and everything. Other children maintain confident control over their environment and take responsibility for events. Based on these observations, some cognitive social learning theorists equate internal locus of control with children's coping ability, the "bouncing" back of the sense of control and competence.

The social cognitive theorists Nowicki and Strickland (1973) drew on Rotter's social learning theory (1966) to develop a child locus of control scale. Locus of control theory is based on the assumption that behavior reinforcement has special significance for developing children's learning of appropriate social and personal behaviors. The scale can be self-administered, and it measures the generalized locus of control of reinforcement in children in grades 3 through 12. As expected, internal scores increase with age and are positively correlated with achievement. According to the developers, scores are not significantly related to social desirability or intelligence. The questions asked in the locus of control scale are shown in the box.

Locus of Control Scale

1. Do you believe that most problems will solve themselves if you just don't fool with them? (Yes) *, †
2. Do you believe that you can stop yourself from catching a cold? (No)
3. Are some kids just born lucky? (Yes)
4. Most of the time do you feel that getting good grades means a great deal to you? (No)
5. Are you often blamed for things that just aren't your fault? (Yes) †
6. Do you believe that if somebody studies hard enough he or she can pass any subject? (No)
7. Do you feel that most of the time it doesn't pay to try hard because things never turn out right anyway? (Yes) *, †
8. Do you feel that if things start out well in the morning that it's going to be a good day no matter what you do? (Yes)
9. Do you feel that most of the time parents listen to what their children have to say? (No) *, †
10. Do you believe that wishing can make good things happen? (Yes) *
11. When you get punished does it usually seem it's for no good reason at all? (Yes) †
12. Most of the time do you find it hard to change a friend's (mind) opinion? (Yes) †
13. Do you think that cheering more than luck helps a team to win? (No)
14. Do you feel that it's nearly impossible to change your parents mind about anything? (Yes) *, †
15. Do you believe that your parents should allow you to make most of your own decisions? (No)
16. Do you feel that when you do something wrong there's very little you can do to make it right? (Yes) *, †
17. Do you believe that most kids are just born at being good at sports (Yes) *, †*
18. Are most of the other kids your age stronger than you are? (Yes) *
19. Do you feel that one of the best ways to handle most problems is just not to think about them? (Yes) *, †
20. Do you feel that you have a lot of choice in deciding who your friends are? (No)
21. If you find a four leaf clover do you believe that it might bring you good luck? (Yes)
22. Do you often feel that whether you do your homework has much to do with what kind of grades you get? (No)

Modified from Nowicki S and Strickland BR: A locus of control scale for children, J Consult Clin Psychol 40:150, 1973.
*Items selected for abbreviated scale for Grades 1-6.
†Items selected for abbreviated scale for Grades 7-12.

Continued

STRESS SCALES AND NURSING INTERVENTIONS

Life change and locus of control scales provide valuable screening tools for assessment of children's stress level. The scales are also useful for case finding of children at high risk for physical and/or mental illness and provide directions for initiating stress-reducing strategies based on health status and developmental tasks and not on

---

Locus of Control Scale — cont'd

23. Do you feel that when a kid your age decided to hit you, there's little you can do to stop him or her? (Yes) *, †
24. Have you ever had a good luck charm? (Yes)
25. Do you believe that whether or not people like you depends on how you act? (No)
26. Will your parents usually help you if you ask them to? (No)
27. Have you felt that when people were mean to you it was usually for no reason at all? (Yes) *, †
28. Most of the time, do you feel that you can change what might happen tomorrow by what you do today? (No) †
29. Do you believe that when bad things are going to happen they just happen no matter what you try to do to stop them? (Yes) *, †
30. Do you think that kids can get their own way if they just keep trying? (No)
31. Most of the time do you find it useless to try to get your own way at home? (Yes) *, †
32. Do you feel that when good things happen they happen because of hard work? (No)
33. Do you feel that when somebody your age wants to be your enemy there's little you can do to change matters? (Yes) *, †
34. Do you feel that it's easy to get friends to do what you want them to? (No)
35. Do you usually feel that you have little to say about what you get to eat at home? (Yes) *, †
36. Do you feel that when someone doesn't like you there's little you can do about it? (Yes) *, †
37. Do you usually feel that it's almost useless to try in school because most other children are just plain smarter than you are? (Yes) *, †
38. Are you the kind of person who believes that planning ahead makes things turn out better? (Yes) *, †
39. Most of the time, do you feel that you have little to say about what your family decides to do? (Yes) *, †
40. Do you think it's better to be smart than to be lucky? (No)

---

disease states. They also accomplish the following (Minter and Kimball, 1980):

1. Provide a broader view of children's dimensions to be considered in assessment.
2. Explore beyond the recent, attention-grabbing event and introduce the possibility that the stress may not be a result of the event reported by the family.
3. Provide a broader view of children's recent life changes and the potential interaction of these events. Since personality changes often result from the cumulation of minor events over time rather than from one major event, the potential interaction effects from biologic, social, and physical events become visible.

The normal ranges of life change score expectations have been established, and using these scales, Coddington (1972) found hospitalized children had two to three times more life changes before the onset of illness. The scales have been widely used as preventive screens with pediatric clients with chronic physical disorders.

Lazarus (1981) also suggests clinicians consider the following when assessing ways in which children and families cope:

1. Stress responses include all four coping modes.
2. Most people are unable to identify whether they use defenses such as denial or intellectualization.
3. Coping patterns change over the life span as developmental levels are achieved.
4. Because of limitations in understanding stress in children (Rutter, 1984), the effect of development and age/stage on children's vulnerability to stress is not known.

After the severity of stressors and stress diagnosis is established, nursing interventions should be congruent with the stress framework of the GAS. Saxton and Hyland (1975) have developed a nursing care plan based on the GAS in which five levels of adaptation distinguish strengths and needs:

1. First level: Reduction of primary stress by physiologic and/or psychologic adaptation occurs. Rarely reaching the conscious level, these are normal defense responses to stress.
2. Second level: Adaptations requiring a general awareness of the existence of a problem (for example, signal anxiety) occur. Persons use compensatory adaptations to control and limit stress.
3. Third level: Nonspecific responses in which individuals cannot limit, reduce, or control stress occur. These are the signs and symptoms of health problems. Psychologic changes include anxiety conversions, physical symptoms of headache and fatigue; physiology changes include alterations in sleeping habits, weight, and attention.
4. Fourth level: Adaptations are required because of stresses created by third-level adaptations. Without outside interventions to halt GAS, irreversible damage occurs. Physiologically, continued elevated blood pressure causes damage to the heart and blood vessels; in a psychologic state of panic, reality distortions and decreased comprehension result.
5. Fifth level: Stresses are multiple, and nursing interventions must reverse the GAS for the client to survive. Acute phases of illness are seen in the physiologic realm; in the psychologic realm, defenses do not reduce anxiety, and the client cannot cope and withdraws from reality.

Objectives of the nursing approach related to stress are to (1) reduce or limit the extent and intensity of the present stress, (2) prevent additional stress, and (3) provide emotional support using crisis intervention strategies. Objectives related to individuals' level of adaptation are the following:

1. To support first-level adaptations to assist in sustaining and maintaining defensive responses
2. To limit and support second-level adaptations to confine compensatory reactions
3. To alter, limit, and support the third-level adaptations to modify response symptoms

4. To interrupt, alter, limit, and support fourth-level adaptations to intervene in stressors
5. To supplement, interrupt, alter, and limit fifth-level adaptations to complement or replace responses failing to control stress

By controlling life change scores, individuals can achieve growth-facilitating change. The steps for successfully adjusting to change suggested in the book *Shifting Gears* (O'Neill and O'Neill, 1974) are useful for latency-aged children participating in life change group experiences. The book is easily read by the average 9-year-old child. Steps suggested include the following:

1. Explore physical and psychologic responses used to accommodate to change, such as insomnia, overeating, and anorexia. Unify the behavioral-physiologic aspects of behavior with cognitive awareness.
2. Establish positive attitudes, working through blaming others and ruminating on past injustices to assume responsibility for self.
3. "Center and focus" on feelings, identity, and life goals, finding the stable center of self by consciousness raising.
4. Share decision making with others who will help modify and validate accurate perceptions.
5. Organize a plan of action within an achievable time interval.
6. After exploration of alternatives, enjoy some "risk" taking.
7. Gradually release the problem through accommodation to newer, more acceptable attitudes and behavior.

STRESS AND VULNERABILITY

The *stress-vulnerability* hypothesis was an early explanation for stress emerging from research of extreme situations such as combat and concentration camps. It considers the dispositional characteristics of children and the holding and facilitating qualities of the milieu. In contrast to the locus of control model, the stress-vulnerability model (Gore, 1981) holds that interactions are judged using life changes and the buffering provided by measurable social supports. Social supports help mitigate the stress on individuals and release their coping behavior. In this model the focus is on the transactional activities activated by the supportive network, not individuals' resistance. The vulnerability hypothesis was replaced by the theory that psychophysiologic strain was an intermediating variable in response to adverse change, an explanation that continues to be a major focus of pediatric scientific research.

STRESS CONCEPTS AND PSYCHODYNAMICS

Stress concepts have not appealed to psychodynamically oriented clinicians, perhaps because most stress literature fails to examine the distinctions and relationships of stress and psychodynamic concepts of anxiety, ego defenses, and trauma.

The concept of trauma can be traced to Freudian psychodynamics and traumatic neurosis. Freud theorized that the ego avoids trauma by binding and/or organizing it through play and fantasy. Recurrent disturbing situations and the repetitive dreaming clients reported in their posttraumatic phases were viewed as regression to a primitive mode of mastery. By reexperiencing events, individuals slowly reestablish mastery control. The psychoanalytic concept considers trauma as cumulative during development, with periods at high and low risk at different ages and stages (Kahn, 1963). Risk, vulnerability, and resilience are changing constructs.

Freudian theory described anxiety as having two characteristics: one aspect was the *anxiety* reaction to a traumatic situation, often paralyzing, overwhelming, and eliciting a *fright-neurosis*. The other aspect was described as the protective *signal-anxiety* that alerts and guards people against a powerful experience and prepares them for the potentially disturbing anxiety or traumatic encounter. Freudian theory appreciated the situation of risk and interpreted anxiety as a shield against overdoses. In contrast to less biologically analytic explanations, Freud said heredity was responsible for the core buffering mechanisms and described an autonomous system that was highly calibrated, sensitive, and perceptual. The concept of ego resilience also emerged from these Freudian concepts.

Kroeber (1963) claims that ego psychology includes a reorientation and shift away from the classical Freudian preoccupation with pathology and that the ego mechanism can be conceptualized as taking on either defensive or coping functions, thus providing a new concept of mental health. Coping mechanisms are more flexible, purposive, selective, and oriented toward present reality and future planning and involve largely conscious, secondary-process thinking operating with cognitive processes. Individuals can use coping over defense mechanisms; however, the ego function of selective awareness can be distorted through the defenses of denial.

Anna Freud was one of the ego psychologists who emphasized health in her theoretic formulations, stressing healthy, adaptive measures. Sullivan's concept of corrective emotional experiences also focused on health, and the hierarchy of ego mechanisms developed by Semrad (1967) was the basis for the current significance of coping invulnerability.

In contrast, Murphy and Moriatry (1976) state that coping is not a healthy antonym for defense and that children use defenses and autonomous ego functions in a mutually supportive way. The coping process therefore includes cognitive functioning and normal defensive strategies, included in the "new ego" model of Kroeber (Anthony, 1987) and shown in Table 5-3.

After extensive clinical studies of childhood coping, Murphy and Moriarty (1976) developed a Comprehensive Coping Inventory (CCI), which covers cognitive, motor, affective, and self-ego coping capacities. Based on the CCI, clinicians can identify ways in which children defend themselves against excessive stimulations by diverting stimulations from the setting; withdrawing, postponing, and turning to more manageable situations; restructuring the environment; accepting both good and bad as reality; and working toward maintaining optimal conditions in integration, security, and comfort.

The CCI is a lengthy, detailed coverage of almost every area of autonomous functioning, limiting its usefulness for most clinicians. In this definition, coping verges on all areas of competence and creativity. Use of the CCI requires an experienced clinician familiar with its administration. Despite these limitations, it is considered the best instrument available to assess children's coping (Anthony, 1987). The scale developed by Caty, Ellerton, and Richie (1984) modified the framework used by Lazarus and others in their stress and coping paradigm (Lazarus and Folkman,

Table 5-3   Defensive and Coping Ego Functions

Ego function	Defensive response	Coping response
Discrimination	Isolation	Objectivity
Detachment	Intellectualization	Intellectual activity
Symbolization	Rationalization	Logical analysis
Attention	Denial	Forced activity
Sensitivity	Projection	Empathy
Postponement	Procrastination	Heightened frustration tolerance
Remembering	Wishful regression	Regression in service
Impulse diversion	Displacement	Sublimation
Impulse transformation	Reaction formation	Substitute activity
Impulse control	Repression	Suppression

Modified from Kroeber T: The coping mechanisms of the ego functions. In White RW, editor: The study of lives, New York, 1963, Aldine/Atherton Press.

1985) and is useful in clinical nursing, as are the scales developed by Hauter (1981) and McCarthy (1974). The box details the factors affecting resilience and prevention capacities for handling threats.

DISTINCTIONS BETWEEN STRESS AND RISK CONCEPTS

Risk refers to the terrible actualities all humans are subjected to throughout life. The processes involved in risk are both subjective and objective, since the same risk may be comprehended by one person as a trivial event and by another as a personal disaster.

Sociologic risk models study populations prospectively, and these finding are usually not contaminated by knowledge of developmental outcomes. Risk researchers select populations providing the greatest number of outcomes, and psychologists seem better skilled at identifying incompetence (poor outcomes) in their research. Their risk models concentrate on populations in which children are more vulnerable to a particular disorder than the general population. "At risk" children who show good outcomes are called *invulnerable;* those at risk who demonstrate poor outcomes are called *true vulnerable.*

Most risk models are based on a single factor of vulnerability such as parents with mental illness, preterm birth with associated medical problems, and parental social status. An example of this single focus is the risk research on children of alcoholics, which inadequately explains the development of at risk children. Complex models that include the intricacy of the development process are needed for clinicians to understand the interplay of risk and protective factors.

The methods of stress and risk research are also different, distinctions important for the clinician using stress or risk as a theoretic rationale for interventions and drawing on research results for a practice rationale.

To date, stress research is more controlled, empirical, and quantitative and is conducted in research laboratories (Anthony and Cohler, 1987). Critics note that the

Summary of Resilience Model

Biologic and physical factors

1. Rest
2. Biochemical aspects (vitamins, food, drugs)
3. Thalamic-autonomic-hormonal factors
4. Prosthetics and props

Psychologic factors

1. Balance and ego cohesion
2. Reduction of pain, anxiety, or threat using discharge of anger
3. Containment of pain by differentiating life areas
4. Active introduction of pleasure, warmth, love, and soothing, evocative contact
5. Stimulus to recover using promises of results
6. Environmental recovery from family, friends, or culture
7. Expectation, fantasy, and the drive to recover, progress, and grow
8. Stimulation of action (recovery of mastery, struggle capacity, and potency)
9. Conditions supporting action, including symbolic support
10. Integrative capacity and growth capacity restructuring
11. Reward for recovery

Means for coping with threat

1. Action in relation to threat
   a. Reducing threat by postponing, bypassing, retreating, and shifting attention or interest
   b. Controlling threat by changing or transforming limits
   c. Balancing threat by changing relation of self to the threat or to the environment
   d. Eliminating or destroying threat
2. Dealing with or avoiding tension aroused by threat
   a. Discharging tension through action; displacing or projecting via fantasy (dramatics, painting, creative writing)
   b. Containing tension via insight, fantasy, or defense mechanisms

Sequence of coping with threat

1. Preparation of steps toward coping
2. Coping acts
3. Secondary coping using more drastic methods

Modified from Barclay L: Further reflections on resilience. In Anthony EJ and Cohler BJ: The invulnerable child, New York, 1987, The Guilford Press.

focus is usually on retrospective designs and that the parsimonious use of theory, the pinpointing of proximal events, and the use of relatively simple atheoretic inventories of life events occur (Kellam, 1974). It has been suggested that stress researchers move to a "second stage" of development and view existing conceptual frameworks more broadly.

Risk research is more prospective in design, is occupied with broad range assessment procedures, and has focused more exclusively on the concepts of resilience and vulnerability. Risk studies are usually conducted in the field and use grounded theory, providing interesting clinical illustrations and case materials.

RISK, VULNERABILITY, AND RESILIENCE

Current knowledge is more a group of generative ideas than a theory. The emerging information is scattered throughout the theoretic and research literature of child developmentalists, child clinicians, risk researchers, psychophysiologists, and psychoanalysts.

The concept of *invulnerability* emerged from a convergence of risk research (Rutter, 1988) and ego psychology (Erikson, 1964; Loevinger, 1976; Murphy and Moriarty, 1976). During the last 15 years, invulnerability has been placed beside the clinical concept of vulnerability. The addition of these theoretic perspectives follows the shift from disease entities to a focus on healthy psychosocial capacities such as competence, coping, creativity, and confidence. It is a synthesis of evolutionary, ego analytic, and cognitive developmental theories, with an emphasis on adaptation as an active process. It may be possible to predict future adaptation ability based on initial success.

Interest in resilience first arose as a result of epidemiology studies on the susceptibility of adults to coronary heart disease. Unexpected findings suggested that dispositional tendencies influenced risk and vulnerability to coronary disease. Longitudinal study results indicated that some individuals viewed as "high risk" lived through major changes in relationships, deprivations, and dislocations and exhibited little or no overt evidence of illness. This was attributed to two factors: They had no history of any preexisting susceptibilities, and they were "insulated" from detrimental life experiences by certain personality characteristics, an invulnerability called *psychoimmunity* (Hinkle, 1974).

Interest in vulnerability in child and infant psychiatry and psychology was stimulated by newer scientific understandings such as Konut's theory of individuality and identity (1977). Life-span and stress research findings also stimulated this renewed interest in their discovery that people reacted differently to similar events and that these differences were found in individuals' apperceptive mechanism, biologic makeup, and psychosocial setting.

Studies found that heightened susceptibility and resilience are similar in animals and humans. For example, when laboratory rats were put in extreme environments, some not only survived but thrived.

The pediatric seminal text in this area is *Vulnerability, Coping and Growth* (Murphy and Moriarty, 1976), which provided the theoretic focus and framework for contemporary research and clinical studies. The text stressed that *all* children have some zones of vulnerability, which existed on a continuum. Increases in vulnerability were the result of interactions between children and their environments.

Resilience and invulnerability researchers concur that there is no completely invulnerable child and that clinical concerns should focus on the degree and locus of vulnerability in relation to the intensity and quality of stress. If children's most vulnerable areas are confronted by severe stress, some degree of breakdown (somatic or psychologic) or "disintegrative reaction" is likely to occur "even though the child does not become delinquent or mentally ill" (Murphy and Moriarty, 1976).

A topology of the invulnerable child from theoretic and research data shows that invulnerable children display the following:

1. They have a life attitude that is somewhat sociopathic and an uninvolved approach to the world from which they seem strategically estranged (Hinkle, 1974). Invulnerable children develop the defenses of suppression, isolation, and distancing from others early, which may cause alienation.
2. They lead a charmed life, attributed to an overprotective mother. They have a good measure of health and as small children are psychologically attached, dependent, and self-centered and tend to be "avoiders."
3. They are "true heroes" in that they leave when heroism is self-effacing. Invulnerable children perform better under difficult circumstances and show an infantile robustness with "in the world" feelings.
4. They are interpersonally skillful with peers and adults, act on their own behavior, and exhibit a strong sense of personal control and self-regulatory capacities.
5. They are reflective rather than impulsive. Invulnerable children control their emotions but can exercise the full range of normal feelings. They are described as children who "work well, play well, love well, and expect well" (Segal and Yahraes, 1978).

A special subgroup of invulnerables have been identified, children who continue to rebound from high risks and vulnerability. These children begin life being frail, weak, and ailing, gradually developing an implacable resolve not to be broken. They show an extraordinary degree of persistence in struggles with adversity. They also demonstrate a high degree of creativity that tends to be inner directed and agonizingly expressed. They have the capacity to transform intolerable reality through fantasy, relieving their overwhelming sense of vulnerability (Anthony and Cohler, 1987).

The Family as a Social Unit

Studies of the family as a social unit and the connections between environmental factors and mental health are the predominant concerns of social psychiatry. The family has multiple and specific functions and key social roles of clinical concern in child psychiatry, for example, the family's role of protecting and nurturing the young, teaching ways to behave and interact in their society, and inculcating social and cultural values. In the last task, the family link between generations, the continuity of culture, and the introduction of cultural change are critical issues for all health care areas.

The general systems theory is a social psychiatric framework used to view the family. Although the role of the family in personality development is stressed by all classical and life-span models, viewing it as a care agent for sick members has just recently been given attention. The contributions of the family in this capacity are seen in neglect, transmission of defects, and maintainence of a sick member in lieu of seeking health care. The role of family as health promoters and health educators is another recent concern.

The DSM-III-R does not include a family axis because types of psycho-pathology and family system deficiencies have not been studied sufficiently and a consensus in family theory and therapy has not been achieved. Advocates of a family axis in subsequent DSM editions note the need for consideration of and provision for documentation of psychologic and familial dynamics, genograms, and family strength grids (Fleck, 1983). Systems parameters needed for accurate assessment include leadership, boundaries, affectivity, communication, and task/goal performance.

TRANSACTIONAL DEVELOPMENT MODEL AND RISK FACTORS

In contrast to the psychologic models presented in Chapter 4, the transactional developmental model holds that the parent-child-environment is the precursor to and maintainer of influences of mental health and that a consideration of these interrelationships and reciprocal influences is essential. Attention to the context in which children are developing is stressed, and the context includes the constitutional, biologic, and psychologic characteristics of children addressing developmental domains, care givers, and the transactional process through which development occurs. A plan for tracing roots, etiology, and the nature of maladaptations is needed so that interventions will be appropriately timed and guided.

Articulation of the interrelationships among the parent-child-environment factors is inherent to the transactional model. Their effect on the ontogenetic process varies across conditions. Transactions among all areas are stressed, and etiologic considerations are important when planning preventive interventions.

The model reflects developmental changes and the need to vary techniques according to children's developmental level. An exclusive focus on cognitive factors is avoided because this overlooks the important relationships with other domains.

Interventions focus on factors that mediate transactions among the care-givers and child. The effects can be altered by making changes in either the parent (or caregiver) or the child. In early childhood, reinterpretation of parental behavior is not feasible; therefore, the focus is on interventions designed to alter children's behavior, the caregiver's behavior, or the caregiver's interpretation of children's behavior. Sameroff (1983) calls these the "three R's of intervention:"

1. Remediation: Efforts to alter children's effect on the quality of the caregiver environment by changing behavior are undertaken. Biochemical and behavioral approaches are used.
2. Redefinition: When remediation fails, this approach helps caregivers to modify their attitudes regarding children's functioning to a more positive focus.
3. Reeducation: This includes parent skill training and counseling in which concrete information and guidance are provided. These stress the importance of the contextual effects and the impact of the environment on the developing child.

To apply a transactional model to the development of intervention strategies, clinicians need to consider risk factors associated with disorders. Risk factors can be classified into two categories and are either transient or enduring: Potentiating factors increase the probability that psychopathology will emerge. Within the areas of potentiating factors, vulnerability includes relatively enduring characteristics of children, their family, and the environment, and transient factors include challengers. Compensatory factors decrease the probability of the disturbances being manifested. Protective factors are relatively stable and buffers are more transient.

Vulnerability and protective factors must be assessed in relation to individual, familial, social, and environmental contexts. Attachment is viewed as a life-span issue, resulting in lifelong difficulties with relationship formations and intimacy (Antonucci, 1976). Examples of the transactional developmental model interventions for infancy through toddlerhood are shown in Table 5-4, and interventions for toddlerhood through early childhood are shown in Table 5-5.

Children's Social Support and Social Networks

Although humans are social species and the social environment is critical to human adaptation, only during the last 15 years has social support research developed and confirmed the impact of social network characteristics and social support resources on coping, adaptation, and health.

The theoretic foundations for viewing a social support system and larger ecologic system are rooted in Lewin's field theory (1935). The development of the Community Mental Health programs precipitated the study of the concepts and their use in the community treatment context.

Despite children's great need for instrumental and emotional resources from others, most research on social support has been conducted with adult populations. Some explanations for this paradox include the following:

1. Children's social networks have historically been viewed as stemming from their parents' networks and of limited importance in their own right. The focus has been on the relationship central to the child—the mother-child relationship.
2. Child development researchers tend to focus on infancy and preschool years.
3. Most research methods use questionnaires and interviews, more suited to the capacities of adults.
4. Research and clinical interventions concerned with the social networks of mothers have included measures to improve maternal morale and child-rearing competency with the goal of affecting the child indirectly. Social networks affect maternal parenting by providing emotional and material assistance and influence parenting styles through role modeling.

Some experts argue that mothers' social networks also influence children directly (Cochran and Brassard, 1979). Mothers' "significant other" adult relationships provide cognitive and social stimulation, direct care and support, observation models, and opportunities for the development of network-building skills.

Table 5-4   Transactional Developmental Model Interventions:
Infancy-Toddlerhood

Focus	Interventions
Homeostatic regulation	Facilitate parents' understanding of problem; provide information about developmental difficulties; use dyadic modeling, videotapes; employ parent support groups to help parents deal with developmental differences related to parenting infant with problems and associated grief
Management of tension	Recommend parents extend themselves more, help infant generate tension and affect, become emotionally engaged in situations, accept greater delays in child's development of fully differentiated affective expressions; facilitate parents' working with infant to sustain attention and build excitement; videotapes, modeling, fostering parental attuning to infant's arousal state important.
Attachment	Employ psychotherapy, parent skill building, support groups to improve on-going attachment relationships; increase social supports and home-based management programs; use modeling to improve dyadic interaction; facilitate parents' interpretation of weak, confusing signals; encourage positive feelings about infant; maintain emotional availability; address ecologic aspects; help ensure use of available resources; educate family about child development, child care
Autonomy	Avoid labeling child bad; if signs of helplessness and passivity present in child, encourage active, adaptive responses; increase environmental supports
Symbolic presentation	Encourage use of stage-salient intervention strategies to encourage language; provide speech and language therapy; sensitize impact of developing child; use cognitive behavior therapy with parent/child dyad to modify parental statements; avoid overcontrolled child development; modify insecure attachment relationships to improve language

Some researchers believe that child clinicians need to give greater consideration to the larger social context in which children develop (Bronfenbrenner, 1979; Whiting and Whiting, 1975). These scientists found that children from other cultures had social support models that were similar to but also differed from the culturally specific social support concepts of other systems usually encountered in Western societies.

In addition, clinical interest and interventions during the past few decades have focused on the importance of children's father, peers, friends, and siblings. For example, sibling therapy is a recent therapeutic intervention.

Table 5-5   Transactional Developmental Model Interventions: Toddlerhood
through Early Childhood

Focus	Interventions
Peer relations	Provide and facilitate children's development of affective expression and regulation; integrate cognitive developmental considerations with play therapy; consider ontogenetic progressions related to ability to achieve goals and developmental levels; use cognitive control therapy to facilitate evaluation of enduring aspects of cognitive functioning and adaptive style; use peer therapy with more well-adjusted children to change social system, provide opportunities for learning to control aggression, improve perspective-taking abilities, engage in intimate relations; if children withdrawn, employ therapy with younger peers
School function	Work with teacher to attain intrinsic orientation toward school performance; facilitate children's capacity to interact with and trust new adults; create positive adult friends through organizations such as Big Sisters/Brothers
Parent interventions	Educate parents about developmental progression; encourage interaction with child in growth-promoting ways

DEFINITIONS

A social network refers to the cast of characters in an individual's social world, the interrelationships among these people, and the connections between diverse structured social networks and the larger social system. Definitions of social networks address linkages connecting individuals and groups or institutions that can be channels for diverse resources.

Definitions of social support vary in the areas of specificity, transactions encompassed, and the importance attributed to stability. For example, in Caplan and Killilea's seminal text on social support and crisis intervention in community mental health (1976), support systems were defined as "continuing social aggregates that provide individuals with opportunities for feedback about themselves and for validations of their expectations of others."

According to this definition, information and cognitive guidance, tangible resources, and emotional sustenance are provided by supportive others in times of need. Social support therefore includes helping others in mastering emotional distress, sharing tasks, giving advice, teaching skills, and providing material assistance.

Social support has also been defined as information leading people to believe that they are cared for and loved, are esteemed and valued, and belong to a network of communication and mutual obligations. More recent definitions by human developmentalists define social support as resources provided by other people that occur in interpersonal relationships, reaching individuals through their social network connections. According to Belle (1989), supportive resources include information, material assistance, affection, physical comforting, empathic listening, assistance in problem solving, and reassurance of worth.

Lin, Dean, and Ensel (1986) extensively reviewed definitions from sociology, social psychology, and psychiatry and developed an operational definition of social support useful in clinical work with children:

> ... perceived or actual instrumental and/or expressive provisions supplied by the community, social networks and confiding partners. ... Social support can be operationally defined as access to and use of strong and homophilous ties (homophilous ties are those between people similar in nature – in social characteristics, attitudes and lifestyles).

UNIVERSAL ASPECTS OF SOCIAL SUPPORT

Understanding social support for children requires a sense of the cultural context of support and the cultural meaning of behaviors defined as help or support. Children use universally recognized behaviors to signal that help and support are needed or are being provided. Provisions of support include "affection, physical comfortings. . . assistance in problem solving" (Sandler and Bert, 1984), food or other material resources, and protective interventions to prevent aggression or harm. A shared human capacity for recognizing signals of distress in others and for responding to offers for help elicits this support. Universal human features for providing support may result from biosocial evolution and common social and functional requirements. Four support functions likely to be found anywhere are tangible help, positive appraisal, self-esteem enhancement, and a sense of belonging (Cohen and McKay, 1984).

Common cultural dilemmas that result in universal similarities have been identified (Shweder and Bourne, 1981). The following aspects are addressed:

1. Personal boundaries: What is me versus what is not me?
2. Sex identity: What is male versus what is female?
3. Maturity: What is grown-up versus what is childlike?
4. Cosubstantiality: Who is of my kind versus who is not of my kind?
5. Ethnic: What is our way versus what is not our way?
6. Hierarchy: Why do people share unequally in the burdens and benefits of life?
7. Nature versus nurture: What is human versus what is animal?
8. Autonomy: Am I independent, dependent, or interdependent?
9. State: What do I want to do versus what does the group want me to do?
10. Personal protection: How can I avoid worldwide war?

Parents face common problems of socializing and training children in the culturally given answers to these dilemmas. Offering support to children and training children to give support to others overlaps several of the culturally universal problems. For example, teaching children to offer support through sharing resources such as food or toys also gives children experience in cosubstantiality.

All societies must protect the young and helpless, and cultural and biologic evolution have established some patterns for ways in which this occurs. These patterns include signaling and response systems such as crying and comforting. The meaning and resolution of inequality and the dominance of some groups or people over others are also addressed.

In the system for coding social behaviors developed by John and Beatrice Whiting in their seminal study of children of various cultures (1975), social behaviors were coded in a system that included nurturing, prosocial behavior, commands and other attempts to change behavior, aggression, the search for and offering of help, sociability, and other behaviors. Activity settings were defined as the personnel, goals, motives, tasks, and culturally appropriate scripts for conduct constituting children's daily routines. This ecocultural model studies daily pressures to understand cultural differences and interpret social support.

COMPETENCE

Children's ability to cope with stress and make good social and emotional adjustments is an aspect of competence, defined as a set of functional or instrumental skills including intellectual, social-emotional, and practical abilities. From an ecologic perspective, the role of social support systems in the development of children's competence varies according to the "niche" in which children live. Social support systems are influenced by environmental and personal factors as part of a culturally organized ecologic system. The main premise of ecologic theory is that since societies consistently produce individuals who are able to function competently according to the requirements of that culture, societies must also develop a means for producing these people. Children's social support system is an important resource they use to learn the competency relevant to their ecologic circumstances.

The recognition context in which behavior occurs is also important. The American Psychiatric Association (APA) task force on ecopsychiatry (1979) suggested that the term *ecopsychiatry* be used to describe the person-environment, with the environment being considered as a general influence on mental health. Controversy still exists about whether traits within an individual or situations surrounding an individual contribute more to behavior and the clinical process. From a personality dynamics point of view, clinical significance depends on the individual, and the environment provides a stage on which life events unfold. From a strict behaviorist or environmentalist perspective, an organism is reinforced and behavior is modified by contingencies existing beyond the individual. Within a systems framework the focus may address the social network, physical environment, family, culture (the service delivery system or organizational framework), or a specific dyadic relationship.

The first applications of ecologic concepts to human behavior were derived from general ecology and dealt with the concepts of competition and success in a biologic ecosystem. Organismic theories (Lewin, 1951; Whiting and Whiting, 1975) and ecologic psychology were found to have limited application in the clinical areas. Family systems theories, however, provided concrete clinical techniques consistent with the view that children are part of a larger surrounding unit. The family is the most immediately accessible on-going system from which clinicians can assess behavior by isolating the individual from the context.

DEFINITIONS AND ASSUMPTIONS OF ECOPSYCHIATRY

Clinicians' ecologic focus involves observing children in relevant life contexts. Children are considered part of a unit that includes interactions not only with the family and significant others but also with the physical environment, organizational environment, and social and cultural context. For example, children's functioning is determined by family; social relationships; clinical status; access to adequate housing, transportation, and services maximizing healthy functioning (such as education); and the coordination of the total treatment delivery system beyond the specific psychiatric services.

The ecologic perspective does not compete with or replace existing clinical techniques in either assessment or treatment. The primary advantage of the ecologic model is that it conceptualizes both children's individual clinical functioning and broader community health and service delivery processes.

Mental health is defined as a congruent relationship between children and the surrounding environment or system. Thus, children interact with an environment in which the requirements and resources are congruent with their needs and capabilities. Clinicians focus on the interaction and on whether the exchange is acceptable and beneficial to both. In some situations, environments contribute notably to children's mental health problems as seen in the effects of institutionalization on chronicity and the effects of alcoholic parents. Children can also disrupt the functioning of the surrounding system such as the community disturbance caused by children with antisocial behaviors. From a broad systems approach, focusing both assessment and intervention on the specific area of mental disorder is essential.

Once behaviors or symptoms confirm the existence of a psychiatric diagnosis, clinicians must discover the primary sources and contributing context events of stress and the primary areas of the psychopathology that are disrupting the ecosystem. Two key elements are involved: the significance of social system contexts in assessment and management and the level at which interventions should take place. Treatment decisions include whether the child (and family) be provided crisis intervention, inpatient hospitalization, partial hospitalization, outpatient treatment, after-care follow-up, referral to a social agency, and involvement in the interventions.

Ecologic assessments focus on 10 key settings (O'Connor, Klassen, and O'Connor, 1979). Areas such as environmental-interpersonal-social contexts commonly affecting children's behavior present practical problems in community functioning and community reintegration. It is important to note that the effect of an area varies: a particular setting may be a source of stressful life events or may stabilize and support functioning. The 10 areas are the following:

1. Work
2. Education
3. Recreational and other stress-reducing settings
4. Social settings
5. Public organizations (welfare, legal)
6. Physical health settings
7. Mental health settings

8. Commercial settings and practical sources (housing, food)
9. Family transportation
10. Private and intimate relationships

The APA task force on ecology (1979) suggests viewing pathology in the context of the deviation-amplifying or deviation-counteracting process. Levels in the system, from internal physiologic processes to broad social cultural areas, collectively exert constraints on behavior. Thus, a feedback loop occurs in which small variations are progressively amplified, built up as deviations, and separated from the initial condition.

Many examples of the impact of ecology are seen in the literature. For example, the mental health functioning of children from single-parent black families has been related to the mothers' ability to use community networks and the availability of specific and concrete resources. Another example is that many young children identified as having mental health problems only exhibit them in specific environments such as school. Community resources may be localized areas of disturbing interaction, with relatively little generalization to other systems and aspects of children's lives. Populations of alcoholics, middle-childhood children with school-related disturbances, and children discharged from public facilities have also been identified as settings of community functioning critical for specific treatment modalities. Multilevel social and ecologic processes related to the incidence of psychopathology in a population and individual clinical symptoms include the quality of life, stress levels, and the ability to cope in a symptom-free or psychopathologic environment. However, the components of the interaction between the family unit and surrounding community are critical to the mental health of preschool and elementary school children.

In an ecosystem framework, assessment and interventions extend beyond children to their interactions within the ecosystem. Clinicians focus interventions on the dysfunctional processes of the ecosystem rather than on adaptation of children. Adaptation refers to children's attempts to cope with the environmental demands, and optimization refers to both children's adaptation to the environmental demands and their maintenance or modification of their surroundings to better meet their needs.

The appropriateness of existing therapeutic techniques are considered in each clinical situation. Clinicians must choose interventions depending on the time and the client, with both traditional and newer interventions selected according to the ecologic evaluations.

The task force suggests that clinicians help clients structure their environment and their relations to it. Nurses should give children and their families some input into the decision-making process, and overt therapeutic contracts are advocated and often based on the client's identification of the problem.

Assessment may also suggest interventions in other areas of children's ecosystem. Clinicians may work with a family as a system or with other critical networks of interpersonal relationships. The techniques chosen affect the interaction between children and contexts. Group dynamic techniques can induce changes in the way children relate to others outside the therapeutic setting and can modify children's role-related behaviors and reoccurring patterns of interpersonal behaviors.

The ecosystem contract is an intervention aimed at a broader context. The contract is written as a prediction of outcomes based on symptoms and states the changes the culture will support in the behavior of children of a particular age, sex, socioeconomic level, symptom complex, and set of circumstances. To modify the prognostic contract, nurse clinicians must influence children and the extra individual aspects of their ecosystem. This may require altering demographic characteristics, for example, changing to another school or in the case of drug-related problems, cult, or gang memberships, moving to another area of the country. In this consultant role, nurse clinicians may initiate and facilitate agency changes. For example, when a number of referred children attending a day care center began exhibiting similar behavioral problems in a specific setting, professionals started working with adults employed at the agency and uncovered a child molestation ring.

SOCIAL SUPPORT AND SOCIAL NETWORK INTERVENTIONS

According to society the individual continues to be the specific province of the mental health clinician. To justify actions in other eco-units, clinicians must show that an individual is affected by other aspects and that interventions can improve functioning. They must redefine the basic unit of treatment from isolated individuals to related individuals within a clear psychosocial context by using goal attainment scaling methods such as the psychosocial kinship inventory to determine social networks. The social system of normal adults consists of a primary group of 20 to 30 people with approximately 60% interconnectivity. Adults diagnosed with neurosis have a social system comprising 10 to 12 people with a 30% level of social connectivity. Psychotic patients' social system contain 4 to 5 people with 90% to 100% social connections. Interventions for the second and third groups include kinship replacement systems in self-help groups and crisis intervention teams.

There is scant data on the optimal psychosocial environment for satisfaction and productivity in mental health systems. Ecologic units in mental health systems include team treatment systems, continuity of care tracking, transfer systems, standardized treatment assignments, and routine procedures, all which can reduce children's individuality even though the goal of treatment is to achieve the most personal and individual human relationship possible. Mental health professionals have dual commitments: to the unique child and the integrity of each child-professional interaction and to the community.

Ecologic Model for Human Development

The theory that the organization of children's social support systems reflects influences from the ecologic context is based on Bronfenbrenner's ecologic model for human development (1979, 1986). In this model, development is defined as the product of the reciprocal interaction of the individual and the environment over time, consistent with other developmental perspectives. Other aspects of the model include the following:

1. Children's traits and characteristics influence the nature of the social support they experience.
2. This influence is likely to increase as children grow older and become more active "niche builders."
3. Children's personal characteristics may be determined by both genes and environmental influences.
4. Children at different developmental levels need and have the capacity to form and maintain diverse social support networks. Different ecologic factors may be associated with disparate developmental needs.

In this model, environment is conceptualized in four nested or hierarchical structures (Figure 5-2).

MICROSYSTEM INFLUENCES

Microsystem influences are defined as the setting in which children experience and create day-to-day reality. Children's microsystems are generally universal and include the family, school, neighborhood, and community. Each of these settings is a potential source of supportive relationships, and their structure and the patterns of social interactions within them influence the nature of children's experience of social support.

The microsystem has been studied more than other ecologic levels. It is the most accessible and easiest to operationalize clinically and has the most immediate and direct influences on children. Structural factors, such as family size and neighborhood density, and system dynamics, such as patterns of parent-child interactions and changes in the system because of divorce or birth of a child, and transitions between systems, such as moving to a new school or neighborhood, have been areas of considerable research and clinical case analysis (Moos and Ruhst, 1982).

Characteristics of children's microsystem influencing the form and content of their social support networks are summarized in Table 5-6.

SUPPORTIVE FRIENDSHIPS

Although Sullivan (1953) and other developmental theorists claim friendships have beneficial effects on the adjustment and development of children and friendship measures are used to assess "social development," there is limited scientific knowledge available. Most concepts defining children's friendships have been derived and applied from the research on adults' relationships (Cohen and Syme, 1985), a questionable assumption in some experts' view. Measures of adult social support are more theoretically based than the current research on children. Researchers studying children's friendships tend to ask children open-ended questions such as, How can you tell that someone is your best friend? From these responses, they have developed categories of supportive friendships.

Despite differences in methodologic approach, independence of research areas, descriptions of children's friendships and supportive relationships, friendships in adulthood and childhood appear to be substantially the same. Childhood friendships also parallel developmental changes; for example, Sullivan hypothesized that friendships are more supportive relationships between middle childhood and early

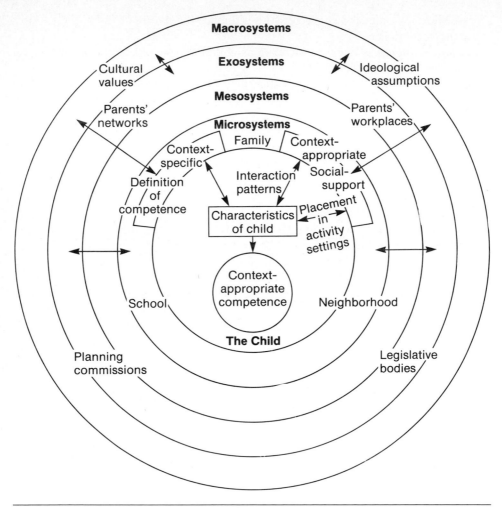

Figure 5-2 An ecologic model for the development of context-appropriate competence in children through social support. (From Tietjen AM: The ecology of children's social support networks. In Belle D, editor: Children's social networks and social supports, New York, 1989, Wiley-Interscience.)

adolescence, and research findings have concurred (Figure 5-3). Instruments measuring social support are shown in Table 5-7.

Health, Stress, and Life Changes and the DSM-III-R

AXIS IV

The DSM-III-R V codes classify problems that are not attributed to a mental disorder but do represent areas causing personal and social distress leading to referral. Although treatment may be indicated, coding these conditions as mental disorders may result in overdiagnosis.

Table 5-6   Ecologic Factors Influencing Social Support Systems:
             Microsystem Influences

Factor	Effect
Family size	In most non-Western societies, adults other than parents available to children, and adult roles and activities learned early; larger family size (three or more children) may decrease risk for social support deficits; in most Western societies, primary adult activities usually not accessible to children; larger family size may result in low levels of some social support; siblings rely on each other and peers more than on adults; influence varies with age: 1. Preschool children in large families have more siblings in networks but no more peers or adults than children from smaller families. 2. Children 5 to 7 years of age from larger families contact fewer people outside nuclear family than children from small families (reverses at school age). 3. School-aged children from large families have more extensive contact with peers and more intimate contacts with grandparents than children from small families.
Parents in the home	School-aged boys have peer interaction problems and disrupted relationships up to 2 years after divorce; when noncustodial parent remarries, contact between children and parent decreases.
Parental relationships	Relationship between parents affects relationship between children; high level of conflict between parents detrimental to interaction between child and mother.
Parenting styles	Children with parents who respect their point of view and enforce clear standards are more socially competent in peer interactions; children securely attached to mother during infancy more well adjusted and popular with peers in preschool than children insecurely attached (Waters, Wippman, and Sroufe, 1979).
Parent-child relationships	Emphasis in United States on cooperative parent-child interaction, democratic decision making, and mutual affection fosters self-regulation, high levels of esteem; after indulged infancy and toddlerhood, children have little interaction with parents or adults in other cultures; interactions occur only when negotiation of parental demands necessary, resulting in authoritarian pattern with heavy demands made on children; children more competent to take on roles in their own societies, more adaptive for developing sense of integration within groups (Whiting and Whiting, 1975).

Continued

Table 5-6   Ecologic Factors Influencing Social Support Systems: Microsystem
Influences — cont'd

Factor	Effect
Sibling support	Sense of interdependence fostered; direct experience in being cared for and caring is provided.
School	Geographic proximity of school to home and ethnic mix of classmates influence supportive relationships; children develop friendships with school mates residing near them and of same race; small schools offer more opportunites to participate in school activities, develop leadership skills, and sense of belonging; large schools provide more challenges in forming and maintaining relationships, fostering development of integration and individuation (Tietjan, 1989).
Neighborhood	Possible primary social contest for development of specialized and differentiated relationships (Bryant, 1982).

	Infancy (0 to 2 yrs.)	Childhood (2 to 6 yrs.)	Juvenile Era (6 to 9 yrs.)	Preadolescence (9 to 12 yrs.)	Early Adolescence (12 to 16 yrs.)
SEXUALITY					Opposite-sex partner
INTIMACY				Same-sex friend	Opposite-sex friend/romance Same-sex friend
ACCEPTANCE			Peer society	Friendship gang	Heterosexual crowd Friendship gang
COMPANIONSHIP		Parents	Compeers Parents	Same-sex friend Parents	Opposite-sex friend/romance Same-sex friend
TENDERNESS	Parents	Parents	Parents	Same-sex friend Parents	Opposite-sex friend/romance Same-sex friend

Figure 5-3   Neo-Sullivanian model of developing social needs. (From Furman W: The development of children's social networks. In Belle D, editor: Children's social networks and social supports, New York, 1989, Wiley-Interscience.)

Table 5-7   Instruments to Measure Social Support

Scale and authors	Dimension of support measured	Scores
Nurturance Scale (Belle and Long-fellow, 1984; Saunders, 1977)	Social embeddedness	Confiding Mother Father Sibling Friend No one
Neighborhood Walk (Bryant, 1985)	Social embeddedness	Network size Knowledge and interaction Intimate talks Ten most important individuals
	(above scores computed separately for peer, parent, and grandparent generations)	
		Special talks with adults
Social Support Rating Scale (Felner and others, 1985)	Quality	Family support Formal support Informal support
Berndt and Perry's Inventory (1986)	Enacted	Play, prosocial Intimacy, loyalty, Attachment Absence of conflicts
	Hybrid of social embeddedness and quality	Play Prosocial Intimacy Loyalty Attachment Absence of conflicts
Inventory (Wolchik, Beals, and Sandler, 1989)		Nurturance Maintenance
Child's section	Social embeddedness Enacted	Recreation
Parent's section	Social embeddedness Quality Enacted	Total network size Closeness of relationship Recreation Occasional maintenance Daily maintenance Nurturance

Modified from Wolchik SA, Beals J, and Sandler JN: Mapping children's support networks: conceptual and methodological issues. In Belle D, editor: Children's social networks and social supports, New York, 1989, Wiley-Interscience.

Continued

Table 5-7   Instruments to Measure Social Support — cont'd

Scale and authors	Dimension of support measured	Scores
Network Relationship Inventory (Furman and Buhrmester, 1985)	Quality	Satisfaction with relationship Reliable alliance
	Enacted	Affection Enhancement of worth Companionship Instrumental help Intimacy
	(Separate scores computed for mother, father, grandparent, older brother, younger brother, older sister, younger sister, best friend, and teacher.)	
Buhrmester and Fuhrman's Inventory (1987)	Enacted	Companionship Intimacy
Social Relations Questionnaire (Blyth, Hill, and Thiel, 1982)	Social embeddedness	
	Hybrid of enacted support and quality	Intimacy
Hirsch and Reischl's Inventory (1985)	Social embeddedness	Cognitive guidance Emotional support Tangible guidance
	(Separate scores are derived for family and school problems.)	Boundary density Reciprocity (for friendships only)
	Enacted	Activities with friends Confiding in friends
Arizona Social Support Interview Schedule	Social embeddedness	Total network size

The inclusion of Axes IV and V facilitated recording the severity of children's psychosocial stressors and introduced social and culturally mediated stress factors into the DSM-III-R diagnostic procedure. Axis IV gives clinicians a scale to list psychosocial stressors and the level of the experience encountered by children during the 12 months before evaluation. Two stress scales were developed, one for rating children and adolescents and the other for rating adults. In addition to occurring during the previous year, the stress must have contributed to: (1) the development of a new mental disorder, (2) the recurrence of a previous mental disorder, or (3) the exacerbation of an on-going mental disorder.

Levels of severity of psychosocial stressors are rated according to clinicians' assessment of the stress as compared to the expected response of a "normal" person.

GAF Scale

Code*

90	Absent or minimal symptoms (e.g., mild anxiety before an exam), good functioning in all areas, interested and involved in a wide range of activities, socially effective, generally satisfied with life, no more than everyday problems or
81	concerns (e.g., an occasional argument with family members).
80	If symptoms are present, they are transient and expectable reactions to psychosocial stressors (e.g., difficulty concentrating after family argument); no more than slight impairment in social, occupational, or school functioning
71	(e.g., temporarily falling behind in schoolwork).
70	Some mild symptoms (e.g., depressed mood and mild insomnia) OR some difficulty in social, occupational, or school functioning (e.g., occasional truancy or theft within the household), but generally functioning pretty well, has some
61	meaningful interpersonal relationships.
60	Moderate symptoms (e.g., flat affect and circumstantial speech, occasional panic attacks) OR moderate difficulty in social, occupational, or school
51	functioning (e.g., few friends, conflicts with co-workers).
50	Serious symptoms (e.g., suicidal ideation, severe obsessional rituals, frequent shoplifting) OR any serious impairment in social, occupational, or school
41	functioning (e.g., no friends, unable to keep a job).
40	Some impairment in reality testing or communication (e.g., speech is at times illogical, obscure, or irrelevant) OR major impairment in several areas, such as work or school, family relations, judgment, thinking, or mood (e.g., depressed man avoids friends, neglects family, and is unable to work; child frequently
31	beats up younger children, is defiant at home, and is failing at school).
30	Behavior is considerably influenced by delusions or hallucinations OR serious impairment in communication or judgment (e.g., sometimes incoherent, acts grossly inappropriately, suicidal preoccupation) OR inability to function in
21	almost all areas (e.g., stays in bed all day; no job, home, or friends).
20	Some danger of hurting self or others (e.g., suicide attempts without clear expectation of death, frequently violent, manic excitement) OR occasionally fails to maintain minimal personal hygiene (e.g., smears feces) OR gross
11	impairment in communication (e.g., largely incoherent or mute).
10	Persistent danger of severely hurting self or others (e.g., recurrent violence) OR persistent inability to maintain minimal personal hygiene or serious
1	suicidal act with clear expectation of death.

Modified from American Psychiatric Association: Diagnostic and statistical manual of mental disorders, ed 3, rev, Washington, DC, 1987, American Psychiatric Association.
*Use intermediate codes when appropriate.

This involves the amount of change in the person's life caused by the stress, the degree to which the event is desired and under control, and the number of stressors present. The DSM-III-R makes a distinction between acute stress, defined as stress that lasts less than 6 months, and enduring circumstances, defined as stress that lasts 6 months or more. Catastrophic stress extends beyond the experiences of normal people, and these responses include disengagement from the environment, social relations, and activities.

AXIS V

Axis V provides clinicians a rating of children's overall level of functioning and can be coded according to the Global Assessment Functioning (GAF) scale (Schaffer and others, 1983), a composite index that considers psychologic, social, and occupational functioning (see box). Two ratings are developed: The first assesses children's current level of function, establishing a baseline against which results of therapeutic intervention can be measured. The second rating is the highest level of function during the year before the evaluation, which may have prognostic significance.

Critics of the DSM-III-R note that clinicians are influenced by cultural biases in rating stress and identifying the average person's reaction. Also, Axis IV implies that stress is causative in producing disorders, a supposition that is difficult to demonstrate. Results from field trials using Axes IV and V in children have also shown little agreement with expected outcomes.

Summary

Recent knowledge in child development and child psychiatry in the past 20 years has paralleled the paradigm shift to health and prevention and has resulted in reevaluation, modification, and radical changes in many long-established and influential theoretic formulations. Some newer theoretic perspectives are refinements of the older themes, but others, such as life-span development, developmental psychopathology, risk, stress, coping, and invulnerability, are innovative theories. The challenge of current research is to integrate the early perspectives with the contemporary views.

REFERENCES

American Nurses' Association: Standards of child and adolescent psychiatric and mental health nursing practice, Kansas City, Mo, 1985, The Association.

American Psychiatric Association Task Force on Ecopsychiatric Data Base: Relating environment to mental health and illness: the ecopsychiatric data base, Washington DC, 1979, American Psychiatric Association.

American Psychiatric Association: Diagnostic and statistical manual of mental disorders, ed 3, rev, Washington, DC, 1987, American Psychiatric Association.

Anthony EJ: Risk, vulnerability and resilience. In Anthony EJ and Cohler BJ, editors: The invulnerable child, New York, 1987, The Guilford Press.

Anthony EJ and Cohler BJ, editors: The invulnerable child, New York, 1987, The Guilford Press.

Antonucci T: Attachment: a life span concept, Hum Dev 19:135, 1976.

Arnold M: Memory and the brain, Hillsdale, NJ, 1984, Lawrence Erlbaum Associates, Inc.

Barclay L: Further reflections on resilience. In Anthony EJ and Cohler BJ: The invulnerable child, New York, 1987, The Guilford Press.

Belle D: Studying children's social networks and social support. In Belle D, editor: Children's social networks and social supports, New York, 1989, Wiley-Interscience.

Belle D and Longfellow C: Confiding as a coping strategy, Unpublished paper, 1984.

Benner MH: Mental illness and the economy, Cambridge, Mass, 1973, Harvard University Press.

Berndt TJ and Perry TB: Children's perceptions of friendships as supportive relationships, Dev Psychol 22:640, 1986.

Blyth DS, Hill JP, and Thiel KS: Early adolescents' significant others: grade and gender differences in perceived relationships with familial and nonfamilial adults and young people, J Youth Adolesc 11:425, 1982.

Bower E: KISS and KIDS: a mandate for prevention, Am J Orthopsychiatry 42:556, 1972.

Brim OG: Types of life events, J Soc Issues 36:148, 1980.

Bronfenbrenner U: The ecology of human development, Cambridge, Mass, 1979, Harvard University Press.

Bronfenbrenner U: Ecology of the family as a context for human development: research perspectives, Dev Psychol 22:723, 1986.

Bryant BK: An index of empathy for children and adolescents, Child Dev 53:413, 1982.

Bryant BK: The neighborhood walk: sources of support in middle childhood, Monographs of the Society for Research in Child Development, No. 210, 1985.

Buhrmester D and Furman W: The development of companionship and intimacy, Child Dev 58:1101, 1987.

Caplan G: Support systems and community mental health, lecture, New York, 1974.

Caplan G and Killilea M, editors: Support systems and mutual help: multidisciplinary approaches, New York, 1976, Grune & Stratton, Inc.

Capra F: The turning point, New York, 1982, Simon and Schuster, Inc.

Caty S, Ellerton MI, and Richie JA: Coping in hospitalized children: an analysis of published case studies, Nurs Res 33:277, 1984.

Cochran M and Brassard J: Child development and personal social networks, Child Dev 50:609, 1979.

Cockerham WC: Sociology and psychiatry. In Kaplan HI and Sadock BJ, editors: Comprehensive textbook of psychiatry/IV, vol 1, ed 4, Baltimore, 1985, Williams & Wilkins.

Coddington RD: The significance of life events as etiological factors in children, J Psychosom Res 16:17, 1972.

Cohen F and Lazarus R: Coping with the stresses of illness. In Stone G, Cohen F, and Adler N, editors: Health psychology, San Francisco, 1979, Jossey-Bass, Inc, Publishers.

Cohen S and McKay G: Social support, stress and the buffering hypothesis: a theoretical analysis. In Baum A, Singer JE, and Taylor SE, editors: Handbook of psychology and health, vol 4, Hillsdale, NJ, 1984, Lawrence Erlbaum Associates, Inc.

Cohen S and Syme SL, editors: Social support and health, Orlando, Fla, 1985, Academic Press, Inc.

Colton JA: Childhood stress: perceptions of children and professionals, J Psychopathol Behav Assess 7:155, 1985.

Danish SJ, Smyer MA, and Nowak CA: Developmental intervention: enhancing life-event process. In Baltes PE and Brim OG, editors: Life-span development and behavior, New York, 1980, Academic Press, Inc.

Dohrenwend BS and Dohrenwend BP: What is a stressful life event? In Selye H, editor: Guide to stress research, New York, 1981, Van Nostrand Reinhold Co, Inc.

Dohrenwend BS and others: Exemplification of a method for scaling life events: the PERI life events scale, J Health Soc Behav 19:205, 1978.

Durkheim E: Suicide, New York, 1951, Free Press.

Erikson EH: Growth and crises of the "healthy personality." In Kluckhom C, Murry HA, and Schneider DM, editors: Personality in nature, society and culture, New York, 1955, Alfred A Knopf, Inc.

Erikson E: The golden rule and the cycle of life. In White RW, editor: The study of lives, New York, 1964, Atherton Press.

Everly GS and Sobelman SA: Assessment of the human stress response, New York, 1987, AMS Press, Inc.

Felner RD and others: Adaptation and vulnerability in high-risk adolescents: an examination of environmental mediators, Am J Comm Psychol 13:365, 1985.

Felsman JK and Vaillant GE: Resilient children as adults: a 40-year study. In Anthony EJ and Cohler BJ: The invulnerable child, New York, 1987, The Guilford Press.

Fleck S: A holistic approach to family typology and the axes of DSM-III, Arch Gen Psychiatry 40:901, 1983.

Furman W: The development of children's social networks. In Belle D, editor: Children's social networks and social supports, New York, 1989, Wiley-Interscience.

Furman W and Buhrmester D: Children's perceptions of the personal relationships in their social networks, Dev Psychol 20:277, 1985.

Gelles RJ: Family violence, Newbury Park, Calif, 1987, Sage Publications, Inc.

Gore S: Stress-buffering functions of social support: an appraisal and clarification of research methods. In Dohrenwend BS and Dohrenwend BP, editors: Stressful life events and their contexts, New York, 1981, Prodist.

Hanlon JJ and Pickett GE: Public health administration and practice, St Louis, 1984, The CV Mosby Co.

Hauter S: The perceived competence scale for children, Child Dev 53:87, 1981.

Havighurst RJ: Developmental tasks and education, New York, 1962, David McKay Co, Inc.

Hinkle LE: The effect of exposure to culture change, social change, and changes in interpersonal relationships on health. In Dohrenwend BS and Dohrenwend BP, editors: Stressful life events, New York, 1974, John Wiley & Sons, Inc.

Hirsch BJ and Reischl TM: Social networks and developmental psychology: a comparison of adolescent children of depressed, arthritic and normal parents, J Abnorm Psychol 94:272, 1985.

Hollingshead AB and Redlich FC: Social class and mental illness, New York, 1958, John Wiley & Sons, Inc.

Holmes TH and Rahe RH: The social readjustment rating scale, J Psychosom Res 11:213, 1967.

Kahn MM: The concept of cumulative trauma, Psychoanal Study Child 18:286, 1963.

Kellam S: Stressful life events and illness. In Dohrenwend BS and Dohrenwend BP, editors: Stressful life events, New York, 1974, John Wiley & Sons, Inc.

Konut H: The restoration of the self, New York, 1977, International Universities Press.

Kroeber T: The coping mechanism of the ego functions. In White RW, editor: The study of lives, New York, 1963, Aldine/Atherton Press.

Lazarus RS: The stress and coping paradigm in models for clinical psychopathology, New York, 1981, Spectrum Publications.

Lazarus RS and Folkman S: Coping and adaptation. In Gentry WD, editor: The handbook of behavioral medicine, New York, 1985, The Guilford Press.

Lazarus RS and Launier R: Stress-related transactions between person and environment. In Pervin LA and Lewis M, editors: Perspectives in interactional psychology, New York, 1978, Plenum Publishing Corp.

Levinson DJ: The seasons in a man's life, New York, 1978, Alfred A Knopf, Inc.

Lewin K: A dynamic theory of personality: selected papers, New York, 1935, McGraw-Hill, Inc.

Lewin K: Field theory in social science: selected theoretical papers, New York, 1951, Harper & Row, Publishers, Inc.

Lin N, Dean A, and Ensel WM, editors: Social support, life events and depression, New York, 1986, Academic Press, Inc.

Loevinger J: Ego development, San Francisco, 1976, Jossey-Bass, Inc, Publishers.

McCarthy D: The McCarthy scales of children's abilities, New York, 1974, Psychological Corp.

Mead GH: Mind, self and society, 1964, Chicago, University of Chicago Press.

Mechanic D: Mental health and social policy, ed 2, Englewood Cliffs, NJ, 1980, Prentice-Hall, Inc.

Minter RE and Kimball CP: Life events, personality traits, and illness. In Kutash IL and Schlesinger LB, editors: Handbook on stress and anxiety, New York, 1980, Jossey-Bass, Inc, Publishers.

Moos RH and Ruhst R: The clinical use of social-ecological concepts: the case of an adolescent girl, Am J Orthopsychiatry 52:111, 1982.

Murphy LB and Moriarty AE: Vulnerability, coping and growth, New Haven, Conn, 1976, Yale University Press.

Neugarten B: Adaptation and the life cycle, Counseling Psychologist 6:16, 1976.

Nowicki S and Strickland BR: A locus of control scale for children, J Consult Clin Psychol 40:145, 1973.

O'Connor WA, Klassen D, and O'Connor KS: Evaluating human service programs: psychosocial methods. In Abmed P and Coelho G, editors: Toward a new definition of health, New York, 1979, Plenum Publishing Corp.

O'Neill N and O'Neill G: Shifting gears, New York, 1974, Avon Books.

Peplau H: Interpersonal relations in nursing, New York, 1952, GP Putnam.

Perlmutter FD, Vayda AM, and Woodburn PK: An instrument for differentiating programs in prevention: primary, secondary, and tertiary. In Perlmutter FD, editor: New directions for mental health services: mental health promotion and primary prevention, New York, 1982, Jossey-Bass, Inc, Publishers.

Rigier DA and Burke JD: Epidemiology. In Kaplan HI and Sadock BJ, editors: Comprehensive textbook of psychiatry/IV, vol 1, ed 4, Baltimore, 1985, Williams & Wilkins.

Rook KS and Dooley D: Applying social support research: theoretical problems and future directions, J Soc Issues 41:5, 1985.

Rotter JB: Generalized expectancies for internal versus external control of reinforcement, Psychological Monographs, No. 609, 1966.

Rutter M: Prevention of children's psychosocial disorders: myth and substance. In Chess S and Thomas A, editors: Annual progress in child psychiatry and child development, New York, 1984, Brunner/Mazel, Inc.

Rutter M: The role of cognition in child development and disorder. In Chess S, Thomas AS, and Hertzig ME, editors: Annual progress in child psychiatry and child development, New York, 1988, Brunner/Mazel, Inc.

Sameroff AJ: Developmental systems: contexts and evolution. In Mussen B, editor: Carmichael's handbook of child psychology, vol 4, New York, 1983, John Wiley & Sons, Inc.

Sandler I and Bert M: Toward a multimethod approach to assessing the effects of social support, Am J Comm Psychol 12:37, 1984.

Sarason IG and Sarason BR, editors: Social support: theory, research and applications, The Hague, 1985, Martinus Nijhoff.

Saunders EB: The nurturance scale, Unpublished report, 1977.

Saxton DF and Hyland P: Planning and implementing nursing interventions, St. Louis, 1975, The CV Mosby Co.

Schaffer D and others: A children's global assessment scale (CGAS), Arch Gen Psychiatry 40:1228, 1983.

Scheff T: Labeling madness, Englewood Cliffs, NJ, 1975, Prentice-Hall, Inc.

Segal J and Yahraes H: A child's journey: forces that shape the lives of our young, New York, 1978, McGraw-Hill, Inc.

Selye H: The stress of life, New York, 1956, McGraw-Hill, Inc.

Semrad E: The organization of ego defenses and object loss. In Moriarity DS, editor: The loss of loved ones, Springfield, Ill, 1967, Charles C Thomas Publisher.

Sheehy G: Passages, New York, 1976, Bantom Books.

Shweder R and Bourne E: Does the concept of person vary cross-culturally? In Marsalle AJ and White G, editors: Cultural conceptions of mental health and therapy, Boston, 1981, D Reidel.

Sullivan HS: The interpersonal theory of psychiatry, New York, 1953, WW Norton & Co, Inc.

Tietjen AM: The ecology of children's social support networks. In Belle D, editor: Children's social networks and social supports, New York, 1989, John Wiley & Sons, Inc.

US Department of Health, Education, and Welfare, Surgeon General's Report on Health Promotion and Disease Prevention: Healthy people, Pub No 79-55071, Washington, DC, 1979, US Government Printing Office.

Vaillant GE: Adaptation to life, New York, 1977, Little, Brown & Co, Inc.

Vaillant GE and Milofsky E: Natural history of male psychological health IX: empirical evidence for Erikson's model of the life cycle, Am J Psychiatry 137:1349, 1980.

Veroff J and Veroff JB: Social incentives: a life span approach, New York, 1980, Academic Press, Inc.

Waters E, Wippman J, and Sroufe LA: Attachment, positive affect, and competence in the peer group: two studies in construct validation, Child Dev 50:821, 1979.

Whiting BB and Whiting JWM: Children of six cultures: a psychocultural analysis, Cambridge, Mass, 1975, Harvard University Press.

Wolchik SA, Beals J, and Sandler IN: Mapping children's support networks: conceptual and methodological issues. In Belle D, editor: Children's social networks and social supports, New York, 1989, Wiley-Interscience.

Zeitlin S: Assessing coping behavior, Am J Orthopsychiatry 50:139, 1980.

Chapter 6

Psychocultural Theories and Child Psychiatric Nursing

There has been a growing emphasis on the need for clinicians to provide culturally sensitive care because of the increasing number of clients from different backgrounds. Transcultural psychiatry has received renewed attention, and the concept of ethnic groups has expanded to include both subculture and minority groups.

The NIMH (Fields, 1979) and the President's Commission on Mental Health (1978) noted the inadequacy of mental health services provided to bicultural and bilingual minority groups and recommended a concentrated professional effort to develop culturally relevant theoretic and clinical practice theories, methods, and research. In response to these mandates, task forces were established that provided clinically valuable literature. For example, the APA's task force on ecopsychiatry (1979) identified a data base of cross-cultural counseling needs and clinical issues; they stated that counseling of persons of culturally diverse backgrounds by clinicians who are not specifically trained to work with such groups is unethical and developed recommendations for cross-cultural curriculum content and ethical research standards (APA, 1981; Taft, 1978). The Association for Advancement of Behavior Therapy has also developed ethical guidelines directing clinicians to provide the rationale and cross-cultural considerations in their practice documentation (Fields, 1979).

The *Code for Nurses with Interpretive Statements* (ANA, 1956) initially mandated two principles of culturally sensitive practice: (1) "The nurse provides services with respect for the dignity of man, unrestricted by considerations of nationality, race, creed, color, or status." (2) "The nurse works with members of health professions and other citizens in promoting efforts to meet health needs of the people" (Peplau, 1974). Psychiatric nursing leaders emphasized the need for cultural content in nursing education in 1979 at the ANA Commission on Human Rights hearings, cautioning: "At the minimum, we need to sensitize every health care professional to the cultural aspects of client care. At the other end—the large, complex social arena—we need to influence the government's expenditure of dollars to support theoretical studies of culture and the impact it has on health care" (Henderson and Primeaueux, 1981).

Cross-cultural mental health practices contribute to professional practice development by enhancing nurse clinicians' clinical sensitivity and repertoire of practical strategies. By acknowledging ethnocultural differences and similarities, clinicians heighten their clinical astuteness and gradually adopt a practice style addressing the effect of certain cultural elements on the process and outcome of psychiatric care.

Anthropology and Psychiatry

MEDICAL ANTHROPOLOGY

Most culturally specific mental health concepts and therapies are derived from anthropology, described as the most scientific of the humanities and the most humane of the sciences. Anthropology is concerned with the holistic study of mankind, including human origins, development, social and political organizations, religions, languages, art, and artifacts. Medical anthropology includes archaeology, paleontology, genetics, serology, primate behavior, and ecology, as well as studies of art, artifacts, and tools. Medical anthropology addresses ways in which the causes of ill health are explained, the types of medical treatment used, the sources of medical care, the relationship between different beliefs and health and disease, and the reasons for disease diversity in human populations.

The clinical application of anthropologic concepts is most evident in the rapprochement of medicine and psychiatry in the new medical model and in the use of behavioral medicine perspectives and other biologically oriented theories, such as psychobiologic resilience, and concepts of wellness, prevention, and culture. The last focus is viewed by some experts as an emerging major health care paradigm (Capra, 1982).

SOCIAL AND CULTURAL ANTHROPOLOGY

There is no consensus on a definition of culture, but dominant perspectives have emerged. The *world view* concept (Sue, Ito, and Bradshaw, 1982) has stronger support among anthropologists. It addresses the ways groups view the world and the phenomena in it and permeates every aspect of life. Locus of control contrasts with locus of responsibility, and clients' perception of access to power and social responsibility relating to their environment is emphasized. Although some theorists separate the three dominant world views—the magico-religious (Hautman, 1979), the holistic, and the scientific (Boyle and Andrews, 1989)—clinicians find that most people use combinations of these views.

Thinking emerges from people's world view because each culture provides symbols to use and tools for expressing thoughts. World views also account for the "national origin" references used to distinguish between different anthropologic schools. In Britain, social anthropology is predominant; it emphasizes the social dimensions of human life. People are organized into groups that regulate and perpetuate themselves, and their experience as members of society shape their world view. Culture is seen as a way to organize and legitimize society and provides the basis for social, political, and economic organizations. Anthropology and psychiatry define normality in a particular society, are part of the etiology of certain diseases, influence the clinical presentation and distribution of mental illness, and determine the ways that mental illness is recognized, labeled, explained, and treated (Helman, 1984). In contrast, cultural anthropologists in the United States focus on systems of symbols (ideas and meanings that compose a culture), with social organization considered as one aspect of individual expression. This school originally focused on minority groups and immigrants. The American culture was considered dominant, and the customs of people of other cultures were compared to it—a *deficit-deficient* approach. In the 1960s the ethnic humanism movement altered many cultural traditions, such as the segregation of elementary schools. Integration in schools profoundly altered the educational and social experiences of children from other cultures, and the term *ethnic minority children* was conceived to designate children who were Black, Hispanic-American, American Indian, or Asian American.

Initially, transcultural psychiatry included the study and comparison of mental illness in different cultures from the perspective of Western-trained psychiatrists and social anthropologists. Social anthropologists were interested in the psychologic, behavioral, social, and cultural dimensions associated with the cultural perceptions of mental illness and not the organic aspects of psychologic diseases. Although the two approaches had different views, they both focused on the diagnosis and treatment of mental illness when the clinician and client had different cultural backgrounds and the effect on mental health of migration, urbanization, and other social change.

CULTURAL PSYCHIATRY

Cultural psychiatry was initially a subspecialty that focused on care for minority group members with mental disorders. Early theories were culture-related, often detailing exotic conditions of little practical significance to clinicians. Interventions consisted of enculturation through Americanization.

Although the use of communication techniques such as verbal therapies in psychotherapy was an American scientific intervention for treating mental disorders, folk healing and primitive and magical rituals of some other cultural groups residing in the United States were viewed as primitive social interventions and as superstitions that were nonscientific and that were generally discredited. Psychosocial concepts blended and obscured the importance of culture in many theories that stressed the social dimensions of development and psychopathology. The need to disentangle these components in clinical practice and discard the deficit explanatory model was first identified by workers in the Peace Corp in the 1950s and later by clinicians and researchers who were often members of minority groups.

Focus of Transcultural Psychiatry

Cultural changes occurring in American society during the last few decades have altered the dominant White Anglo-Saxon Protestant (WASP) life styles. Social movements, such as the feminist movement and sexual liberation, and changes in "traditional" values demonstrated by "reconstituted" families and religious affiliations have affected behavior, behavioral disorders, and treatment approaches. Cultural psychiatry no longer focuses on small ethnic groups or unique cultural practices; the modern goals include learning more about humanity and its ills and the coping mechanisms used by majority groups and mass populations and investigating the cultural adaptations required with social change.

The APA listed the specific purposes of the field as the following (Tseng and McDermott, 1981):

1. To study ways in which culture interrelates with personality development, behavior patterns, and adaptive styles
2. To explore culture-related stresses, problems, and coping mechanisms
3. To investigate cultural influences on symptom formation, manifestations of pathology, clinical pictures, and frequency of certain mental illnesses
4. To understand the ways in which clients perceive, conceptualize, present their problems and seek help, including the available healing systems and their use
5. To sharpen awareness of the impact of culture on psychiatry in evaluation, diagnosis, and treatment
6. To examine the cultural influence on psychiatric theory and the universal applicability and culture-specificity of psychiatry
7. To improve cross-cultural research methods
8. To work with health scientists, social scientists, and political and community groups to change damaging patterns of life

Effective cross-cultural practice models need to address the interaction of ecology, human behavioral problems, competence building, and cross-cultural helping processes. Current models avoid ethnocentric evaluations of practices and beliefs and emphasize positive features of cultural variation and the cultural context of development.

Society has shown an intense fascination in learning about people of other cultures and cultural differences. For example, books by the British anthropologist Ashley Montague on touching, territory, and nonverbal communication have been widely read by the lay public and translated into 20 languages (1977). Desmond Morris's books, such as *The Naked Ape,* have contributed to society's understanding of cross-cultural differences. *The Human Zoo, Intimate Behavior,* and *Manwatching* are useful resources when clinicians work with children experiencing minor perceptual "dominant cultural" adaptations.

Cross-Cultural Practice Theories

LIFE SPACE THEORY: LEWIN

Lewin's theory of life space is based on concepts of cultural relativity and uses pattern development, which refers to the appearance of similar actions and outcomes in separate contexts. The relationship between patterns often discloses unexpected identities and correspondences and expected discontinuities, thus identifying cultural specifics and universals. The theory refers to the place individuals occupy at a particular moment and assesses the forces acting on them within a developmental context. According to this theory, psychologic structures become increasingly complex and differ from one time to another. To understand human development does not require using personality type, traits, developmental, or dynamic theories; life themes make up human development. The pattern recognition component of Martha Roger's nursing theory (1970) is an implementation of Lewin's theory.

CULTURAL CONTEXT OF HUMAN DEVELOPMENT THEORY: VYGOTSKY

Developed in the 1930s, Vygotsky's theory (1978) integrates social and cognitive processes within a cultural context. Assumptions include: (1) human development is inseparable from human social and cultural activities, (2) both institutional and interpersonal levels of social context must be considered, (3) individuals' cultural history provides the organization and tools useful to the development of cognitive activities, and (4) practices and interventions need to facilitate socially appropriate solutions to problems. Thus, problems and cognitive problem-solving strategies are culturally specific.

Vygotsky's theory holds that the cultural structuring of social interactions provides the essential context for development. Interpersonal situations guide children in their development of the skills and behaviors considered important in their culture. Information regarding tools and practices is transmitted through interactions with more experienced members of society, and patterns of interpersonal relations are organized by institutional conventions and the availability of cultural tools. *Zones of proximal development* refer to children's capacity to use environmental cues to solve problems, a process defined by Cole and Brunner (1971) as "where culture and cognition create each other." This cognitive capacity is determined by attention, flexibility, and persistence. Vygotsky's theory is clinically useful for understanding the relationships between culture and the developing child and has been emphasized in special education literature.

Culture and Child Psychiatric Nursing

MIND-BODY DUALISM AND PSYCHOSOMATIC SYMPTOMS

The world view emerged from the Cartesian doctrine stating that the mind—or psyche—exists on one level and cannot be reduced to matter or to the physical (Flaskerud, 1987). The body or soma is a separate area, and specific terms and language divide the two entities. This mind-body distinction is not held by other theories, nor does the varied, descriptive language exist for psychologic problems.

When translating the present state examination from English to seven other languages, researchers found differences in the words available for emotional expressions and proposed a theory linking the degree of individualism fostered by a culture to the degree of language available for differentiation of emotional expression. These differences can be placed on a continuum, with the least individuated cultures (characterized by strong group orientations with highly extended family and kin obligations) being most likely to register emotions in somatic terms and having the least number of words to describe emotional or psychologic states. As cultures moved toward greater individualism, expressions of emotions combined bodily experience terms and psychologic experience terms to a final position in which highly differentiated body-mind words were available.

The inability of clients from other cultures to talk about their feelings has been paralleled with the psychosomatic disorders of clients from the Western culture. A combination of child-rearing practices and world views fostering the development of verbal unexpressiveness may explain the reason for children of other cultures not responding to established child therapies with the success of children from Western cultures (Dahl, 1989). However, psychosomatic symptoms are frequently seen in children of all cultures following periods of excessive emotional strain. For example, neurasthenia is the most frequent diagnosis Chinese psychiatrists report in children with school problems (Lin and Finder, 1983).

Cross-cultural and epidemiologic research show that the manifestations of psychopathology change within different cultures as world views change, and some psychiatric disorders disappear (Mollica and Redlich, 1980). For example, the neurasthenia and hysterical paralyses commonly found in American veterans after World War II are seldom encountered in Vietnam veterans, and posttraumatic stress disorders are "new" DSM-III diagnoses, frequently used for Vietnam veterans.

Changes in ways in which different cultures express mental diseases are most noticeable in the major psychiatric disorders. In the United States, frank psychosis is seen less often clinically, and psychotics that appear for treatment are less disturbed than psychotics seen in the past. Epidemiologic data indicate catatonic and hebephrenic subtypes of schizophrenia are less common than they were a decade ago, while paranoid subtypes appear more often. The increase in borderline states implies that although bodily manifestations of psychoses are less severe, the more intellectual manifestations require longer and different treatments.

It has been suggested that psychotic manifestations progress from body to mind as cultures become more civilized and complex and that manifestations of the subtypes of schizophrenia are culture-related, even though the basic disorder is primarily identified with biologic factors (Tseng and McDermott, 1981). These shifts have also been observed in the Third World nations as they become more Westernized. Primitive societies have a greater incidence of subtypes of schizophrenia in which disturbances take the form of psychomotor expressions. In these societies the body most clearly exhibits the ills of the mind.

People who reside in psychiatrically sophisticated cultures with a highly verbally expressive life style differ from people residing in ritualistic cultures with many restrictions on behavior. People from the latter express their mental diseases in elaborate ways. In cultures free of emphasis on rules, expression of psychologic conditions usually occurs in simpler forms.

CULTURE-BOUND PSYCHOLOGIC DISORDERS

Culture-bound disorders are groups of symptoms indicative of specific illnesses that do not exist in Western societies, Europe, or the United States. Most of these disorders occur in children and infants and are a way for cultures to provide for the expression of emotion and distress. Culture-bound disorders present a constellation of symptoms that are somatic, psychologic, social, and spiritual, and members of the culture attribute the causes of the disorders to natural, supernatural, physical, psychologic, social, and moral factors.

Examples of disorders found in Hispanic cultures that have no counterpart in Western medicine include: *susto* (supernatural fright), in which an indigenous therapist, the *curandero,* provides support, attention, and relief. *Caida de molleras* (fallen fontanel) is attributed to an excessively rapid removal of the nipple from an infant's mouth. Symptoms include diarrhea, vomiting, and the inability to suck or eat adequately. Folk medicine interventions include pushing up on the palate while holding babies by their feet over a pan of water. Found predominantly in Carribean cultures, *mal ojo* is based on the belief that children are highly vulnerable due to their immature status and are subject to "evil eyes." Victims are usually admired by adults with "strong vision" who "cast their eyes" on them. Symptoms include fever, diarrhea, vomiting, crying, and restlessness. The *curandero* performs several treatments, such as rubbing a raw, broken egg over children's body while praying, passing an unbroken egg over their body, or rubbing their body with an egg to draw out the fever.

Folk disorders are usually treated by indigenous therapists (Torrey, 1969), and collaboration with them is essential for clinicians working in transcultural community mental health care settings (Hautman, 1979). Cultural brokers (representatives from the culture of the client acting as an advocate) facilitate health care negotiations for interventions (Weidman, 1975).

PSYCHOCULTURAL CONCEPTS AND THE DSM-III-R

Research has shown that findings in clinical research and studies in psychiatry and psychology need to be qualified by their culture of origin. This is especially true of the minor psychiatric disorders that are closely related to culture and social conditions.

Triandis and Draguns (1980) propose that culture be included as a parameter in the construct of all new theories and that the identification of cultural dimensions be the focus of interdisciplinary research. Scientific efforts toward unpackaging the concept of culture are critically needed to ensure that ethically appropriate, scientifically based care for people of other cultures is possible. Because of the lack of methods to identify dimensions of cultural variation that have clinical and practical implications, limitations in the DSM-III-R disorders were noted with a caveat:

Many persons live in, or come from, cultures different from those of the evaluating clinician or that on which most of the DSM-III-R criteria are based. A clinician involved in transcultural assessments should understand both normal and psychopathological aspects of individuals in the "foreign" group and be sensitive to the possibility of misunderstanding, even when he or she has considerable experience with it. This caveat applies even to traditionally distressing symptoms (e.g., certain hallucinations or experiences during bereavement in some Native American cultures) (Reid and Wise, 1989).

Some critics believe that the DSM-III-R criteria are culturally biased. For example, although the DSM-III-R criteria for antisocial personalities may appear abnormal to clinicians from white, middle-class America, the behaviors may not be considered deviant by members of other cultures and other socioeconomic groups. In contrast, many sociopathic behaviors exhibited by the educated elite white collar groups, such as tax evasion, sexual harassment of employees, stealth in business dealing, broken commitments, backbiting, and slander, are not included in the DSM-III-R (Shea, 1988).

Clinical Process in Cross-Cultural Child Psychiatric Nursing

Clinical models used in psychiatric cross-cultural counseling with parents and adapted for clinical work with school-aged children include the following (Pederson, Lonner, and Draguns, 1981):

1. Kleinmans's ethnomedical model favors the contextually more complex *illness* perspective of clients over the simple *disease* perspective of physicians. According to the theory, when people become ill, they identify, communicate, and manage symptoms with the assistance of friends, family members, and social support networks. When people seek professional help for their illness, it becomes a disease and is assigned a diagnosis by health professionals or indigent therapists.
2. Goldstein's structured learning theory emphasizes a proactive *reformity* prescription requiring therapy with a less adequate, reactive *conformity* prescription.
3. Prince's self-righting theory contrasts exogenous and endogenous approaches to mental health and emphasizes the mobilization of endogenous resources of a self-righting mechanism, self-healing with minimum outside intervention, and the importance of subjective and objective knowledge.
4. Goffman and Harris focus on patterns of cultural shock and expand on the idea of role sets, making generalizations from phenomena of cultural shock to experiences of deinstitutionalization.
5. Ruiz and Casas' bicultural counseling model seeks cultural variables in multicultural groups. It emphasizes counselors' bicultural skill as a mediating link between clients and the troublesome environment.
6. Sue contrasts locus of control with locus of responsibility to emphasize the complex interaction of clients with their environment.
7. Meyer and Engel's biopsychosocial model stresses the importance of every level of human behavioral interaction in terms of community, family, interpersonal, individual, psychologic, biochemical, psychoanalytic, physiologic, genetic, and constitutional factors.

ASSESSMENT

Clinicians need to include the cultural assessment components as part of the initial diagnostic interview whenever cultural difficulties contribute to or have caused the chief complaints or reasons for referral. Cultural assessments are also indicated whenever children and their family belong to a different cultural group. This applies to all first- and second-generation immigrants, except when behavioral or brief therapies highly focused on noncultural or family-related problems are indicated. Cultural assessment is also appropriate for evaluation and diagnosis with third, fourth, and later generation children when treatment issues are unclear, long-term psychotherapy is used, ethnocultural issues are a presenting complaint, or children and their family are in a transcultural situation.

Many questions on the standard MSE are misleading for children of other cultures, and it needs to be adapted to the specific situation or discarded altogether. For example, proverbs vary from culture to culture and are not useful in determining older children's thought processes.

Guidelines for cultural assessment suggest that this component be completed during different phases of contact, for example, while obtaining the standard history. However, if clinicians perceive that children and parents are highly sensitive to issues of ethnic identity, it may be clinically appropriate to defer part of the assessment until the therapeutic alliance has been established.

The purpose of the psychocultural assessment is to place children and their family within a cultural contextual framework. Questions explore the intellectual and emotional understanding of several historical stages contributing to the evolution of the ethnocultural identity.

Most cultural assessment tools found in psychiatric literature implement concepts emphasized by the different clinical models discussed on p. 154. They are useful when interviewing the parents of preverbal children and can be adapted to school-aged children's level of verbal and cognitive development. The following culture status exam is based on the ethnomedical model for working with children with psychiatric problems as the major concern (Pfiffeling, 1980):

1. What do you think has caused your problem?
2. Why has this happened to you?
3. How long have you had this problem? Why do you think it started when it did?
4. What do you think your sickness does to you? How does your sickness work?
5. What do you think should be done to help clear up or get rid of your problem? What kind of treatment do you think you should receive?
6. Who can help you get better?
7. What are the most important results you hope to receive?
8. What concerns you most about your sickness? What are the chief problems your sickness has caused you?

The assessment interview should convey interest in the family and help foster a safe atmosphere in which conflicts in ethnocultural identity may be disclosed. Jacobsen (1988) suggests including additional questions to discern the stages of the ethno-cultural status. Although recommended for use in mental health settings, the guidelines shown in the box have application in other areas of medicine and public health.

CROSS-CULTURAL DIAGNOSES

Presenting behaviors and complaints commonly reported in children in cross-cultural settings include anger, tantrums, irritability, depression, sadness, loneliness, anxiety, psychomotor and verbal hyperactivity or retardation, school adjustment problems, social withdrawal, and somatic complaints. In preverbal children, eating problems and regressive behaviors are frequent concerns.

Formulating a cross-cultural diagnosis begins with defining normality and abnormality by examining the child-rearing practices and expectations of children in the native culture. Clinicians need to be aware of the following factors (Helman, 1984):

1. The extent to which cultural factors affect some of the diagnostic categories and techniques of Western psychiatry
2. The role of the family's culture in helping children to understand and communicate their psychologic distress
3. The ways in which children's behavior are viewed by their parents and other members of their cultural group

---

Ethnocultural Assessment

Stage I

Obtain information about children's ethnocultural heritage, that is, the culture of origin for both maternal and paternal lines of the family and delineation of ethnic heritage. The place of geographic origin is insufficient to understand a complex multicultural-multiethnic background. A single, readily identifiable attribute of a person, such as family name or native language, is not useful and implies stereotyped cultural characteristics.

Stage II

Obtain information about the circumstance leading to the ethnocultural problem. Do the children understand the events leading to the transitions from the culture of origin? If the culture of origin is in a state of sociopolitical transition leading to the move, what are the family's thoughts and feelings about these events?

Stage III

This stage is based on children's and parents' intellectual and emotional perception of development of the family's niche in the host society since the translocation. Have family members stayed together or are they dispersed? What has the family's relationship been with other members of its original ethnoculture? How have they fared financially? Are they better or worse off than before translocation? Have the children internalized the family's sagas?

Stage IV

This stage addresses the children's view of cultural adjustment as an individual and distinct from the family. Clinicians should ask about their feelings regarding ethnocultural integration. Are they striving to become more American, disavowing the norms and customs of their ethnocultural background? Are they resisting acculturation?

Stage V

Clinicians should recognize that children of other ethnic groups may have no knowledge of the process of psychotherapy and are likely to need detailed explanations and reassurance.

Modified from Jacobsen FM: Ethnocultural assessment. In Comas-Diaz L and Griffith EEH, editors: Clinical guidelines in cross-cultural mental health, New York, 1988, John Wiley & Sons, Inc.

---

4. The interpretation of the specific cluster of symptoms, signs, and behavioral changes by the family and their community as evidence of a culture-bound psychologic disorder

CULTURALLY RESPONSIVE SERVICES

Once a diagnosis has been made and the need for interventions established, engaging families of other cultures in treatment is especially challenging. Even when available, services for families of other cultures are underused, and these clients are often crroneously labeled "noncompliant." Culturally responsive services are those in which the clients and therapists share the same cultural view of illness (Sue and Morishima, 1982) and are usually located in the client's community.

Some experts believe that only therapists with the same ethnicity as the client should perform psychotherapy (Torrey, 1969); others hold that cross-cultural counseling can be done with a certain amount of training, skill, and empathy (Kinzie, 1978). Therapists' ethnocultural identity may cause counter-transference difficulties in treating clients with the same background, and children and their family may leave therapy. Allen (1988) has developed a list of 12 commandments for engaging clients of other cultures in therapy that have been adapted to child psychiatry (see box).

Specific Cultural Diagnoses and Interventions

FRAGMENTED ETHNOCULTURAL IDENTIFICATION

Ethnocultural identity may be influenced by migration and changes in a group's social, political, economic, or health status. As a therapeutic tool, it can assist clinicians in helping children progress through the five stage developmental framework of adjusting to cross-cultural transitions (Adler, 1975):
1. Initial contact with a second culture: Children are insulated by their culture of origin.
2. Disintegration: Children's awareness of being different results in depression and withdrawal.
3. Reintegration: Children reject the second culture by expressing anger and rebellion.
4. Autonomy: Children can negotiate different situations culturally and survive new experiences.
5. Independence: Children accept and enjoy ethnocultural, social, and psychologic differences. They exercise choice and responsibility and can discern the cultural aspects of everyday interactions and circumstances age appropriately.

When ethnocultural assessment confirms that older children's self-identification is fragmented, therapists actively foster identification with their ethnocultural origin by using three major therapeutic functions (Jacobsen, 1988):
1. Reflection: Therapists mirror the ethnocultural pieces of the fragmented self and acknowledge the pervasive influence of ethnicity and culture. Therapists underscore aspects that reveal ethnocultural identity conflict: "It is difficult for you to see yourself as Cuban," or "You avoid people from your community because they remind you of being Cuban."
2. Education: Therapists guide children through a reformation of ethnocultural identity, providing a "safe" environment where children can examine conflicted identity. By using direct approaches, therapists help them to examine inconsistencies in aspects of their ethnic background, other ethnocultural values, and values of the second culture.
3. Mediation: Therapists help children integrate their ethnocultural self into a consolidated sense of self by connecting different aspects of the self. Restoring a sense of identity may require resolving cultural conflicts within the family, between the family and community, and between children and the wider

Cross-Cultural Therapy

1. Clinicians should avoid assuming that children and their parents are absolutely certain to have or not have any particular life problem, personality disorder, illness, mode of presentation, or attitude to therapy; that is, stereotyping is not appropriate.
2. Assessment of their understanding of psychiatry and psychotherapy and the extent to which they were adequately prepared by the referring agent is important. Clinicians should try to understand the model the family is using and the effect of cultural conditioning and intrapsychic defenses.
3. After a proper clinical assessment is made, clinicians should help the family understand the link between nonpsychologic and psychologic models.
4. Assessment of the cultural influences, socialization patterns, and culturally determined adaptive traits affecting children is essential.
5. Cultural issues should be approached while assessing cultural awareness, openness, flexibility, general defensiveness, and other ego strengths of the child and family. Clinicians should share interest in and knowledge of the culture or subculture.
6. Clinicians should avoid being judgmental and show respect for the strengths of the cultural background. Condescending, overenthusiastic, phony, or prescribing attitudes should also be avoided.
7. A degree of formality dependent on the cultural relatedness and counter understanding that develop between clinician and client should be used.
8. If the family has a strong religious affiliation, suggesting a member of the clergy as a mediator is appropriate. Information about the use and views of nontraditional healers should be elicited tactfully. Clinicians should collaborate with nontraditional healers and rely on cultural brokers if necessary. If the child is school aged, parents should be encouraged to become involved in parent-child school activities and the child's formal educational experiences.
9. Learning as much as possible about the ethnic group and culture, especially the group's preferences is essential. Clinicians should learn the expressions to enhance empathy and understanding and become acquainted with the culture's children's literature.
10. Arranging for separate interview opportunities so that the father, mother, and child can ventilate grievances, explore values and roles, and help discover means of conflict resolution between and across generations without loss of pride is important. Children should not be used as an interpreter in family sessions.
11. Clinicians should search for the meaning and form of cultural confusion, stresses, coping mechanisms, and secondary gains in children.
12. If working with migrants and relocated families who wish to return to their original residence, suggesting the move as a solution to adjustment problems should be avoided.

Modified from Allen EA: West Indians. In Comas-Diaz L and Griffith EH, editors: Clinical guidelines in cross-cultural mental health, New York, 1988, John Wiley & Sons, Inc.

context in which they and their family function. Therapists encourage children to verbalize existing identity conflicts. Enunciations such as "It is confusing to you because at times you feel like a Cuban, and at other times you feel like an American," help children name the identity conflict and initiate the reintegration process. The following case example illustrates a child's "cultural reeducation for life."

Case Example

John, an 8-year-old boy with Oriental parents, came for therapy acting sullen, with band aids on his hands and scratches on his face. He gave the following account of his experience:

John was riding his new bicycle on the pavement in front of his home with his parents' permission when the bicycle tire caught a loose stone as he was crossing the neighbors' driveway. John was thrown onto the gravel — his elbow was painfully but not deeply bruised. While John sat on the grass adjacent to the drive to "stop crying" and "settle down," a man came out of the neighbors' house and walked toward his car, which was parked in the driveway. Seeing John, the man waved and called several times to "watch your bicycle"; John waved back to the man and did as advised. After several moments, the man suddenly seemed "mad," shouting and waving at John again to "watch your bicycle." John waved again, and while he sat and watched his bicycle, the man got "more angry" and shouted, "OK, kid, you asked for it." He got into his car and backed out, driving over John's bicycle, and went on his way down the highway.

John was shocked; now uncontrollably crying, he picked up his mangled bike and ran home to his mother. When John's father called the neighbor for clarification and found the man, the neighbors' friend noted that he had heard John was a "case," and his behavior that day seemed additional proof that the "kid needed help." Hearing that John had been rude and defiant, John's father punished him for disregarding and taunting an adult's request and for being a neighborhood troublemaker.

CULTURAL REORIENTATION

Children requiring assistance in cultural reorientation are frequently seen in multicultural health care settings, providing opportunities for primary prevention interventions. The outline shown in the box illustrates a process of cultural reorientation for clinicians to use with clients as part of the traditional psychotherapeutic interventions (Allen, 1988). It provides a guide for nurse clinicians beginning to develop cross-cultural counseling skills and for child psychiatric nurses consulting with community agencies in which conducting individual, sibling, and "life change groups" is a productive intervention.

CULTUROGENIC STRESS

Culture stress or shock is defined as an abrupt, disorganizing reaction resulting from exposure to a new culture. Culture or reality shock is familiar to most nurses from

---

Culturally Sensitive Child Psychotherapy

1. Cultural self-assessment and insight information: Clinicians help children identify the following:
   a. Areas of psychocultural confusion
   b. The relationship between evident features of history, social disintegration, and psychologic disorder
   c. Universalism and openness, that is, the extent to which their cultural cognition includes timeless values and represents an open system
2. Cultural reevaluation by reviewing cultural strengths: Clinicians help children discover and analyze the following:
   a. Positive survival strengths throughout their national history involving their ethnic group
   b. Daily individual social manifestations of coherence-producing values
   c. Cultural traits, such as humor, old world-new world contrasts, cosmopolitanism, hospitality, articulateness (oral traditions), high achievement motivation (social mobility), and strong interpersonal values (commonality)
   d. Common face-to-face indigenous support systems, for example, friending (Mintz, 1971) extended family tenement yards, religion, and friendly societies such as scouts, church activities, and after school sports
   e. Specific cultural folklore and arts
   f. Achievements of individuals and the region affecting the world
3. Cultural reevaluations by establishing criteria of adaptiveness of cultural values: Clinicians assist children in evaluating the role of cultural values in the following:
   a. Promoting physical, psychologic, and spiritual health
   b. Promoting human rights, self-esteem, and dignity
   c. Promoting universalism and openness
   d. Promoting social integration
4. Cultural goal settings: Clinicians help children set goals for achieving the following:
   a. Newly desired adaptive versus maladaptive cultural values and behaviors
   b. Internality versus externality

Modified from Dahl C: Some problems of cross-cultural psychotherapy with refugees seeking treatment, Am J Psychoanal 49:19, 1989.

---

the work of the nurse anthropologist Kramer, whose research related the concept to the experiences of recently graduated nurses when entering the hospital work setting and confronting the conflicting realities of the values mastered "idealistically" in preparatory programs and those encountered in the work place (Kramer and Schumalenberg, 1978).

Culture shock occurs when people adhere rigidly to old, familiar ways. Migration causes many additional traumas: not only are old cultural values in conflict with values in a new culture or setting, changes often include changing roles and loss of sources of support. Many children experience these reality shocks when they enter junior high school or move to a different community, for example, from a rural to an urban setting.

In some instances, cultural values protect people from culturogenic shock, and different cultural groups exposed to similar stress display different responses because of these value protections. For example, in cultures valuing extended family relationships, there is less stress in child rearing because family members help the new parents.

Engle (1968) has described a *giving up, given up complex* in which death was proceeded by the inability to cope. In cultures where females were subservient, overly protected, and highly dependent on males, the wife "gave up" after the death of her husband, and her death was highly likely within the next 2 years.

Sociocultural death has also been attributed to the culturogenic stress incurred by some diagnoses. Some cultures view certain physical disorders as "death labels," and once patients are assigned these labels, death becomes a self-fulfilling prophesy. Cultural beliefs are frequently given as explanations for the same clinical condition resulting in death for some people but not for others.

Posttraumatic stress disorder is also culturally influenced, dependent on ways in which different cultures deal with and express stress. Initially this diagnosis was limited to military personnel and refugees, especially those who had resettled following major traumas. Currently, this diagnosis has been expanded to include adults and children who have been victims of rape, incest, and severe accidents involving the death of others.

PSYCHOANALYTIC PSYCHOTHERAPY

Anthropologically oriented psychotherapists have emphasized that differences in culture affect the treatment of emotionally caused symptoms and disorders. Prince (1987) has commented extensively on the limits of verbal therapies and diagnostic labels, theorizing that only a small minority of clients benefit from verbal therapies:

Proposed reasons . . . a lack of psychologic mindedness; lack of interest in introspection; shame over acknowledging psychological difficulties; reluctance to speak of family problems beyond the confines of the family; and of course, the broad cultural notions about the causes of psychiatric disorders, which, except in the West, seldom include psychological causes, and particularly psychological causes dating back to childhood.

Experts in the analytic disciplines counter these claims with suggestions that negative opinions of psychotherapy are often based on personal views and experiences, not systematic research. Dahl (1989) suggests that differences in relating feelings to emotional conflicts in different cultures is not due to deep-seated developmentally based differences and character traits but to differences in expressive styles and codes of interpersonal conduct between cultures. Using therapy founded on psychoanalytic theory is advisable, but it does require alterations in therapeutic techniques and therapeutic relationships that are considered meaningful by clients. Role expectations and culture-specific communicative interactions are the central elements to be explored, and cultural empathy includes acceptance of clients' cultural self-image.

Regardless of culture, clinicians need to evaluate children's and their family's psychologic strengths and adaptations and monitor indicators of developmental progress and signs of stress. Understanding the parents' and children's world view and expectations, combined with clinicians' identification with their own body of professional knowledge, experience, and accountability, is essential in the provision of safe care.

CULTURALLY SENSITIVE NURSING PSYCHOTHERAPY: SOMATOPSYCHIC THERAPY

Somatopsychic therapy was designed specifically for work with Vietnamese and Philippine clients in the United States (Flaskerud, 1987). It has been successfully adapted and applied to children of other cultural groups, especially when somatization is a major symptom. The aim of this nursing psychotherapy is to provide therapy congruent with clients' beliefs about health and illness, deemphasizing the stigma associated with mental illness and reintegrating children into the family and social group.

The following factors in somatopsychic therapy have been adapted to the psychiatric nursing of children:

1. Therapists are clinical specialists with master's in child psychiatric nursing who share children's language and culture and are called nurse-counselors to avoid the stigma associated with mental disorders. They possess the physical and mental assessment skills and specific child intervention knowledge and experience needed to function as therapists. Their education is congruent with clients' expectations of health professionals.
2. Assessment of children includes psychiatric, functional, developmental, and physical areas, with attention given to those areas in which somatic complaints are focused. This attention legitimizes somatization as an appropriate means of expressing distress.
3. Pharmacotherapy specific to the client's diagnosis is prescribed and instructions are given by nurse-counselors to children and their family.
4. Brief family center therapy is the treatment approach, focusing on current problems and using situational or crisis-oriented family techniques. Families are told the probable length of treatment on the first visit, and the reason for referral is discussed and treated as the family's problem.
5. Therapy is active and directive and includes giving advice and guidance. Nurse therapists are viewed by the family as knowledgeable authorities, and the family is given special roles and is involved in the regime.
6. Therapy includes encouraging children to conform with family values and the family to forgive children's transgressions and accept them back into the family. The family is reassured that the problems are manageable and is given specific directions on managing behavior problems. Working with other social systems such as schools and teachers, helps the family develop a strong support network with others.
7. Referrals are made for social, economic, and legal problems that often accompany psychologic distress.
8. Families are asked about self-treatment measures and are encouraged to follow these customs. When folk remedies are incongruent with prescribed medications, clinicians and families seek alternatives that meet both value systems. Families are encouraged to continue consulting traditional healers.

NONSPECIFIC CULTURAL INTERVENTIONS

Before 1975, clinicians exclusively endorsed one theoretic perspective, but since then nonspecific interventions have become predominant. Research in adult therapies has repeatedly shown that all major schools and forms of therapy are equally effective. In child therapies, multimodal interventions have been traditional because of children's multiple lines of development, and several interventions may be used simultaneously. For example, a hyperactive 7-year-old boy whose family is of another culture experiencing relocation difficulties could be treated with medication, individual therapy (to assist with low impulse control and enhance ethnoidentity), group therapy (to enhance interpersonal skills), and parent and sibling sessions (to direct and air parental ethnocentric adaptation conflicts and to cope with the demands of "two worlds"). A bilingual clinician or tutor may assist children with language difficulties impeding school performance.

Cultural Dimensions of Verbal Communication

Studies show that the more people communicate, the more often they develop a language of their own. For example, many families develop a shorthand communication style evolving from shared past experiences and verbal discussions. This is especially true among mothers and young children who are just learning to speak. When adults invent words with unique, personal meanings, the word is *autistically* created and referred to as a *neologism*. Small children who invent words through poor enunciation when mastering language are not autistically creating words but are responding to reinforcement by the mother.

The special use of words has important implications for nurse clinicians, especially when the family is from another culture. Clinicians need to ask mothers about special words and terms their small child uses, the meaning of these words for the child, and ways in which mothers are moving their child toward conventional usage. Clinicians also need to ascertain whether the private mother-child language indicates difficulties in resolving the attachment process. Under normal circumstances, most parents encourage children to use words that have conventional meanings and recognize their need to master the language used by others in their expanding social world.

Studies indicate that people seldom use all the words available to them. Of the over 600,000 words in the English language, the average American adult uses about 500 in daily communication, and school-aged children use about half that many. However, the 500 most frequently used words have more than 14,000 possible definitions, explaining the reasons for adults and children who share the same culture and language frequently misunderstanding each other. Clinicians should use words that are commonly used with standard meanings, especially with clients who are bilingual or of other cultures.

Gender differences in the number of times words are spoken in an average day are also present. American adult men say about 500 words each day, and American women speak about 2500 words per day. The kinds of words men and women use also differ. Women use words describing feelings and thoughts, and men use more "action-oriented" words and phrases to avoid "talking like a sissy." The emotional language content differences may partially explain the excess of words women use because words describing emotions are less precise and thus require more talk to convey.

The theory of the anthropologists Whorf and Sapir (1956) posits that because language mediates thought and culture influences thinking, changing a person's language will change a person's thoughts. There is a static, unchanging nature in the grammar of different cultures, and people regard people and objects as unchanging. Although it has been found that people and languages do change, the Whorf-Sapir hypothesis led to the development of the subdiscipline of psycholinguistics and seminology, whose area of scientific focus is the use of symbols, language, and communication, theories emphasized in child psychiatric nursing. Because thoughts govern behavior, changing language will change behavior. A nonverbal anthropologic theory of special relevance to child psychiatric nursing is Walder's seminal theory of play (1990). He posits that emotions and their expression exist before the development of language and can be used therapeutically through symbolic actions such as play.

LANGUAGE BARRIERS

Language barriers within the structure of a culture's language perpetuate cultural and social norms and values. For example, the English language does not have words denoting both sexes, and *them* and *they* can refer to more than one member of the same sex or a combination of both sexes. The pronoun *he* generally refers to both sexes, reemphasizing a male-dominated English-speaking culture and affecting the ways women think, know, and problem solve (Belenky and others, 1986).

Clinicians should be aware that children and families whose language of origin includes both female and male pronouns are often confused by language differences and *he and she* transpositions such as *he/she* or *s/he*. References to males as *she* should not be interpreted as an identity crisis if children are using English as a second language. Clinicians should also be aware that parents who accept only parts of the new culture often conflict with their school-aged children who readily adapt to the new culture.

Changes in language are seldom assimilated immediately (or ever, in some cases) by all members of a group. People usually adhere to the most comfortable aspects of their culture while adjusting to the expectations of the larger culture, often without internal commitment, which weakens the group. For example, interprofessional disagreements over the meaning of the term *learning disabilities* were finally resolved by lay legislators.

The "new language of psychiatry" was introduced a decade ago with the publication of the DSM-III. Previously there was a lack of appropriate words in the English language to describe people with mental diseases. Traditional psychiatric words had negative, stigmatizing, labeling effects. The language of the DSM-III was specifically selected to initiate a "new way of talking" and thinking about mental disorders and to eliminate negative words such as *emotionally ill, emotionally handicapped, emotionally disturbed,* and *mentally ill,* words that "hearken back to the dark ages of psychiatry" (Levy, 1982).

BILINGUAL LANGUAGE BARRIERS

In the United States, English is not the primary language in the home of over 30 million people. Of these, 2.5 million are school-aged children, a number that is expected to double by the year 2000. In many states, including Arizona, California, Colorado, Florida, New Mexico, New York, and Texas, the rate is approaching 25%.

Research indicates that a second language does not interfere with the first language of origin. Development is guided by common principles across languages and are part of the human cognitive system. The rate of learning a second language is also highly related to the proficiency level of the first language. The two languages build on and expand a common underlying base and do not compete for the resources of cognition.

Snow (1987) has documented two different dimensions or task domains of language proficiency in bilingual children—contextual and decontextual—which function independently. The contextual language skill dimension refers to the use of language in face-to-face communication settings, and decontextualized language skills are those removed from contextual supports.

Recent research findings argue against earlier data showing bilingualism as harmful to children's cognitive development. Higher degrees of bilingualism are associated with higher levels of cognitive attainment, including such areas as cognitive flexibility, metalinguistics awareness, concept formation, and creativity. These findings were from studies conducted in settings in which a second language was an enrichment to the native language.

Adeptness in shifting from one language to another depends on the conversational situation and is called *code switching* by ethnographers. One function of code switching is to establish and regulate the social boundaries of the two worlds. Because language is social, some scientists believe that questions about language use are really questions about social contexts.

Clinical work with bilingual children is challenging and requires special supervision and an understanding of ways in which bilingual children think and express themselves symbolically. A linguistic mismatch between home and school does not account for children's school failure, and larger social and cultural issues embedded in the histories of different linguistic-minority groups need to be considered. The learning styles of different cultures that interact efficiently with instructional approaches need to be identified and modified when teaching about health and stress reduction techniques.

Studies have found that when different languages are used, more pathology is reported. This increase has been attributed to the lack of linguistic competence in children that impedes the flow of thought, misinterpreted by clinicians as cognitive slippage. Other mistaken interpretations include illogical, incoherent speech, diminished concrete thinking, and impoverishment of thought.

If possible, ethnocultural assessment should be conducted in children's native language because the stress of speaking in a less familiar idiom can accentuate discomfort, frustration, and misunderstanding by clinicians and children. If translators are required, clinicians need to be aware of possible problems and therapeutic impasses. Family members are not good as primary interpreters because their presence often inhibits the child's communication, and content may be changed to their own interpretation. Paralanguage is also required, and cross-cultural mental health practitioners need to be familiar with the work of experts in this area such as Paul Ekman (1982), who has demonstrated that nonverbal equivalents of many basic emotions are constant across a wide range of cultures.

Cultural Dimensions of Nonverbal Communication

According to Hall (1966), communication is approximately 10% words and 90% nonverbal, hidden cultural grammar, an "amalgamation of feelings, feedback, local wisdom, cultural rhythms, ways to avoid confrontation, and unconscious views of how the world works." Nonverbal communication refers to an actual attempt to communicate a message using an accepted code between the sender and receiver or encoder and decoder. In contrast, a nonverbal sign represents a behavior by which an observer infers meaning. All behaviors displayed other than speech content, such as tone of voice and pacing of speech, are considered nonverbal communications.

Most emotional states are conveyed nonverbally, and troubling emotions usually occur below people's conscious, cognitive level. Through denial, repression, and other defenses, people are often not "in touch" with their emotions, and the task of the nurse is to facilitate congruence and awareness between verbal and nonverbal communication.

Analysis of nonverbal communication is based on the assumption that individuals are constantly maneuvering to accommodate others and that nonverbal behaviors are culturally learned and analyzable. Much of the science and art of nursing relies on nurses identifying clients' problems using nonverbal cues.

Nonverbal communication is of special importance in assessment when psychiatric disorders are present. Children's skills needed to maintain social interaction processes are often lost and thus not identified, and clinicians need to determine whether children have developed age-appropriate social interaction skills, the age level at which these skills failed to develop, and whether change, developmental disability, or reversal to earlier states has occurred.

Children display these difficulties through idiosyncrasies in verbal and nonverbal communication styles. For example, children's conversation may be pressured or punctuated by long pauses, or children may seem distracted and muddled in verbal responses. There may be flat, unanimated speech, a monotone voice, a distracted manner, and a lack of "visual touching" during the conversation. Markers of speech such as hand gestures may be missing.

Unfortunately, there are inadequate terms to describe these kinds of nonverbal cues, and clinical practice opportunities and supervision are necessary for nurses to learn the application of nonverbal cues and interventions with children. Clinical learning is achieved through role models and draws on the imprecise science of *semiology,* a term from communication sciences referring to the diagnosis of diseases from symptoms (Ashcraft and Scheflen, 1976). Semiology addresses three broad questions: (1) How does the use of signs affect or influence perceptivity (pragmatics)? (2) What is the system of the code employed or the form of statements received by observers (syntactics)? and (3) How are signs interpreted to mean specific things or sets of things-ideas, events, or attitudes (semantics)?

Pragmatics includes ways in which the use of signs influence people's actions, thoughts, and feelings (Reusch and Bateson, 1951). Advertising is a highly developed example of pragmatics in our culture in that it commercially manipulates people's response to symbols. Pragmatics are culturally specific and include nonverbal appearances, vocal tones, facial expressions, eye contact, and body language.

Syntactics are the formats of senders' statements as perceived by receivers, and appearance or behaviors often confuse receivers' ability to ascribe meaning. For example, nurses coming to work in an intensive care unit dressed in blue jeans or children arriving for play therapy in their best clothes are syntactic statements that are in conflict of the purpose of the contextual encounter.

Semantics include three areas:
1. Icons: Signs implying meanings that cannot be taken at face value because the intended meaning, if any, and the inferred meaning may be very different
2. Indexical signs: Signs in which the index of an event can be inferred from signs that are caused by another event (for example, a bent fender implying that the damage resulted from an accident)
3. Symbolic signs: Symbols that help people infer meaning through arbitrary use of cultural convention and custom (for example, school lunch boxes and girl scout uniforms)

Speechless messages are sent by vocal, facial, and gesturings signals and are received through the sense organs. Although all senses are involved in nonverbal communication, visual perception has received the most emphasis and is frequently used interchangeably with the term *observation*. However, observation is the objective assessment of behavior, and nonverbal communication also includes sensing (detecting), identifying (differentiating), and cognitive interpreting:
1. Much nonverbal communication occurs outside the focus of attention and impinges subliminally on the observer.
2. Language does not have the descriptive terms to label, describe, and quantify forms of nonverbal behaviors.
3. Nonverbal communication modes are combined or "patterned" for receptive inferences.

The classification system of nonverbal behaviors developed by Ruesch and Kees (1972) has provided a basis for most work in the science of communication field and is frequently used in basic nursing texts. The system includes three categories:
1. Sign language: Gestures and conveying signals
2. Action language: Walking, body posture, and other acts with dual functions
3. Object language: Intentional and nonintentional displays of material objects

Another nonverbal classification system frequently used in clinical practice and in nonverbal communication research was developed by Ekman and Friesen (1969, 1974; Ekman and others, 1987) and is based on the origin, circumstances of usage, and interpersonal significance of nonverbal behavior. This system has five generic classes of nonverbal behavior: emblems, illustrators, affect displays, regulators, and adaptors. In contrast, Mehrabian's system (1972) uses a three-dimensional framework of nonverbal communication that includes evaluation, potency, and responsiveness. A recent system identifies the dimensions of cultural variation applicable to the study of nonverbal communication of emotion as power distance, uncertainty, avoidance, individualism, and masculinity.

As these frameworks indicate, the science of communication is an evolving field, and classification systems vary widely, with no agreement on a theoretic model or classification system that covers all aspects of nonverbal communication.

PROXEMICS

Proxemics are the "interrelated observations and theories of man's use of space as a specialized elaboration of culture" (Hall, 1966). The *body buffer zone* or *personal space* refers to the area surrounding people that moves with them from place to place, and *territoriality* is the drive to defend and hold exclusive right to property or abstract domain.

Personal space is related to feelings and emotions and varies according to situations: the more intense the feelings, the more limited the perceptual field and people's life space. Hall (1966) identified four spatial interaction zones:

1. Intimate zone or zone of physical contact: This area's boundary is 18 inches from the body. Olfactory and thermal experiences are transmitted at this level, and touching predominates. This zone is usually reserved for lovers and children. Invasion of the intimate zone occurs when people are crowded on an elevator or in public transportation. Most Americans dislike being "packed" and respond with immobile, rigid bodies and eyes. Most nurses have observed this same response when attempting to comfort or provide physical care to children with whom they have not established rapport.
2. Personal zone: This area is between 18 inches and 4 feet from the body and is the "bubble" people keep between themselves and others. Personal distance is usually maintained in nurse-patient interactions.
3. Social distance: This area is approximately 4 to 12 feet from the body and is the business or professional distance. Although touch and body contact are insignificant at this distance, eyes and voices take on a critical importance.
4. Public distance: An area of 12 to 25 feet from the body, this distance is for formal occasions, separating public figures from the public. Visual and auditory channels predominate.

The intimate zone is of special importance in child psychiatry, especially when children perform self-intimacy behaviors to provide comfort. These behaviors are unconsciously mimed acts of being touched or held by someone else (Morris, 1977). Autocontact behaviors include self-touching, self-intimacies (holding their hand and sitting with their hand on their chin), and self-stimulation behaviors (sucking their fingers, rocking, banging their head, and other repetitive acts). These behaviors are viewed as indications that children are pained or anxious and are a method to reduce tensions.

In the management of child inpatient milieus, clinicians should note children's interpersonal movements and distancing as they affect their emotional stability. Claustrophobic, panic, and anxiety attacks by potentially acting-out children may be prevented by anticipatory proxemic interventions. Acting out may be triggered by spatial confinement because crowding in small areas stimulates perceptions of the threat of depersonalization when weak ego boundaries are a problem. Anticipatory interventions include monitoring children's stress levels with traffic flow, providing wide body buffer zones, identifying children's specific trigger factors, and estimating distances various children require to not feel pressured.

KINESICS

Kinesics include the ways people use body parts to communicate and include: (1) eye behaviors such as blinking and gaze direction, (2) pupil changes, (3) facial expressions, and (4) posture, positions, and movements. Birdwhistell, an anthropologist and pioneer in kinesic analysis, spent 25 years developing a kinesic notation system in which hundreds of elements of behavior were identified using slow motion film analysis (1970). Birdwhistell's conceptual system of classifying body movements and positions has become generally accepted body language reading content and includes the following interpretations: (1) extended, loose limbs convey relaxed, open states, (2) contracted, restricted, "close to the body" limb positions convey fear, anxiety, and self-protection, (3) a slumped posture with sagging muscles conveys being burdened with the "weight of the world" or the need to "get something off the chest," and (4) a stiff-backed, upright posture conveys strict propriety. Current American usage of the word *posture* also refers to a position taken toward an abstract concept.

The kinesic scientist Paul Ekman used Birdwhistell's slow motion film technique to analyze communication encounters and found that speakers and listeners perform a *conversation dance* with elaborate feedback in conversation concert. The listener indicates synchrony (agreement) by moving in harmony or demonstrates disharmony, which he termed *interactional synchrony,* the coordinated *in tune* or *out of tune* kinesic movements and adjustments exchanged between persons in verbal and nonverbal interactions (Ekman, 1982). Ekman also found that while synchronous movements may be directed by speech, the coordinating movements of social interaction can be done without eye contact or words.

Studies of nonverbal behavior of infants indicate that kinesic synchrony is first learned during mother-child interactions and that normal infants have highly developed nonverbal communication repertoires forming the essential foundations for speech development (Condon, 1973). These findings provide the rationale for early infant stimulation programs for children with congenital and cognitive deficits. Kinesthetic and verbal communication protocols stressing early interactional synchrony between infants and parents enhance children's later verbal learning. *Benjamin,* a commercially available film, is useful in teaching these techniques because it illustrates infants' nonverbal mirroring and the influences of parents' body positioning on the preverbal child (Condon and Ogstoon, 1976). It has been postulated that faulty parent relationships during infancy result in kinesic disruptions and partially explain the "bizarre" unsynchronized behavior patterns evolving autistically.

Kinesic synchrony provides compatible, productive interactions and preliminary opportunities for getting in tune with the client. Empathic synchrony can be established by the nurse consciously mirroring clients' kinesic gestures and body language.

Children's use of symbolic behavior and nonverbal or limited verbal communication is highly pertinent to clinicians. The use of videotapes is a highly effective and efficient way of teaching and learning child psychiatric nursing and also enhances self-awareness and self-monitoring in clients.

PARALINGUISTICS

Paralanguage refers to the context of communication in contrast to the content. Voices convey the state of an interpersonal interaction: repetitions, slurs, stuttering, hesitations, and silences are all paralinguistic indications of affects. Paralanguage is of special importance when working with children learning to speak, and research shows first approximations of words are molded and structured by significant others (Goldman-Eisler, 1968).

Chronemics is a form of paralanguage referring to the nonverbal use of time, for example, who waits for whom and for how long. People who talk the most view themselves as the most important person in the interaction. Silences can indicate boredom or be attention getting. Time pauses can mark the conclusion of a topic or punctuate an important message such as "Listen for the following important announcement."

Cross-cultural differences affect paralanguage expressions. Sue and Sue (1977) noted that variations in paralanguages can interfere with the assessment process when clinicians work with children outside their culture. Silences are frequently interpreted as moments when clients, for conscious or unconscious reasons, are holding back. These moments, however, may also signal that clients are ready for a new question:

Although silence may be viewed negatively by Americans, other cultures interpret and use silence much differently. English and Arabs use silence for privacy, whereas Russians, French, and Spanish read it as agreement among parties. In Asian culture, silence is traditionally a sign of respect for elders. Furthermore, silence by many Chinese and Japanese is not a floor yielding signal inviting others to pick up the conversation, rather it indicates a desire to continue speaking after making a particular point. Often silence is a sign of politeness and respect rather than lack of desire to continue speaking. Clinicians uncomfortable with silence may fill in and prevent the client from elaborating further. An even greater danger is to impute false motive to the client's apparent reticence (Sue and Sue, 1977).

Timing is another form of paralanguage that is usually attributed to natural impingements beyond people's control. *Poor timing* is a rationalization for out of sequence errors. Timing also refers to taking turns while talking, for example, talking at the same time creates embarrassment generally viewed as a social error.

EYE BEHAVIORS

Oculesics are characterized by traditional language attributing mystery and power to eyes through expressions such as *windows to the soul* and the *evil eye*. The *mind's eye* is linked to verbal recall, and the commonly used *I see* means *I understand*. Freudian insight differs from the third eye insight, which is earned by adhering to certain Eastern religious practices.

Eye contact is used to show attention, but when people are engaged in abstract thought, the gaze is often directed elsewhere (Reismer, 1949). Americans interpret eye contact as a sign of mental health: the averted shifty gaze and the inability to look someone in the eye are signs of dishonesty. In comparison to other cultures, higher status Americans get more visual attention than they give (Exline, 1972).

Many cultural differences are related to eye contact. For example, Blacks often do not consider eye contact important in conveying attention to listener; just being in the room may be enough to convey attention. Direct eye contact is considered disrespectful in certain cultures such as Mexican-American and Japanese. Clinicians should not misinterpret poor eye contact as an indication of rudeness, boredom, lack of assertiveness, or poor blending.

Developmental psychologists have extensively studied mother-infant eye contact as a major aspect of evolving emotional interaction in dyads, and mutual mother-infant gaze behavior has been viewed as the initial force forming preverbal affective ties, providing insights into preverbal relatedness (Morris, 1977). Visual recognition by young children has also been studied extensively. Mothers' or caretakers' face and eyes reflect praise, indifference, or displeasure at the sight of their child, and children respond to this visual facial expressiveness. Most experts agree that eye-to-eye contact is a precondition to smiling.

By 2 months of age, infants smile when there is social eye-to-eye contact, and by 3 months, infants look soberly and searchingly at unfamiliar faces as if they notice a difference. At 6 to 8 months, infants cry, withdraw, and show wariness, thus displaying visual awareness of unfamiliar faces or *stranger anxiety*. This response is usually alleviated when mothers touch and hold their children. Stranger anxiety decreases as children have more contacts with adults and learn that others will respond positively and comfortingly toward them.

Infants and small children show high sensitivity to visual stimuli (Mahler, 1975), and by the age of 6 months, infants can distinguish between faces but not facial expressions. The visual cognitive skills required to distinguish between smiling approval and frowning in anger unfold between 12 and 18 months of age.

Infants' ability to read their mother's face coincides with their locomotion. Infants respond to their mother's facial and eye responsiveness and messages, which restricts roaming toddlers. Thus, eye contact and facial expressions are first used as educational protective and socialization tools.

Visual prohibition has a more disturbing effect on the infants than verbal prohibition. When mothers withdraw eye contact from their infant, the infant is left frightened and bewildered in a world depleted of the lifegiving force of the mother's eye and emotional availability. Early intensity on eye contact is superseded by verbal communication, but prohibitive glances continue throughout childhood.

Children may show averting glances during therapy with the nurse clinician. For some children, to look directly at clinicians is the same as looking at their mother's eye, which would create more anxiety. An averted glance avoids memories of their mother's facial threats and is a defense with an isolating effect.

Visual trauma experienced by children in the relationship with their mother may later present as academic difficulties because of children's need to look elsewhere for confirmation (Riess, 1987). Morris (1977) has developed terms to describe *visual cutoffs* frequently encountered in therapeutic relationships that stem from early infant contacts:

1. Evasive eyes: Clients shun eye contact by looking distractedly across their shoulder or at the floor.
2. Shifty eyes: Clients glance away and back.
3. Stuttering eye: Clients' eye lids waver as if they were swatting away another's glance.
4. Stammering eye: Clients shut their eyes with an exaggerated blink.

Pupillometric effects include pupil changes from autonomic nervous system responses, such as dilation of pupils when pleased (wide-eyed) and constriction of the pupils when disturbed (narrow or angry eyes). In contrast to other nonverbal communication signs, these responses are unconscious.

FACIAL EXPRESSIONS

Facial expressions are the most commonly used index of nonverbal communication and are the most unreliable and culturally different. Because physiognomic structures vary, a face is a recognized individual characteristic, as unique as fingerprints. People distrust their facial control and will not show their face to prevent emotions from being unwittingly conveyed. Freud (1904) stated that facial expressions, slips of speech, omissions, blushing, and symptomatic responses reflect unconscious conflicts between the ego and superego.

Blushing or turning white happens only when face and body surfaces are exposed to observing eyes. Blushing occurs below the level of awareness, and the body message sent is that the blusher is having psychic discomfort.

Discrepancies between verbal statements and nonverbal blushing may cause anger in receivers, who may perceive that the sender is trying to deceive them. When discrepancies between verbal and nonverbal messages occur, credence is given to the nonverbal signal.

ORGANISMICS

Organismic characteristics refer to appearances and physical traits such as sex, race, age, and personal attractiveness. Impressions conveyed organismically often overwhelm simultaneous verbal messages. Human rights movements protest discrimination on organismic grounds.

In contrast, adornments refer to conscious efforts to alter or enhance the physical image through cosmetics, jewelry, and clothing. Self-presentations convey moods by style and color selections, reflect the aspired image of the wearer, and have status-signaling functions. The blurring of masculine-feminine adornments is confusing to older Americans and immigrants who have traditionally relied on adornment for nonverbal indices of sex-role status.

Objectics are personal belongings used as extensions or expressions of the self-image. Coffee cups, briefcases, motorcycles, home furnishings, sports cars, and designer clothes convey people's selection, choice, and emotional investment in objects. Clinicians should avoid reacting with nonverbal communication to elements in clients' house and home life that are different or new to them. Their response may be perceived as negative by the family, straining the therapist-family relationship (Dodds, 1985).

HAPTICS

Touch is the most basic form of human interaction. The self-system has its roots in parental handling, which fosters feelings of acceptance and recognition. Instinctual bonds of attachment are formed through sight, sound, and touch, the essential framework for later ego separation and individuation (Rubin, 1989), and infant studies suggest that early tactile experiences determine later intellectual and emotional development.

Although maternal bonding weakens as children mature, mothers need to be available as a tactile safety reinforcer. Long after ego boundaries are defined, children regressively run to their mother to "kiss away" a cut or bruise or hold them close to take away the pain of hurt feelings or anxiety.

Touching is especially important in child psychiatric nursing. Some therapies of the Human Potential Movement are based on the premise that in becoming adults, many people deny this important avenue of communicating warmth and affection in interpersonal and sexual relationships. Embraces, tightly squeezing another's hand, reassuring pats on the back, and jovially pushing others nonverbally communicate feelings through body contact.

The deliberate and judicious use of touch is part of the art of nursing. Clients sometimes regress to acting like sick, frightened children when they experience pain and anxiety. For some clients the fear of losing their independence and separate identity is terrifying, stirring sentiments of past ties and dependencies. In these cases, nurses' use of touch is counterproductive to clients' self-actualizing defenses. By demonstrating courtesy and respect and conveying that they are emotionally able strangers, clinicians can initiate the professional closeness inherent in a nurse-client relationship. Nursing actions should sustain clients in their efforts to maintain ego differentiation or should communicate support. For child psychiatric nursing, clinicians should be sensitive to children's initial pattern and responses to strangers and adjust their behavior, reactions, and touching accordingly.

Nonverbal Communication in Therapy

The following list summarizes suggestions from Dodds (1985), Ginott (1964), Barker (1990), Boyle and Andrews (1989), and Jones (1972) for using nonverbal and paralanguage communication therapeutically when working with children of other cultures:

1. Tone of voice: Clinicians should avoid assuming a condescending or distinctive tone of voice. Using a childish tone when talking to children is also counterproductive. Clinicians should slow their speech rate, and if children give no response to a question or comment, they should rephrase or try the question later. Avoiding insistent "answer me" attitudes is also important.

2. Displacement activities: Clinicians' displacement behaviors may distract children. Children's displacement actions may increase therapists' anxiety and be interpreted as signs of being hyperattentive to the environment. To alleviate initial conversation blocks, clinicians should give children a pad to doodle on while talking with them.

3. Note taking: This displacement activity is distracting to children and should be limited. Children are more responsive if direct interest is shown in them, and explaining the need for note taking while providing them with an alternate activity is productive for children of 9 or 10 years of age.

4. Spatial interaction: Clinicians should mirror children's nonverbal actions and posture, provide an introductory period and a sufficient body buffer zone area, and reduce differences in size when possible.

5. Anger: Clinicians need to learn signals of submission and signs of poor impulse control in children to avoid temper tantrums. Recognizing cultural and individual differences in expressing frustration and aggression is also important. Clinicians should avoid speaking loudly or authoritatively and should decrease eye contact. If children are working toward regaining their self-control, clinicians should avert their gaze and not touch them.

6. Self-awareness: Clinicians should avoid direct confrontation seating arrangements and watch for signs of being too physically close. The desk should not be between clinicians and their client, and signs of acknowledgement, encouragement, understanding, and agreement should be provided. Clinicians need to be aware of their natural preverbal style. Videotaping sessions regularly will raise clinicians' consciousness.

7. Touching: Clinicians should not touch children without their permission. Shaking hands with children helps to break initial tensions, especially with boys.

Spirituality in Children

Margaret Burkhardt

Spirituality has received little attention in transcultural nursing, perhaps because it is the least understood area with no clear and consistent definition (Burkhardt, 1989). The literature indicates that spirituality is an essential factor in a people's health and well-being, and it has been described as the vital principle and unifying force integrating all manifestations of people. Spirituality is individual, experienced and expressed by each person in a unique way. Expressions of spirituality are influenced by culture, experiences within the family and with others, experiences within organized religious structures, and self-experiences.

SPIRITUALITY AND RELIGION

Until recently, discussions of spirituality in nursing texts and much of the nursing literature have focused primarily on religion and religious practices and beliefs, particularly reflecting a Western Judeo-Christian orientation (Miller, 1985; Reed, 1987). It is important to recognize that although religion often relates to the expression and experience of spirituality, spirituality is more inclusive than religious beliefs and practices. Religion refers to an organized system of beliefs and experiences addressing fundamental problems of existence and usually includes worship and prescribed rituals. Religion involves the conceptualization of spiritual experiences by forming them into a system, and it is a "social institution in which a group of people participate rather than an individual search for meaning" (Steiger and Lipson, 1985). Religious development may include spiritual awakening or may remain external and symbolic. Religion may enhance or inhibit healthy development.

CHARACTERISTICS AND EXPRESSIONS OF SPIRITUALITY

Spirituality refers to the life principle that pervades and animates a person (Dombeck and Karl, 1987). Green (1986) describes it as "the information nexus which binds things and people and the world together and informs a thing of its nature and context." Through spirituality, people can experience transcendence — a moving beyond their usual limits — and understand and experience their existence in direct and personal ways.

Common characteristics of spirituality noted in nursing and health-related literature include a unifying force within persons, a source for discovering and struggling with meaning and purpose in life, relatedness to and connectedness or bonding with all of life (including self, others, nature, and often God or Universal Force), a sense of peace and harmony with the universe, awareness, consciousness, sense of self, and inner strength.

SPIRITUALITY AND MORALS

Morals relate to individual perceptions of right and wrong actions or behaviors, and ethics refer to codes that govern the implementation of morals. Morals can also be related to religious and humanistic teachings and beliefs. These perceptions are influenced by people's experience in family and society. Kohlberg's research (1971) indicates that moral judgments are also influenced by cognitive factors such as the ability to reason, types of knowledge, and experiences with problem solving. Spirituality cannot be addressed solely through morals because the presence of spirituality is not dependent on people's level of cognitive development. Similar to other expressions of spirituality, moral development can vary depending on age, abilities, and experiences.

SPIRITUALITY AND VALUES

Values are common beliefs shared by members of a group or society. They may be learned through formal and conscious teaching or through informal role modeling. Values that are highly esteemed, such as love, trust, forgiveness, and hope, hold a central place in the teachings of the major world religions and in humanistic writings.

Stoll (1989) notes that the supreme value for people can vary from a loving and trusting relationship with a personal God to science, money, or trust and hope in themselves. Clinebell (1984) suggests that individuals' development of creative images and values to use as guidelines reflects a spiritual need.

Love has been described as the core of spirituality and has been recognized throughout the ages as the essential healing agent. Depending on its application, love contributes to health or to illness. Highfield and Cason (1983) state that giving and receiving love is a spiritual need. Clinebell (1984) suggests that basic spiritual needs include enhancement of self-esteem, an awareness of being valued by God, and development of the higher self to the center of being.

FACTORS INFLUENCING SPIRITUALITY IN CHILDREN

Because spirituality is the essence of being from the beginning of life, it influences and is influenced by all aspects of development. Researchers have usually approached the subject from a developmental framework within the context of basic needs and developmental tasks as they relate to developing beliefs and concepts of God (Betz, 1981; Carson, 1989). These approaches can give insights into children's spirituality; however, most theories of development reflect a Western world view and values and may not apply to persons in all cultures.

Piaget's stages of cognitive development (1958, 1963) reflect the progression of abilities of thinking, perceiving, forming concepts, and abstraction. These abilities are needed for learning and understanding aspects of a belief system and relate to developing a sense of self and position.

Erikson's stages (1963) are traditionally used to describe the needs and developmental tasks of each age, which can be related to characteristics and expressions of spirituality during development. Fowler (1981) discusses faith in light of psychosocial development. He views it as a human universal that is more fundamental than religion or beliefs and is present in all people. Faith is an orientation involving a quest for meaning in life and relates to transcendence.

NURSING CONSIDERATIONS

Nurses need to be attentive to the spirituality of parents, from providing opportunities for bonding at birth to assessing the quality of parent-child interactions as children develop. Clinicians should examine patterns of touch, verbal interactions, and nonverbal communication and should provide information to parents or caregivers to encourage healthy development in all areas and to set realistic expectations. If children's pattern of development has been affected by limitations in abilities or does not meet the expectations of the parents, clinicians need to address the associated feelings of anger, guilt, or concerns about the parents' abilities.

Parents should maintain important connections in their lives and incorporate their child into meaningful patterns of relating. If a child is hospitalized, clinicians should arrange for the parents to be present and to share in the care as much as possible and provide continuity with important connections such as favorite toys, music, stories, and religious practices. Nurses need to consider the values, beliefs, and expressions of spirituality of the parents and child.

Nursing actions during the time of pregnancy and infancy include providing information to allay fears, supporting the parents in their questioning and searching, and helping them to connect with their sources of support. For toddlers, nurses should encourage parents to provide their child with experiences of connectedness and to be affirming while setting reasonable limits. Discussing normal development and behaviors assists parents in forming realistic expectations supportive of healthy self-concept development. Discipline focusing on distraction rather than punishment should be encouraged.

Children need support in appreciating awe and reverence for all creation, including themselves. They continue to need guidance in finding the meaning in each new experience and in giving expression to experiences of the numinous. Parents should make religious experiences enhance feelings of belonging, acceptance, and personal adequacy.

Some clinicians suggest that children sense a need for hearing their inner selves and that moments of silence can be helpful to them. Asking children to listen to or find the silence is different from not talking or merely being quiet. Silence expands their creativity, self-satisfaction, and concentration. Insights into children's spirituality can also be gained through play, drawings, discussion of dreams, and stories about their lives and family.

Early experiences and expressions of spirituality lay the groundwork for the questioning and reappraisal of self and life's purpose occurring throughout adolescence and young adulthood. Expressions may be internalized, altered, or discarded. Children's experiences of connectedness and belonging, of feeling valued and having a place in the world, and of comfort with the unknown and acceptance of self will influence expressions of spirituality in later years.

The following case example illustrates nurses' role as it relates to the spirituality of children and their parents.

Case Example

Connie is a 9-year-old girl who has just learned that she has cystic fibrosis. The disease was first diagnosed in Connie's 3-year-old sister Aileen, which led to the testing of the other four siblings.

During the initial meeting, the nurse finds that Connie is a quiet person with a gentle spirit—a contrast to Aileen. Helping Connie to express her feelings about herself, her family, and what is happening to them is an appropriate starting point. Because Connie is comfortable with silence, simply being with Connie is an important intervention. As Connie and the nurse become comfortable with each other, the nurse may ask, "I wonder how you feel about . . . ?" The question is asked without a demand for an answer but as a sharing of the nurse's wondering and willingness to listen at any time.

This family will be dealing with the issues of mystery and uncertainty as they face the acute and chronic aspects of cystic fibrosis. An important aspect of their support is their Roman Catholic faith. They are active participants in their parish and speak easily of God, hope, faith, and suffering. As the nurse listens to the way they use these words and what they mean to them, the nurse can apply them to be helpful and meaningful to this family.

Because the nurse encourages Connie to share her own story in the context of an on-going and supportive relationship, she can share her feelings about herself—her fears, hopes, and questions. The nurse begins to see ways in which Connie experiences herself in her relation to the illness, her place in the family and world, and her value as a unique person. The nurse may find that Connie is more comfortable with her situation than the clinician. Children are often intuitive and accept aspects of life that adults want to explain. Initial and continuing involvement with Connie and her family is directed to learning ways in which they view and experience themselves and others. The nurse's initial role is to simply be with them.

After continued contact, the nurse recognizes a sense of awe and reverence for life in Connie. Although she may be described as quiet, Connie is very much alive and involved. She describes each of her siblings with humor and love, telling stories about each of them with enjoyment. When asked about her illness she says simply, "Well, we don't know much about it — even the doctors don't. I know I won't ever get all well unless they find something new to help, but there are medicines that help." She seems matter-of-fact and thoughtful as she says this. The most difficult aspect for her is seeing how sick Aileen is sometimes, requiring hospitalization, an oxygen tent, intensive antibiotic therapy that includes shots at home, and painful respiratory treatments. Initially Connie does not compare her own treatments with Aileen's or articulate a connection between what is happening to Aileen and what may happen to her in the future.

By encouraging Connie to talk about the significant relationships in her life, the nurse helps Connie to feel those relationships and connections that anchor her and to recognize her effect on others. Connie experiences a part of who she is — an important member of this family unit. While listening, the nurse may remark to Connie about some special aspects of her relationships with others or may respond to something particularly humorous, touching, or outstanding.

The nurse's attention to and support of Connie's parents is a major role. Parents influence a child's response to any situation because the interpretations they give to events and situations color the child's understanding. Recognizing and pointing out the strength and wisdom of their parenting skills gives them an understanding of who they are in this situation. The nurse reinforces the positive parenting skills by noting the family member's nonverbal support of each other and acknowledging the energy and strength they demonstrate in encouraging the other siblings' activities and interests. The nurse shares with the parents the observation that the caring of the children for each other reflects the caring and teaching of their parents. As these observations are articulated, the parents see themselves in new ways and experience affirmation of themselves in a difficult situation.

The parents share their feelings of puzzlement and pain with the children and the nurse. They acknowledge that they also wonder why this is happening but that much about life is mysterious. The nurse helps the parents identify and use their support system, including family, friends, and professionals.

More specifically, the parents are encouraged to strengthen those connections that give them support. They are urged to ask questions when they need more information from health care professionals. The importance of letting people who love them help is noted. When the parents seek advice, the nurse listens to their perceptions and understandings, recognizing that affirming their ability to deal with the situation is an important part of helping them experience themselves as valuable.

The nurse assists the parents in developing each child's potential. The nurse listens as members of the family express their questions of purpose and meaning. Connie's fraternal twin may wonder why this did not happen to her and feel guilty that she is well. The oldest child may feel responsible for other aspects of the situation, and the 18-month-old child may sense the stress in the family and respond behaviorally. Each person may ask, "Why is this happening? Is someone to blame? How can I help? What help do I need? Who or what can I trust?" Providing spiritual care often consists of the nurse's intentional presence with persons as they express and explore the meaning of a situation for themselves. In this process people more clearly recognize who they are and value their unique response and experience in the situation.

When the mother hugs Connie and says, "You know, you've helped me understand so much and I can be a better mom for Aileen because of you," Connie's picture of herself is deepened and broadened. When the nurse says to the parents, "Even with all the tough treatments and things to do, you guys never seem to lose track of each of your kids . . . and you seem to understand what this is like for each of them," it adds to their appreciation of themselves and affirms who they are as parents. When the mother listens quietly to Connie as she talks about where she would like to be buried one day, she offers herself in a relationship allowing her daughter to explore some of the mystery and pain of loss associated with this illness without offering false hope or premature reassurance. When the family participates in the activities of the other children in school projects and church bazaars, they affirm that life is bigger than cystic fibrosis. The nurse facilitates the family's connections with others, encourages and affirms their expression of feelings and concerns, and enhances their experiencing of themselves as active participants and valuable individuals.

REFERENCES

Adler PS: The transitional experience: an alternative view of culture shock, J Human Psychol 15:13, 1975.

Allen EA: West Indians. In Comas-Diaz L and Griffith EH, editors: Clinical guidelines in cross-cultural mental health, New York, 1988, John Wiley & Sons, Inc.

Ashcraft N and Scheflen AG: People space: the making and breaking of human boundaries, New York, 1976, Doubleday-Anchor Press.

Belenky MF and others: Women's ways of knowing, New York, 1986, Basic Books, Inc, Publishers.

Betz CL: Faith development in children, Pediatr Nurs 7:22, 1981.

Boyle JS and Andrews MM: Transcultural concepts in nursing care, Glenview, Ill, 1989, Scott Foresman & Co.

Burkhardt MA: Spirituality: an analysis of the concept, Holistic Nurs Pract 3:69, 1989.

Capra F: The turning point, New York, 1982, Bantom Books.

Carson VB: Spiritual dimensions of nursing practice, Philadelphia, 1989, WB Saunders & Co.

Clinebell H: Basic types of pastoral care and counseling: resources for the ministry of healing and growth, Nashville, 1984, Abingdon Press.

Cole M and Bruner JS: Cultural differences and inferences about psychological processes, Am Psychol 26:876, 1971.

Condon WS: Movement of awake-active neonates demonstrated to synchronize with adult speech. Paper presented at the meeting of the Society for Research on Child Development, Philadelphia, March 1973.

Condon, WS and Ogstoon WD: Sound film analysis of normal and pathological behavior patterns, Cambridge, Mass, 1976, Cambridge University Press.

Dahl C: Some problems of cross-cultural psychotherapy with refugees seeking treatment, Am J Psychoanal 49:19, 1989.

Dodds JB: A child psychotherapy primer, New York, 1985, Human Sciences Press, Inc.

Dombeck M and Karl J: Spiritual issues in mental health, Journal of Religion and Health 26:183, 1987.

Ekman P: Emotions in the human face, New York, 1982, Cambridge University Press.

Ekman P and Friesen WV: The repertoire of nonverbal behavior: categories, origins, usage and coding, Semiotica 1:49, 1969.

Ekman P and others: Universals and cultural differences in the judgments of facial expressions of emotion, J Pers Soc Psychol 53:712, 1987.

Engle JG: A life setting conducive to illness: the giving up-given up complex, Ann Intern Med 69:293, 1968.

Erikson EH: Childhood and society, ed 2, New York, 1963, WW Norton & Co, Inc.

Fields S: Mental health and the melting pot, Innovations 6:2, 1979.

Flaskerud JH: A proposed protocol for culturally relevant nursing psychotherapy, Clin Nurse Spec 1:150, 1987.

Fowler JW: Stages of faith, New York, 1981, Harper & Row, Publishers, Inc.

Freud S: The psychopathology of everyday life, New York, 1904, WW Norton & Co, Inc.

Ginott HG: The theory and practice of "therapeutic intervention" in child treatment. In Haworth MR, editor: Child psychotherapy, New York, 1964, Basic Books, Inc, Publisher.

Goldman-Eisler F: Psycholinguistics: experiments in spontaneous speech, New York, 1968, Academic Press, Inc.

Green R: Healing and spirituality, The Practitioner 1422:1087, 1986.

Hall ET: The hidden dimension, New York, 1966, Doubleday & Co.

Hautman MA: Folk health and illness beliefs, Nurse Practitioner 4:23, 1979.

Helman C: Culture, health and illness, Bristol, UK, 1984, Wright & Sons, Ltd.

Highfield MF and Cason C: Spiritual needs of patients: are they recognized? Cancer Nurs 6:187, 1983.

Jacobsen FM: Ethnocultural assessment. In Comas-Diaz L and Griffith EEH, editors: Clinical guidelines in cross-cultural mental health, New York, 1988, John Wiley & Sons, Inc.

Jones NGB: Non-verbal communication in children. In Hinde RA, editor: Non-verbal communication, London, 1972, Cambridge University Press.

Kohlberg L: Recent research in moral development, New York, 1971, Holt, Rinehart & Winston, Inc.

Kramer M and Schumalenberg C: Bicultural training and new graduate role transformation, Wakefield, Mass, 1978, Nursing Resources.

Levy R: The new language of psychiatry, Boston, 1982, Little, Brown & Co, Inc.

Lin KM and Finder E: Neuroleptic dosage for Asians, Am J Psychiatry 140:490, 1983.

Mahler MS: The psychological birth of the human infant: separation and individuation, New York, 1975, Basic Books, Inc, Publishers.

Mehrabian A: Nonverbal communication, Chicago, 1972, Aldine/Atherton.

Miller JF: Assessment of loneliness and spiritual well-being in chronically ill and healthy adults, J Prof Nurs 1:79, 1985.

Mollica R and Redlich F: Equity and changing patient characteristics: 1950–1975, Arch Gen Psychiatry 37:1257, 1980.

Morris D: Manwatching: a field guide to human behavior, New York, 1977, Harry N Abrams, Inc.

Pedersen PB, Lonner WJ, and Draguns JG, editors: Counseling across cultures, Honolulu, 1981, University of Hawaii Press.

Pfiffeling JH: A cultural prescription for medico centricism. In Eisenberg L and Kleinman A, editors: Relevance of social science for medicine, Dordrecht, 1980, Reidel.

Piaget J: The growth of logical thinking from childhood to adolescence, New York, 1958, Basic Books, Inc, Publisher.

Piaget J: The origins of intelligence in children, New York, 1963, WW Norton & Co, Inc.

Prince R: Alexithymia and verbal psychotherapies in cultural context, Transcultural Psychiatry Review 24:107, 1987.

Reed PG: Spirituality and well-being in terminally ill hospitalized adults, Res Nurs Health 10:335, 1987.

Reid WH and Wise MG: DSM-III-R training guide, New York, 1989, Brunner/Mazel, Inc.

Reismer MD: The averted gaze, Psychoanal Q 23:108, 1949.

Reusch J and Bateson G: Communication, the social matrix, New York, 1951, WW Norton & Co, Inc.

Riess AS: The mothers eye, Psychoanal Study Child 33:29, 1987.

Rogers ME: An introduction to the theoretical basis of nursing, Philadelphia, 1970, FA Davis Co.

Rubin N: Family rituals, Parents Magazine, p 105, Mar 1989.

Ruesch J and Kees W: Nonvervbal communication, Berkely, Calif, 1972, University of California Press.

Shea SC: Psychiatric interviewing: the art of understanding, Philadelphia, 1988, WB Saunders Co.

Steiger N and Lipson J: Self-care nursing: theory and practice, Bowie, Md, 1985, Brady Communications.

Stoll RI: The essence of spirituality. In Carson VB, editor: Spiritual dimensions of nursing practice, Philadelphia, 1989, WB Saunders Co.

Sue DW and Sue D: Barrier to effective cross-cultural counseling, J Counseling Psychology 24:420, 1977.

Sue S and Morishima JK: The mental health of Asian Americans, San Francisco, 1982, Jossey-Bass, Inc, Publishers.

Taft R: Statement on ethics, July 29, 1978, International Association for Cross-Cultural Psychology.

Torrey EF: The case for the indigenous therapist, Arch Gen Psychiatry 20:365, 1969.

Triandis H and Draguns J, editors: Handbook of cross-cultural psychology, Boston, 1980, Allyn & Bacon, Inc.

Tseng WS and McDermott JF: Culture, mind and therapy: an introduction to cultural psychiatry, New York, 1981, Brunner/Mazel, Inc.

Weidman H: Concepts as strategies for change, Psychiatr Ann 5:17, 1975.

Whorf BL: Language, thought and reality. In Carroll JB, editor: Selected readings of Benjamin Lee Whorf, New York, 1956, John Wiley & Sons, Inc.

Part II

Intellectual, Developmental, and Behavior Disorders

Chapter 7

Infant Psychiatry and Mental Health

Megan McKee

One may say that instincts are transmitted through genes, and values are transmitted through traditions, but that meanings, being unique, are a matter of personal discovery.

VICTOR FRANKL

Many professionals recognize the developmental challenges and environmental dependencies of infants and are conducting research, developing assessment tools, and building models and frameworks to guide assessment, diagnosis, and intervention. Infant psychiatry is dominated by the medical model and classification system, but current thought emphasizes the importance of a multidisciplinary approach, which includes nurse clinicians. This chapter presents some recent theories and familiarizes child psychiatric nurses with this emerging field.

Greenspan (1989) prefers the term *infant mental health* to *infant psychiatry* and stresses the multidisciplinary approach. Fraiberg, Adelson, and Shapiro (1975) advocate the development of a clinical subspeciality in infant mental health for all professionals who serve babies and their parents, including psychiatrists, pediatricians, pediatric and psychiatric nurses, psychologists, and social workers.

Origins of Infant Psychiatry and Infant Mental Health

Social and cultural attitudes toward infants have changed throughout time, influencing parents' and professionals' treatment of children (see box). However, parents have long demonstrated their interest in understanding their infants and in learning ways to care for them. The more recent concepts of bonding, failure to thrive, attachment, and separation and individuation are found in most child-rearing books read by the general public, providing additional impetus to parents' quest for information and clarification. The demand for infant psychiatric research and infant psychiatrists originated when parents requested help from professionals, who found a dearth of models for infant assessment and practice.

Social and Cultural Attitudes toward Infants

300 BC. In response to a corrupt society, Plato recommended that the state provide communal living in which children would have equal educational opportunities and would be molded into worthwhile citizens and leaders. Aristotle agreed with the concept of building an ideal society and a state-directed educational system but did not believe that the state should take over the responsibility of parenthood. He thought children should be educated and molded to suit the political system. Unlike Plato, Aristotle believed that individuality should be fostered and that the family unit composed society and was a better environment for enculturation than state communes. He agreed with Plato that children should have equal opportunities regardless of their social standing or gender (de Mause, 1974).

300 AD. From antiquity to 300 AD, infanticide was common. Infants were not perceived as humans with souls and were often viewed as a financial burden. Parents had minimal emotion involvement with their infants (de Mause, 1974).

1300 to 1600. Infants were considered wicked because of the doctrine of original sin. To counteract the "wickedness," parents used strict instruction and punishment.

1700 to 1800. A more liberal interpretation of original sin promoted the belief that children were innocent, and child care improved.

1800 to 1950. Children were valued but were expected to conform to rigid expectations. The adage "Children are to be seen and not heard" was consistent with that era. Child rearing became preplanned, fathers became involved in child rearing, and the emphasis was on self-control and satisfying strict expectations.

1950 to present. Children are viewed as unique individuals and encouraged to develop their potential—they are even considered to be wise. Parents guide and facilitate their childrens' development and do not insist that a specific mold be filled (de Mause, 1974).

PHILOSOPHIC AND THEORETIC CONTRIBUTIONS TO INFANT PSYCHIATRY

Scientists have studied the development of infants through childhood from different perspectives. The central question has always been whether children develop established personalities, ideas, and behaviors from an innate blueprint or from the affect of caregivers. In addressing this question, many philosophers and scientists have contributed elaborate explanations about the process of development and have given advice about child rearing (see box).

During the 1900s, behaviorism, humanistic psychology, psychoanalytic theory, learning theory, systems theory, and social learning theory were all being explored as explanations for human development. Binet developed an effective intelligence test, and institutes for the study of children's development were established. Freud described development focusing on psychosexual stages, levels of consciousness, and object relations, and Erikson addressed psychosocial stages and the importance of parental and peer relationships. Piaget identified the manner in which infants learn and ways in which the perception of cause and effect evolve as children grow older. He maintained that the inherited tendencies for children to organize experiences and

Contributors to Infant Psychiatry

Darwin. Darwin's theory of evolution introduced a shift in scientific study of human development. It appeared conclusive that if nature could be conquered through technology, human nature could be improved with the right tools. Using this assumption and the beliefs of philosopher Locke that children are born with a "blank slate" and that knowledge is acquired through experience, psychologists began searching for ways to mold personality (Biehler, 1981).

Pavlov. Pavlov described conditioning response in dogs, and psychologists believed that humans might respond in similar ways.

Watson. Drawing on Pavlov's conditioning technique, Watson established a theory of human development and proposed that the role of parents is to shape their children's behaviors by reinforcing positive behaviors and extinguishing negative behaviors. He introduced behaviorism and was one of the first scientists to study infants. Watson also contributed the experimental model in which individuals are exposed to a stimulus and the response is noted objectively. All judgments were based on observable data (Watson and Rayner, 1920). Results from scientists testing this line of study indicated that behavior conditioning was not based purely on observable causes, that behaviorism had limited application, and that other explanations of behavior and the order of infant development needed to be identified.

Gesell. Gesell promoted the concept that growth and behavior occur in sequential intervals at certain stages of maturation. This principle contradicted the earlier belief that infants are born without any direction. Gesell eventually developed assessment tools for children from birth through childhood to measure age-specific abilities (Ilg and Ames, 1955).

Continued

adapt to their environment resulted in self-directed, goal-oriented behavior. New experiences were understood within the context of the old, and as new information was gained, it was accommodated. He also proposed that children do not require staged learning experiences to use newly acquired abilities (Elkind, 1974).

Learning theorists identified the importance of guiding infant activities, especially learning. Their theories explained ways in which infants generalize responses from one situation to another. Social learning theory focused on the move from dependence to independence and the role of imitation in learning and proposed that different approaches to child rearing may influence personality.

From theory development and empirical research, three theoretic approaches became dominant: psychoanalysis, self-psychology, and ethology. Psychoanalytic theory emphasizes the importance of object relations and the process used by infants to develop relationships with others and themselves. It concentrates on the inner conflict of instinctual feelings. Self-psychology identifies two components of self: the grandiose self, which is modified through interactions with others and is responsible for individual ambition, and the idealized parent amago, which is the internalizing of parents' power and strength, contributing to self-actualization. Self-psychology recognizes the importance of the parents' interaction with their

Skinner. Demonstrating the possibility of operant conditioning, Skinner refocused the scientific community on the concept of free will versus conditioning. He did not ignore the inherited influences on behavior but asserted that because those influences could not be altered, it was more productive to focus exclusively on environmental experiences that could be arranged and changed. Skinner also contributed the concept and method of behavior modification (Skinner, 1948).

Bandura. Recognizing the importance of operant conditioning, Bandura (1974) proposed that "humans do not simply respond to stimuli; they interpret them." He claimed that humans were capable of judgment and could determine the outcome of their behavior by weighing several alternatives and choosing their response accordingly.

Rogers. A psychotherapist, Rogers did not believe that behavior was determined by societal conditioning. He felt that predetermination was an incomplete explanation and counterproductive in the mental health field (Rogers, 1963).

Maslow. Maslow (1968) supported humanistic psychology, which emphasized the significance of qualities such as thoughts, feelings, and attitudes. Maslow believed that children should be encouraged to develop in their unique way within a safe, nurturing, and stimulating environment. He also proposed a hierarchy of needs.

Lorenz. Lorenz developed *imprinting*, a term for the attachment that forms between a gosling and its mother. This concept was extrapolated to human infants. Findings indicated that early interaction between the mother and infant resulted in a stronger investment from the mother and that human infants do not have a critical period of attachment (Lorenz, 1970).

Harlow. Harlow (1958) tested the hypothesis that attachment is a learned response driven by receiving food from the mother. Baby monkeys were provided two inanimate substitute mothers. One was a cloth-covered figure, the other a wire-mesh form. The food was provided by the wire-mesh form. The baby monkeys only spent time with the wire-mesh figure while they were eating. The rest of the time they explored or clung to the cloth mother. When the babies were frightened, they ran to the cloth mother. This experiment discounted the belief that maternal-infant attachment is a conditioned response, showing that a comforting presence is more important.

infant, believing that poor interactions result in infant disorders. Ethology evolved from biologic research and is based on a stimulus response model, focusing on conditioned and learned responses.

MARASAMUS

The effects of maternal deprivation were an early infant psychiatric concern. While diagnosing and treating infants at Boston Children's Hospital, Ribble (1943) first identified the condition of *marasmus*. The diagnosis applied to infants with behavior disorders that were not traceable to organic causes. They were listless and unresponsive and refused to eat. The common factor was the lack of mothering (Biehler, 1981). Spitz (1965) concluded that early deprivation had an irreversible impact on infants.

As cultural attitudes toward children changed and public support for social reforms increased, treatment for children in institutions improved. Once the problem was identified, many international studies were conducted on infants separated from their mothers and institutionalized. Continued research in this area also showed that survivors from concentration camps overcame similar negative experiences (Freud and Dunn, 1951).

Ainsworth (1962) proposed that with the right support, infants can recover from interruption of attachment:

1. Infants seem capable of recovering from a single, brief separation experience but may become vulnerable to future threats of separation.
2. Even after children have a fairly prolonged deprivation experience in early infancy, provision of stimulation before they are 12 months old will often lead to rapid and dramatic improvements. Language development may lag behind intellectual and personality functioning.
3. Prolonged and severe deprivation that begins early and continues for as long as 3 years often results in severe retardation in intellectual, personality, and language functioning. The longer the deprivation experience, the greater the retardation and the poorer the prognosis for recovery.
4. Impairments in language and in the capacity for strong and lasting interpersonal relationships resulting from maternal deprivation are not easily reversed. Intensive therapeutic efforts early in life may be successful.

Developmental Structuralist Theory

Some problems seen in infancy requiring professional help included delayed development, aggressive disorganized behaviors and withdrawal, and apathy. Other difficulties that needed to be addressed were the pervasiveness of child abuse and neglect; the extent of infant and child sexual molestation; and the implications of abuse, inadequate parenting, and teenage pregnancy. Health care providers lacked the tools and framework to assess the needs and a mental health model that could be operationalized. As a result, the interactional model was replaced with a transactional model — the developmental structuralist theory. This theory draws on the hypotheses of cognitive, social, and physical development and describes them and emotional development in a sequential, integrated fashion. It provides parents and professionals with the tools to recognize and respond to infants' needs.

Developmental Structuralist Classification

Greenspan and Lourie (1981) developed a classification approach based on the developmental structuralist theory of infant mental health. Evolving from clinical experience and longitudinal studies, the system describes chronologic personality organization of experience and behavior in infancy and early childhood. Using the concept of adaptation, the framework guides assessment and intervention of infants who do not successfully adapt to their environment. The focus is on preventive intervention and considers developmental milestones of physical, cognitive, and affective pathways (Table 7-1). Greenspan and Lourie believed that

Table 7-1   Developmental Structural Delineation of Stage-Specific Capacities

Stage	Age	Illustrative adaptive capacities	Illustrative maladaptive (pathologic) capacities	Adaptive caregiver	Maladaptive caregiver
Homeostasis	0-3 months	Internal regulation (harmony) and balanced interest in the world	Unregulated (e.g., hyperexcitable) or withdrawn (apathetic) behavior	Invested, dedicated, protective, comforting, predictable, engaging, and interesting	Unavailable, chaotic dangerous, abusive; hypostimulating or hyperstimulating; dull
Attachment	2-7 months	Rich, deep, multisensory emotional investment in animate world (especially with primary caregivers)	Total lack of or nonaffective, shallow, impersonal involvement (e.g., autistic patterns) in animate world	In love and woos infant to "fall in love"; effective, multimodality, pleasurable environment	Emotionally distant, aloof, and/or impersonal (highly ambivalent)
Somatopsychologic differentiation	3-10 months	Flexible, wide-ranging, affective, multisystem contingent (reciprocal) interactions (especially with primary caregivers)	Behavior and affects random and/or chaotic or narrow, rigid, and stereotyped	Reads and responds contingently to infant's communications with a range of senses and affects	Ignores or misreads (e.g., projects) infant's communications(e.g., is overly intrusive, preoccupied, or depressed)
Behavioral organization, initiative, and internalization	9-24 months	Complex, organized, assertive, innovative, integrated behavioral and emotional patterns	Fragmented, stereotyped, and polarized behavior and emotions (e.g., withdrawn, compliant, hyperaggressive, or disorganized behavior)	Admiring of toddler's initiative and autonomy, yet available, tolerant, and firm; follows toddler's lead and helps organize diverse behavioral and affective elements	Overly intrusive, controlling; fragmented, fearful (especially of toddler's autonomy), abruptly and prematurely separate

| Representational capacity, differentiation, and consolidation | 1½-4 years | Formation and elaboration of internal representations (imagery); organization and differentiation of imagery pertaining to self and nonself, emergence of cognitive insight; stabilization of mood and gradual emergence of basic personality functions | No representational (symbolic) elaboration; behavior and affect concrete, shallow, and polarized; sense of self and "other" fragmented, undifferentiated, or narrow and rigid; reality testing, impulse regulation, mood stabilization compromised or vulnerable (e.g., borderline psychotic and severe character problems) | Emotionally available to phase-appropriate regressions and dependency needs; reads, responds to, and encourages symbolic elaboration across emotional and behavioral domains (e.g., love, pleasure, assertion) while fostering gradual reality orientation and internalization of limits | Fears or denies phase-appropriate needs; engages child only in concrete (nonsymbolic) modes generally or in certain realms (e.g., around pleasure) and/or misreads or responds noncontingently or unrealistically to emerging communications (i.e., undermines reality orientation); overly permissive or punitive |
| Capacity for limited extended representational systems and multiple extended representational systems | Middle childhood through adolescence | Enhanced and eventually optimal flexibility to conserve and transform complex and organized representations of experience in the context of expanded relationship patterns and phase-expected developmental tasks | Derivative representational capacities limited or defective, as are latency and adolescent relationships and coping capacities | Supports more complex, phase- and age-appropriate experiential and interpersonal development (i.e., into triangular and posttriangular patterns) | Conflicted over child's age-appropriate propensities (e.g., competitiveness, pleasure orientation, growing competence, assertiveness, and self-sufficiency); becomes aloof or maintains symbiotic tie; withdraws from or overengages in competitive or pleasurable strivings |

Modified from Greenspan S and Lourie R: Developmental structuralist approach to classification of adaptive and pathologic personality organizations: infancy and early childhood, Am J Psychiatry 138:725, 1981.

achieving a comprehensive understanding of infant development and the maladaptive responses requiring professional intervention necessitated integrating all aspects of development.

The first stage in growth and development is homeostasis, which involves two simultaneous challenges. The first is to feel regulated and calm, and the second is to use the senses to interpret the environment.

The attachment phase occurs between 2 and 7 months of age. Infants interact with their parents by initiating actions that will elicit a response from them. Infants begin to understand cause and effect and to distinguish individuals. Between 3 and 10 months of age, infants learn somatopsychologic differentiation. Some experts have also delineated a separation stage in infants that occurs between 6 months and 3 years of age. During this phase, infants begin to recognize their ability to affect the environment. Successful resolution of the autonomy versus dependency conflict occurs when infants successfully communicate their needs to their caretaker. The next stage is characterized by behavioral organization, initiative, and internalization and occurs between 9 and 24 months of age, concurrent with the separation phase. Infants connect feeling and social behavior into complicated patterns, demonstrating their understanding of the meaning of objects. Infants may hold a play telephone to their ear or pretend to be brushing their hair. This is the beginning of a conceptual view of the world in which objects have functions and parents have unique attributes.

Between the ages of 18 and 48 months, children's organization of internal representations advances to imagery — the ability to create objects in their mind's eye and remember people when they are not present. Curiosity about sights and sounds translates into interest in people, growing into love and emotional dialogue, the communication of emotions, and reception of communication of others' emotions. The development of imagery leads to imagination.

FEEDING DIFFICULTIES

Infants respond to stimuli in a calm manner, a disorganized, upset manner, or some gradation between the two extremes. Infants who find multiple stimulations overwhelming, unpleasant, or frightening may respond by withdrawing or displaying irritable behavior, and eating and sleeping pattterns may be affected.

Caretakers have an important role in facilitating the establishment of homeostasis. They must provide a supportive emotional and physical environment for infants to balance the inner state and external stimuli. When caretakers can interpret infants' cues, adequate stimulation occurs without overstimulating or overwhelming infants. If infants have constitutional or medical problems that interfere with establishing a regular pattern, their difficulties may be intensified by mothers' anxiety and disorganization. Early identification of difficulties interfering with homeostasis and timely intervention are essential to prevent problems that impede physical growth (Drotar, 1985).

Nursing management. The goals of intervention are that the infants will develop sleep, feeding, and elimination patterns allowing them to interact with their environment. Mothers will read their infant's cues and respond supportively. To accomplish these goals, clinicians should do the following:

1. Observe parent-infant interaction to identify reciprocity of cues.

2. Determine from history and observed interaction what measures, cues, and responses are effective in engaging and calming the infant
3. Assess for stimuli that result in aversive behavior, for example, being passed around from person to person, averting eyes when held face to face, crying and affecting a rigid posture when mother talks in high-pitched tones
4. Support the mother by reassuring her and empathizing as she relates her difficulties.
5. Educate the mother about the infant's need to achieve self-regulation. Explain her role in regulating the infant's environment. Teach her to identify her infant's signals and respond appropriately. Provide general guidelines for feeding schedules when hunger cues from the infant are absent.
6. Identify incontiguous behaviors using videotape role modeling and written material. Give the mother an opportunity to identify her learning needs and the needed behavioral changes.
7. Assess the mother's resources: intellect, affect, finances, knowledge base, experience with infants, knowledge of resources available to her, and social support system. Make referrals when needed.

FAILURE TO THRIVE

According to Klaus (1982), the progression of infant growth involves the integration of biologic, cognitive, sensorimotor, and affective factors. An impediment of one area will have a deleterious effect on the others. Neglect of the infant, impaired parenting, maternal deprivation, environmental factors, and severe stress on families have been identified as determinants of failure to thrive (FTT). Mitchell, Gorrell, and Greenberg (1980) cited studies that compared children who failed to thrive with a normal group and found that the FTT children had altered intellectual abilities and numerous psychosocial problems. Early intervention programs have developed in communities in response to the critical need for timely intervention.

FTT is used to describe the growth of infants and children that lies consistently below the third percentile for age or decreases rapidly from a higher percentile (Berwick, Levy, and Kleinermann, 1982). Frequently associated with delayed developmental milestones, FTT generally means a failure of physical growth with malnutrition, and the symptoms may be organic, psychogenic, or interrelated (Holmes, 1979). Although usually an attachment disorder, FTT can be related to separation, as illustrated in the case example.

Case Example

Jena, an 18-month-old girl, was admitted to the hospital with gastroenteritis, scabies, and FTT. Jena had been brought to the emergency room by her father who implied concern about his wife's ability to care for their child.

On admission, Jena was below the fifth percentile for weight and height and was developmentally delayed in speech, motor, and social development, functioning at approximately the 10- to 12-month level. She was indiscriminate in her appeals for physical closeness with adult strangers. She was without either an externally imposed or internally developed schedule for eating, sleeping, or other activities.

Hospital staff speculated that Jena had become used to snacking all day and never felt sufficient hunger or satiety to ensure adequate caloric intake. Jena also shook her head "no" vehemently when her mother pried her mouth open to force food.

Her parents did not visit for the first few days but did come in after some coaxing. Frightened, confused, and emotionally labile, Jena's mother was difficult to communicate with initially. She projected her own feelings of anger onto the hospital staff and Jena. Mrs. Z's history showed a 30-year-old woman with limited intellectual functioning, poor social skills, and low self-esteem. Her relationship with her own mother was characterized by frequent rejection and unavailability. Mrs. Z revealed that she had been unable to provide a structured routine or a consistent caring relationship for her child. She teased Jena or pushed her away and alternately felt angry and rejected by Jena because of the child's approaches for affection to strangers. Mrs. Z was overwhelmed by her child's needs.

Mr. Z, a grocery store clerk, was also the product of a troubled abusive childhood. Although he professed great willingness to cooperate with the hospital staff and with his wife, he left her to cope with the child while he spent much of his time in the local bars. The marital relationship was very troubled with frequent mutually abusive verbal behavior, anger, rejection, and tension. Nevertheless, both parents appeared interested in maintaining the relationship.

In this case, both issues of attachment and separation were prominent. From the beginning the mother-infant attachment was fragile due to the mother's deprivation, which limited her capacity to nurture Jena and understand her needs. The concomitant separation difficulties arose as a result of the poor attachment, Jena's thwarted initiatives for individuation, and the limited opportunity for obtaining maternal assistance in developing autonomy. As Jena learned means-end differentiation, provoking her mother became more important than satisfying her own hunger.

The treatment of this FTT child and her family consisted of the in-hospital treatment of mother and toddler, the development of an after-care plan, and long-term, outpatient follow-up. Hospitalization was aimed at enhancing the functioning of both mother and child. It was necessary to help Jena develop a regular eating and sleeping pattern. Autonomy in self-feeding was emphasized. As this goal was achieved, her weight began to increase. Scheduled activities were geared to foster growth and development of motor, speech, and social skills. Mrs. Z was gently nurtured, and she became less frightened and more open about her fears and her feelings about herself and her child. She became dependent on the social worker and remarked that it was the first time she was ever treated as a "grown-up lady" instead of a "retarded" person. Because of this positive relationship, she began to participate in her daughter's growth and development and then to feel responsible and effective in her own right for Jena's weight gain and improved development.

After a 1-month hospital stay, discharge was achieved with a complicated after-care plan. Mrs. Z and Jena continued to see the social worker-therapist once a week in the outpatient psychiatry department. Mother and child also attended the speech clinic and had close medical (weight) follow-up with the resident physician who had treated Jena in the hospital. Day care outside the home was recommended but was not available. Mrs. Z also attended a therapeutic infant center weekly where mother and baby could be guided through new mutual developmental tasks. All of these plans were held together by a Protective Services' worker who provided both weekly transportation to the hospital and a weekly visit by a parent-aide.

After 2 years of treatment and intervention, Jena's developmental progress was significant in all areas. Her weight was around the tenth percentile, and her eating behavior was more appropriate. Mrs. Z maintained close contact with the extremely maternal and nurturing parent-aide and achieved increased self-esteem and interpersonal maturity in her relationship with the clinical social worker at the hospital. Mrs. Z's growth in these two important relationships was associated with improvements in her interactions with Jena.

Modified from Drotar D, editor: New directions in failure to thrive: implications for research and practice, New York, 1985, Plenum Publishing Corp.

Before it was recognized that FTT can result from psychogenic causes often related to maternal deprivation, evaluations frequently entailed long hospitalizations and a battery of expensive tests, and the cause often remained undetermined. This is not surprising because only a small percentage of cases of FTT have a physical basis.

To reduce invasive and often painful testing of infants and to manage the mounting expenditure of financial and personnel resources, researchers sought the most effective methods to determine the underlying causes of the condition. Berwick, Levy, and Kleinerman (1982) focused on the hospital admission to resolve the diagnostic dilemma in obscure cases of FTT. They compared characteristics of growth in the hospital and laboratory results with the discharge diagnosis. Results revealed nonorganic causes in 9 out of 10 cases; only 0.8% of tests performed substantiated a medical diagnosis. They concluded that a thorough initial history and physical and the observation of mother-infant interactions provide the best diagnostic information. Sills' study of 185 clients (1978) supported the theory that a psychosocial history was the most effective tool in diagnosing environmental deprivation as the underlying cause of FTT. Beal (1987) concluded that direct observation is the most effective method for collecting research data on attachment phenomena. Direct methods include home and laboratory observations, process recording, and videotape analysis.

Studies have produced conflicting results, consistent with the controversy among professionals in the field. One study indicated that of the infants who had FTT but did not have structural abnormalities, gastroesophageal reflux was the most common specific diagnosis (Holmes, 1979). Both reflux and nonspecific diarrhea can have strong environmental components. In a longitudinal follow-up of the study subjects, Holmes reported constitutional growth delay or genetic short stature in some infants following a growth pattern parallel to the third percentile.

Adverse environmental factors have been associated with impaired growth and development; however, addressing FTT as a mother-infant interactional problem is a more efficacious approach than isolating the difficult child or inadequate parent or trying to alter an unsatisfactory environment.

Nursing management. The potential diagnoses for FTT include inadequate caloric and nutrient intake, oppositional feeding behaviors, and caretaker knowledge deficit of infant nutritional needs. The goals of treatment are to promote adequate caloric and nutrient intake and normal growth and development and to help parents develop an interactive feeding routine that responds to their baby's cues and satisfies the child's physical hunger. To accomplish these goals in an inpatient setting, clinicians should do the following:

1. Weigh and establish the infant's position on the growth graph as compared to other same-aged infants.
2. Establish daily caloric needs and decide on the appropriate formula while watching for lactose intolerance.
3. Strictly monitor intake and output and document these findings.
4. Observe and document infant's feeding behavior and patterns. Rule out physical problems such as pyloric stenosis.
5. Assess caregivers' interaction with their infant during feeding and their knowledge of normal infants' nutritional needs. Nurses need to teach proper nutrition, feeding schedules, and effective routines.
6. Gradually allow the caregivers to take over the feedings after the infant has begun gaining weight. This should be continued until the infant is gaining weight at the desired rate, the feeding routine is effective, and the interaction between caregivers and the infant is satisfying.

AUTISM

The symptoms of autism are similar to the signs of other disorders such as altered receptive language ability. The presence of deviance rather than delay is the differentiating factor. The cause of autism has not been determined, although many possibilities have been excluded. "Most autistic individuals are physically normal, do not exhibit any evidence of overt structural brain pathology, and have not experienced hazards known to be likely to cause brain damage" (Rutter, Tuma, and Lann, 1988). Early theories attributed the cause to psychogenic factors, but current concepts of autism consider an underlying abnormality in brain function as the most likely determinant. Biogenic theories related to "genetics, the perinatal period, hemisphere specialization, arousal and neurotransmitters" (Dalton and Howell, 1989) are being investigated.

The three approaches to the diagnosis of autism using standardized rating instruments are based on questionnaires completed by parents or teachers, structured observations of the child, and a standardized interview of the parents (Rutter, 1985). These methods reliably differentiate between autistic, mentally retarded, and normal children. The information gathered is effective in diagnosing, planning treatment, and providing services, but the tools are not sensitive to the cues and departures from normal behaviors that distinguish autism from other syndromes. Another problem is that the boundaries of autism have not been determined. These instruments will need refining once research provides clearer boundaries, distinctions, and assessment practices (Rutter, 1985).

Autism is a separate syndrome from emotional and conduct disorders, schizophrenia, general mental retardation, and specific developmental disorders of speech and language. Autistic children may reveal a mixture of bizarre behaviors, developmental delay, and developmental deviance. Autism is usually identified before the age of 3, and a later onset of the same symptoms may indicate genetic disorders or acquired brain disease (Rutter, 1985).

Another set of diagnostic criteria relate to autistic children's deviance in forming relationships. Cognitive abilities must be assessed in relation to developmental age. Infants must also be assessed for reciprocity of social emotional cues. Common characteristics found in autistic children include: (1) failing to use eye-to-eye gaze, facial expression, body posture, and gesture to regulate social interaction; (2) rarely seeking others for comfort or affection; (3) rarely initiating interactive play with others; (4) rarely offering comfort to others or responding to other people's distress or happiness; (5) rarely greeting others; and (6) failing to develop peer friendships with sharing of interests, activities, and emotions despite ample opportunities (Rutter, 1985).

The use of language for social communication is also affected (Rutter, 1985). Common findings include the following:

1. A delay in or total lack of the development of spoken language that is not compensated for by gesture or mime (often preceded by a lack of communicative babbling)
2. A failure to respond to the communications of others
3. A relative failure to initiate or sustain conversational interchange in which responsivity to the communications of the other person is necessary
4. Stereotyped and repetitive use of language
5. Use of *you* when *I* is meant
6. Idiosyncratic use of words
7. Abnormalities in pitch, stress, rate, rhythm, and intonation of speech

Rigid behaviors are also seen, including an encompassing preoccupation with stereotyped and restricted patterns of interest, attachments to unusual objects, compulsive rituals, and stereotyped and repetitive motor mannerisms. Preoccupations with part-objects or nonfunctional elements of play materials and distress over changes in small details of the environment are also demonstrated by autistic children (Rutter, 1985).

Autism and schizophrenia are dissimilar in the age of onset and in family history. Schizophrenia's peak onset is in adolescence, and the peak age of autism is during infancy. Family histories do not reveal incidents of the other disorder occurring. Delusions and hallucinations are rare in autism and common in schizophrenia. In schizophrenia, episodes of normal or near-normal functioning are common, a finding not seen in autism. In addition, epileptic seizures occur in approximately one fourth of the cases of autism and are rare in cases of schizophrenia (Rutter, 1985). Therefore, schizophrenia and autism do not appear to be variations of the same disorder.

Three fourths of autistic children are also mentally retarded (Rutter, 1985), and they differ from nonautistic mentally retarded children. Seizures occur in approximately one fourth of the children in both diagnostic groups; however, they begin in early childhood in the mentally retarded group and in adolescence in the autistic group. Down's syndrome (the most common cause of mental retardation) is rarely associated with autism. In mental retardation among nonautistic children, slightly more males than females are affected. In autism the sex distribution is four to one males to females. Autistic children are more likely to fail when presented a task that requires abstraction, language, or use of meaning. Discrimination of social motion cues are also impaired in autistic children but not in mentally retarded children.

Autistic children also differ from children who have suffered environmental trauma. Institutionalized children are clingy and indiscriminate in their attachments, and abused children are insecure in their attachments. Autistic children seem to view human beings the same way they view inanimate objects (Rutter, 1985).

Nursing management. Research verifies that autistic children suffer from a basic cognitive deficit underlying language and behavioral problems and that, in many cases, overt organic brain dysfunctions are also etiologic factors. These findings have lead to two different therapeutic directions. One focuses on the medical causes and management of autism and employs the use of drugs and psychopharmacologic agents. The other concentrates on cognitive deficits and associated behavior abnormalities and emphasizes psychologic interventions.

As with any developmental disorder, the first goal is to foster normal development. In the management of autistic children, goals include the reduction of rigidity/ stereotypy, elimination of nonspecific maladaptive behaviors, and alleviation of family distress.

To promote autistic children's cognitive development, clinicians should provide active, meaningful experiences and address deficits in the child's cognitive capacities by using direct teaching at the appropriate developmental level. Interventions specifically addressing the behavioral problems of self-isolation, impaired under-standing, and lack of initiative include planning specific periods of interaction, simplifying communications, selecting and structuring learning tasks, and using direct, individual attention and teaching.

Language development goals are designed to address the autistic child's need for social conversation interchange and to enhance linguistic capacity. Clinicians use planned periods of interaction, promotion of social development, structured reciprocal interchanges, reinforcement, and a focus on communication rather than on speech to manage autistic children's social isolation, lack of reciprocity, and failure to use language socially. When linguistic incapacity is the problem, the use of alternative modes of communication, such as signing, is recommended (Rutter, 1985).

Problems related to autistic children's lack of social approach, social responsive-ness, and social cognitive capacity suggest interventions involving structured interactions with social intrusion and direct social skills training to foster social development. When disruptive behaviors are management problems, avoidance of precipitants, provision of coping skills, differential reinforcement, and feedback with rewards for positive behavior and time out for negative behaviors are recommended. Methods for tackling problems of fear include desensitization, flooding, modeling, and fostering coping skills.

SLEEP DISORDERS

The duration of each stage in sleep in newborns varies from the periods experienced by older individuals. The sleep pattern of a newborn starts with REM sleep. By 3 months of age, infants' sleep pattern will start in non-REM, more closely resembling the adult pattern. After 10 minutes in the first sleep cycle, infants pass through the lighter non-REM stages and enter stage IV, which lasts 40 to 60 minutes. REM sleep may follow, lasting 5 to 10 minutes. Depending on their age, infants may awaken briefly or completely between sleep cycles.

The duration of the stages is longer in the second cycle (Ferber, 1988). After 40 to 50 minutes, infants awaken just before the REM stage, which may last 10 to 40 minutes. Because babies cannot separate reality from dream, they expect to find physical evidence of their dreams after awakening from REM sleep; for example, a person who was present in the dream is expected to be near their bed. They often check their environment before falling back to sleep. Infants will then alternate between REM sleep and stage II non-REM sleep. They experience deeper stage III or stage IV sleep before awakening in the morning (Ferber, 1988).

As infants get older, the time spent sleeping and the number of sleep periods decrease. By 6 months, some babies sleep through the night – a phenomenon termed *settling* (Ferber, 1988). Infants will sleep about 14 hours a day (mostly at night), and a regular morning and afternoon naptime will emerge. The 14 hour sleep requirement will continue for about a year. The morning nap is usually eliminated at 1 year of age, but the afternoon nap continues (Ferber, 1988).

Circadian rhythms are based on a 25-hour period and guide biologic activities such as sleep and waking cycles; hormone secretion; body temperature regulation; and respiratory, cardiac, renal, and intestinal functions. Synchronization of these rhythms is infants' task for the first 2 months of life. Dysynchrony results in a disturbance of homeostasis.

Teething, chronic serous otitis media, and cold or flu symptoms are examples of medical problems that disrupt sleep. Although frustrating to infants and parents, these disrupters are self-limiting and can be alleviated with medical treatment. Neurologic sensory deficit and seizure disorders, medication for asthma, barbituates, and responses to nonprescription medications may also affect sleep patterns (Ferber, 1988).

NIGHTMARES AND SLEEP TERRORS

Nightmares are dreams that represent underlying fears. Although the fears are irrational, the feeling of fear is real, and comforting from the parent provides safety and security. Sleep terrors are related to partial wakening. They occur 1 to 3 hours after the onset of sleep at night when infants or children are aroused from stage IV non-REM sleep. Instead of fully awakening and then returning to sleep, they are suspended between stages and appear awake. Infants may react by showing lack of recognition, crying, screaming, and thrashing. Holding infants may be unsuccessful because they resist feeling restrained during this state, and efforts to awaken them may result in more agitation. These partial wakenings usually last a few minutes, and the onset of fully developed sleep terrors does not usually occur until late childhood or early adolescence (Ferber, 1988).

SLEEP APNEA

Infants subject to sleep apnea may have enlarged tonsils or adenoids and/or recurrent throat or ear infections. Noisy breathing, retractions, and shallow breathing while sleeping are signs of the disorder. Infants fall asleep; the upper airway narrows, limiting air intake; oxygen saturation drops; they awaken, which reopens the airway; they breath deeply and fall back to sleep; and the cycle then repeats. Partial or complete awakening may accompany each cycle, resulting in significant sleep disruption that can be fatal. Careful observation and monitoring of breathing problems at night and reporting any concerns to physicians are crucial for proper evaluation, diagnosis, and intervention (Ferber, 1988).

Nursing management. The goals of intervention are that infants will establish internal organization leading to a regular sleep pattern and that parents will follow a consistent set of conditions at bedtime maintainable throughout the night. After 6 months of age, infants should sleep through the night. To achieve these goals, clinicians should advise parents to do the following:

1. Promote a consistent bedtime ritual with a specific bedtime. This ritual may include sitting with the infant, talking, singing, reading stories, or engaging in any calming activity that provides a peaceful transition between wakefulness and the separation of bedtime.
2. Use a chart to determine their infant's baseline sleeping pattern.
3. Promote consistent mealtimes to help cue sleeping times.
4. Provide comforting familiar objects and surroundings such as pillows, blankets, and stuffed animals.
5. Allow the child to fall asleep in bed so that when the child awakens during the transitions in the sleep cycle, a change in surroundings will not be upsetting. When the child awakens and cries, parents should briefly reassure the child, and then leave the room. Several visits to the child's room may be necessary with sequentially longer intervals between trips.
6. Decrease the amount of fluid before bedtime and increase the time between feedings during the night.

INFANTILE ANOREXIA NERVOSA

Infantile anorexia nervosa (AN) is a disorder of separation and is characterized by FTT and food refusal or extreme food selectivity and undereating. During the separation stage, mothers and infants have an underlying conflict with infants' new thrust for autonomy, especially if mothers have subconscious anxiety, rage, and confusion from not successfully resolving these issues with their own mother. Mothers whose own needs were met will find it easier to allow independence without feeling rejected and will be able to set appropriate limits. For infants, these same developmental issues of individuation and autonomy will resurface during adolescence. The variable that determines the timing of the onset of AN is the temperament of a child. If infants are willful, they will demonstrate AN by refusing food and controlling their eating. Food becomes an emotional issue rather than a physiologic need. As a result, infants have difficulty distinguishing feelings such as anger, frustration, and fear from physiologic signals such as hunger and satiety. If their temperament is compliant and they are not allowed to develop autonomy and individuate, AN will be seen in adolescence. Parental interviews of adolescent anorexic girls consistently reveal descriptions of sweet, compliant children who tried to please (Chatoor and others, 1987a).

In a matched study of 72 infants and toddlers, trained observers used a one-way window and videotapes to observe the feeding and play interactions of infant-mother pairs. Feeding took place for 20 minutes, followed by a 10-minute play period. The study revealed a significant difference between the mother-infant pairs. The most dramatic findings in one group of mothers were their lack of mirroring and their inability to read and respond to their infant's cues. Interviews with them revealed that they wanted to be good mothers and tried very hard but were frustrated, angry, resentful, and unsure of the correct feeding behavior. Some of them even felt paralyzed. These mothers' inability to set appropriate limits led to exaggerated responses in which they expressed anger by force feeding and punishment or permissive limits. These mothers felt guilty about their negative feelings and their harsh or unsupportive behaviors and viewed themselves as bad mothers. Some of them had experienced the same conflicts with their own mothers and had not resolved the control conflict; others felt insecure in their mother role and measured their competence by how well their babies ate. The infants had to struggle to make their wants known and to try new things such as feeding themselves (Chatoor, 1989).

Another significant finding is related to the role of fathers: "The father's psychopathology and involvement with the mother and the infant are important variables that also determine the severity of the separation difficulties and eating disorder of the infant" (Chatoor, 1989). Research results conclude that fathers' mental state and involvement in child rearing can neutralize or intensify the influence of a mother who has shown maladaptive behavior toward a child.

Nursing management. Infantile AN does not match the criteria that appears in the DSM-III-R because of the vast differences in developmental stages between adolescents and infants. It is depicted as atypical AN. The goals of treatment are for infants to differentiate between physical and emotional feelings and eat in response to hunger rather than emotions and for mothers to accurately interpret infants' cues and respond supportively. If infants require hospitalizations, clinicians will be substitute caregivers. To achieve these goals, clinicians should do the following:

1. Explain to the parents about the developmental conflict of autonomy and dependency and the expression of this conflict through food refusal.
2. Provide feeding guidelines by advising parents to do the following:
   a. Facilitate self-feeding by offering finger food and providing a spoon and a bowl.
   b. Feed infant at regular times and not offer snacks between scheduled meals.
   c. Limit meal time to 30 minutes and terminate the meal earlier if the infant refuses to eat, throws food or eating utensils, or plays with the food.
   d. Attend to the child during meals in a neutral manner to allow hunger to determine food intake.
   e. Introduce a play time after the meal to meet the attention and affection needs of their child.
3. Encourage parents to work together and support each other. Stress the importance of not bringing the parents' control conflicts into their approach with the infant.
4. Be sensitive to the concerns of the parents and ask questions, for example, "Are you comfortable with the food guidelines?"

Signs and Symptoms of Lead Poisoning

Hyperactivity	Learning difficulties
Aggression	Short attention span
Impulsiveness	Distractability
Decreased interest in play	Acute, crampy abdominal pain
Lethargy	Vomiting
Irritability	Constipation
Delay or reversal of verbal maturation	Anorexia
Loss of newly acquired motor skills	Headache
Clumsiness	Fever
Deficits in sensory perception	

From Whaley LF and Wong DL: Nursing care of infants and children, ed 3, St Louis, 1987, The CV Mosby Co.

---

5. Teach limit setting.
6. Teach the mother to observe, recognize, and respond to infant cues.
7. Encourage the mother to receive therapy if her issues are reactivated by her infant's attempts to establish more autonomy.
8. Encourage the parents to seek therapy if there is conflict over control issues.

Fraiberg, Adelson, and Shapiro (1975) described intervention during home visits using a goal-specific psychotherapeutic approach as a way to bring resolution to "ghosts from the past." Mothers having difficulty with their infant's move toward autonomy were at risk for abusing their infants as well. This approach was very effective with the efforts of a multidisciplinary team that supported the identified intervener through regular staffings and easy access.

PICA

Pica is the habitual, purposeful, and compulsive ingestion of nonfood substances. Infants and toddlers explore their environments in progressively complex ways, and initially anything that can be grasped and brought to the mouth is tasted and sometimes swallowed. Although many substances that infants may swallow are not harmful, others may cause serious injury, for example, wood chips covered with household insecticides or peeling lead-based paint (see box above). Small objects that can get caught in the trachea causing airway obstruction present another hazard related to pica.

The characteristic feature of pica is the persistent eating (for at least 1 month) of a nonnutritive substance. Infants with the disorder typically eat paint, plaster, string, hair, or cloth. Older children may eat animal droppings, sand, insects, leaves, or pebbles. There is no aversion to food. The age at onset is usually from 12 to 24 months but may be earlier, and pica usually remits in early childhood but may persist into adolescence or, rarely, continue through adulthood (American Psychiatric Association, 1987).

Complications from pica include lead poisoning from the ingestion of paint of paint-soaked plaster and intestinal obstruction from hairball tumors. Toxoplasma or toxocara infections may follow ingestion of feces or dirt.

Mental retardation, neglect, and poor supervision may be predisposing factors of pica, which is rare in normal adults but is occasionally seen in young children and pregnant females. Pica is also associated with autism, schizophrenia, and Kleine-Levin syndrome (American Psychiatric Association, 1987).

Nursing management. The goal of treatment is to prevent infants from ingesting harmful chemicals or objects from the environment. To achieve this goal, clinicians should do the following:

1. Identify potential safety hazards and educate the parents about these hazards.
2. Identify lapses in parental knowledge of infant development and educate parents about age-appropriate behaviors.
3. Explain age-appropriate developmental tasks to parents.
4. Identify the need for adequate supervision and assess for barriers to proper parental supervision.
5. Provide emotional support by praising and reinforcing positive attitudes, behaviors, and knowledge.
6. In the case of lead poisoning or other types of poisoning, infants must receive immediate medical attention. The treatment for lead poisoning is to neutralize the substance by administering a lead-chelating preparation intravenously. Other poisons may require gavage or the use of emetics. Keep the parents with their infant whenever possible. Decrease stimulation as much as possible. Provide on-going explanations of procedures and emotional support. Include them as part of the team to enhance the infant's care.
7. If child abuse or neglect is suspected, additional intervention steps are needed. Every state requires that suspected child abuse or neglect be reported to Child Protective Services. Discuss with the parents the procedure and what will be reported.
8. Document the assessment, intervention, and response to the intervention to provide data for present and on-going care and to account for nursing time and expense.

RUMINATION

Rumination may be a feature of a disorder of attachment and include FTT. The age of onset is usually between 3 and 12 months; however, rumination in children with neurologic impairment or mental retardation may not begin until they are several years old (Chatoor, Dickson, and Einhorn, 1984). It involves regurgitation of stomach contents, but it varies from the projectile vomiting seen with pyloric stenosis. The unique characteristic of rumination is that is self-induced. Infants appear to obtain satisfaction in the process of regurgitation and may eject the food or chew and swallow. Before a diagnosis of rumination can be made, a physiologic basis for vomiting must be ruled out.

There has been considerable controversy over the etiology and treatment of infant rumination disorder. Many studies have attempted to clarify the cause from the symptom and approach the problem in an effective comprehensive manner. The compulsive nature of rumination disorder makes it particularly tenacious. When coupled with failure to thrive, this disorder can be life threatening and difficult for clinicians to treat.

Causation and treatment of infant rumination include biologic, psychodynamic, behavioral, and integrated approaches. Proponents of the biologic approach believe that rumination is a symptom of an underlying medical problem, as demonstrated in the case example. Radiographic techniques employing gamma cameras are used to differentiate between normal reflux and pathologic reflux to validate a physiologic basis for the disorder. (Chatoor, Dickson, and Einhorn, 1984).

Case Example

T, a 6-week-old white male infant, was admitted to Children's Hospital National Medical Center because of vomiting and poor weight gain. He was born prematurely at 34 weeks gestation, weighing 4 lb 4 oz. He was taken by cesarean section because of abruption of the placenta. There were no noted perinatal problems but he remained hospitalized for 18 days to gain weight.

After he went home, the infant had occasional vomiting and frequent loose stools. The vomiting increased, occurring during, after, and between feedings. He became increasingly irritable, failed to gain weight, and cried frequently.

During the infant's present hospitalization, different areas of concern were addressed. The maternal-infant interactions were erratic. The mother was found to have suffered organic brain damage and seizures resulting from a diving accident and a subsequent automobile accident. During his gestation, she had been taking phenobarbital for a seizure disorder.

The infant's autonomic regulation seemed labile. His breathing was irregular, and he was observed to have a few apneic episodes. His stools were frequently loose and watery. His vomiting was so severe that he continued to lose weight in the hospital. The nursing staff finally noted that he initiated the vomiting with voluntary tongue thrusting. Because of his significant irritability and jitteriness, a diagnosis of phenobarbital withdrawal was made and he was treated with phenobarbital. He became less jittery, but the vomiting, diarrhea, and rumination continued. A jejunal tube was inserted for feeding.

T remained poorly related in spite of active nursing efforts to engage him. Because the mother admitted to polydrug usage before and after gestation, the infant was treated with paregoric since the possibility of methadone withdrawal was a consideration. Institution of paregoric therapy was followed by increased availability for social interaction and subsidence of rumination. The vomiting, however, continued. The diagnosis of hiatal hernia was made and a Nissen fundoplication was carried out. After the surgery, T was able to feed orally without vomiting. However, when the paregoric was discontinued, he again tried to thrust his tongue to initiate rumination but was no longer able to bring up food from his stomach. Since he was more socially available, it was decided not to reinstate the paregoric but to engage him in interactions after feedings to deter him from ruminating. Within 2 weeks, efforts at his ruminations subsided, and he gained weight and turned into a smiling, cooing infant.

Modified from Chatoor I, Dickson L, and Einhorn A: Rumination: etiology and treatment, Pediatr Ann 13:927, 1984.

In the psychodynamic context, rumination is seen as an outward expression of a psychic disturbance and as a means to relieve tension resulting from a dysfunctional relationship with the mother (Lourie, 1954). Infants use rumination when they are unable to evoke more supportive nurturing responses. Certain characteristics have been noted in mothers of ruminating infants. They seem immature, dependent, and depressed, rendering them emotionally unavailable to their infants. Other traits frequently seen are personality problems and marital conflict. Maternal psychiatric illness such as schizophrenia, anxiety disorder, addictive disorders, and depression also contributes to infants' maladjustment and resulting rumination.

Advocates of a behavioral approach believe rumination is a learned behavior reinforced by parental attention and inherent satisfaction. Even negative attention in the form of disapproval can be a powerful reinforcer. Based on the learning theory and operant behavior, shock treatment can serve as negative conditioning in response to rumination. Parents and hospital staff are resistant to this method, but other aversive approaches have been developed.

The integrated approach is the prevailing view. It explains rumination in a holistic interactional context, encompassing physiologic factors, developmental tasks and patterns, and repetitive patterns of behavior. Although mothers usually adjust their infant's environment to ensure the right amount of stimulation, infant's cues are sometimes so difficult to interpret that mothers are frustrated. Rumination then becomes the infant's means of self-stimulation and a maladaptive attempt at self-regulation (Chatoor, Dickson, and Einhorn, 1984).

Chatoor and others (1987b) tested the hypothesis that endorphins mediate social attachment and that infants become dependent on their mother for endorphin stimulation. Separation triggers endogenous endorphin withdrawal. Administration of morphine or an opiate antagonist may act as a physiologic substitute, and Bender (1956) suggested that rumination may also stimulate endorphin production. This recent research gives a new perspective on a possible cause of rumination.

Nursing management. Goals in the treatment of rumination include infants achieving self-regulation and mothers providing adequate stimulation and emotional support and protecting their infant from overstimulation. Weight and nutritional status need to be stabilized, which may require hospitalization. To achieve these goals, clinicians should do the following:

1. Assess the infant's eating behaviors and patterns to determine if the interventions are resulting in feeding that meets the infant's emotional needs rather than the infant's physical needs.

2. Intervene as primary caregiver and feed the infant. Limit the number of caregivers to promote consistency and emotional bonding.
3. Record specifics of symptoms and patterns to help determine the approach and focus of intervention efforts.
4. Stabilize nutritional status by providing adequate calories to support growth. Nasogastric feeding tubes and continuous pump feedings may be necessary through the night to catch up or maintain caloric intake.
5. Provide substitute sources of tension release and pleasure through play and quiet interaction. Provide appropriate toys and play simple games while assessing the infant's response to stimulation.
6. Provide nurturing attention to meet the infant's emotional needs.
7. Regulate environmental stimuli.
8. Monitor effectiveness of prescribed medication and aversive approaches such as using lemon juice or tabasco sauce to end the behavior.
9. Establish a program of both social rewards and negative conditioning.
10. Maintain on-going documentation to clarify the course of treatment, communicate between disciplines, and provide data.

POSTTRAUMATIC FEEDING DISORDER

A new feeding problem that has developed in the last decade is an unexpected result of advanced technology life support. Infants requiring special tube feedings for survival may develop complex and often intractable feeding problems. Clients with bronchopulmonary dysplasia, severe neurologic damage, and complex congenital anomalies of the intestines or heart are most susceptible. These infants are often compromised at birth and require intensive intervention, including total parenteral nutrition (Chatoor and others, 1987b).

Infants quickly learn that sucking and swallowing satisfies hunger, and caregivers reinforce their development autonomy by responding to their cues. This autonomy is not established in infants fed through a gastrostomy tube. They are typically fed precise quantities of food at prescribed intervals, without regard to signs of hunger and satiety. Rather than helping infants develop sensitivity to their physiologic needs, tube feeding reinforces passive dependence (DeBear, 1986).

Chatoor and others (1987b) posit the following reasons for feeding disorders in tube-dependent infants: (1) disruption of the biochemistry governing the normal hunger/satisfaction cycle, (2) disruption of the progression from reflex by coordinated sucking and swallowing to learned oral feeding patterns, and (3) abnormal behavior conditioned by the nasogastric or endotracheal tubes through the oral cavity, causing gagging or choking.

Nurses have successfully used nonnutritive interventions to stimulate autonomous feeding behavior. Nonnutritive sucking (NNS) on a pacifier during gavage feedings helps infants associate the sucking with the feeling of food in the stomach (Whaley and Wong, 1987). Nonnutritive feedings (NNF) on sham feedings can be used with conditions such as esophageal atresia. Caregivers feed their infant gastrically and orally at the same time. The feedings begin when infants' cry signals hunger and end when they no longer accept food. In a study of seven infants with esophageal atresia, mothers consistently following this procedure established autonomous feeding behavior in as little as 12 weeks (DeBear, 1986).

Nursing management. The goal of nursing interventions is that infants will reach and maintain their desired body weight through oral ingestion of nutrients. To achieve this goal, clinicians should do the following:

1. Establish the infant's measurements and placement in the norm. It may require several months to determine a pattern.
2. Determine the infant's appropriate weight and the number of calories needed daily to reach the desired weight.
3. Adjust tube feedings to allow the infant to be hungry at mealtimes, if necessary.
4. Increase the tube-feeding infusion rate during the sleeping hours if feedings are insufficient during the day.
5. Begin to desensitize the infant using the principles of behavior modification. Identify the objects or sequence of actions that are most upsetting. In nonthreatening situations, introduce those objects that may trigger anxious and panicky reactions.
6. If acting as the caregiver, role model for the mother and provide praise and explanations to maintain her self-esteem.
7. Introduce food once the infant can mouth toys without fear. Introduce water first and then add juices and milk. Next provide semisolid food that will dissolve in the mouth and progress to jello, applesauce, and thicker food, leaving meat until last. Avoid introducing any food that could lead to choking until the infant demonstrates the ability to chew and swallow. A choking experience could severely impede progress. Role model for the infant and provide positive reinforcement as each new skill is offered.
8. Regulate the tube feedings once the infant has developed good feeding skills and oromotor coordination. Allow the infant to eat until full.
9. Provide documentation to show the pattern of improvement or reflect the need to alter the approach. Stop the tube feedings once the infant is ingesting enough calories to support daily needs.
10. Provide regular checkups to assess the growth pattern and other developmental delays.

Summary

The approach to infant mental health has been reframed in the last 50 years. An appreciation for the unique characteristics of infants has emerged, a sharp contrast to the expectation that they will fit into a prescribed mold and behave as a small adult. Recognition of infants' feelings and the role of significant caregivers in providing physical and emotional nourishment and permission to develop uniquely has also occurred. Professional intervention from the disciplines that encounter and care for infants and parents is critical to families and society.

The most widely known and accepted diagnostic manuals used in infant psychiatry and mental health are the DSM-III-R and *The International Classification of Diseases,* ninth edition (ICD-9), which was sanctioned by the World Health Organization (WHO).

Nursing diagnoses relating to infant psychiatry are included in *NANDA* by Townsend (1983). This manual was developed by nurses for nurses as a reference tool to improve and standardize psychiatric nursing, and it provides descriptions of the DSM-III-R disorders, possible diagnoses, likely goals and objectives, and potential interventions. It is particularly helpful to nurse clinicians working in infant psychiatry because it correlates well with other disciplines when developing multidisciplinary treatment plans. Refinements of the developmental structuralist classifications also continue and, once developed, should be an invaluable aid to child psychiatric nurses.

REFERENCES

Ainsworth M: The effects of maternal deprivation: a review of findings and controversy in the context of research strategy, No 14, Geneva, 1962, World Health Organization.

American Psychiatric Association: Diagnostic and statistical manual of mental disorders, ed 3, rev, Washington, DC, 1987, American Psychiatric Association.

Bandura A: Behavior therapy and the models of man, Am Psychol 29:859, 1974.

Beal J: Use of direct versus indirect methods in attachment research, J Pediatr Nurs 2:72, 1987.

Bender L: Schizophrenia in childhood: its recognition, description and treatment, Am J Orthopsychiatry 26:499, 1956.

Benoit D, Zeanah CH, and Barton ML: Maternal attachment disturbances in failure to thrive, Infant Ment Health J 10:185, 1989.

Berwick D, Levy J, and Kleinerman R: Failure to thrive: diagnostic yield of hospitalization, Arch Dis Child 54:347, 1982.

Biehler R: Child development: an introduction, Boston, 1981, Houghton Mifflin Co.

Chatoor I: Infantile anorexia nervosa: a developmental disorder of separation and individuation, Manuscript submitted for publication, 1989.

Chatoor I, Dickson L, and Einhorn A: Rumination: etiology and treatment, Pediatr Ann 13:924, 1984.

Chatoor I and others: Mother-infant interactions in infantile anorexia nervosa, J Am Acad Child Adolesc Psychiatry 27:535, 1987a.

Chatoor I and others: A multidisciplinary team approach to complex feeding disorder in technology dependent infants. Paper presented at the fifth biennial National Training Institute, Washington, DC, Dec 4-6, 1987b.

Dalton ST and Howell CC: Autism: psychobiological perspectives, J Child Adolesc Psychia Ment Health Nurs 2:92, 1989.

DeBear K: Sham feedings: another kind of nourishment, Am J Nurs 80:1142, 1986.

de Mause L: The history of childhood, New York, 1974, Psychohistory Press.

Drotar D, editor: New directions in failure to thrive: implications for research and practice, New York, 1985, Plenum Publishing Corp.

Elkind D: Children and adolescents' interpretive essays on Jean Piaget, New York, 1974, Appleton-Century-Crofts.

Ferber R: Sleep disorders in children, Ped Consult 7:1, 1988.

Fraiberg S, Adelson E, and Shapiro V: Ghosts in the nursery: a psychoanalytic approach to the problems of impaired mother relationships, Acad Child Psychiatry 14:387, 1975.

Freud A and Dunn S: An experiment in group upbringing, Psychoanal Study Child 6:127, 1951.

Greenspan S: Personal communication, Mar 1989.

Greenspan S and Lourie R: Developmental structuralist approach to classification of adaptive and pathologic personality organizations: infancy and early childhood, Am J Psychiatry 138:725, 1981.

Harlow H: The nature of love, Am Psychol 13:673, 1958.

Holmes G: Evaluation and prognosis in nonorganic failure to thrive, South Med J 72:693, 1979.

Ilg F and Ames F: Child behavior, New York, 1955, Dell Publishing Co.

Klaus M: Presentation to the Academy of Child Psychiatry, San Francisco, 1982.

Lorenz K: Studies in animal and human behavior, 2 vols, Cambridge, Mass, 1970, Harvard University Press.

Lourie R: Experience with therapy of psychosomatic problems in infants. In Hoch PH and Zuben J, editors: Psychopathology of children, New York, 1954, Grune & Stratton, Inc.

Maslow A: Toward a psychology of being, ed 2, Princeton, NJ, 1968, Van Nostrand Reinhold Co, Inc.

Mitchell W, Gorrell R, and Greenberg R: Failure to thrive: a study in a primary care setting epidemiology and follow-up, Pediatrics 65:971, 1980.

Ribble M: The rights of infants, New York, 1943, Columbia University Press.

Rogers C: Learning to be free. In Farber S and Wilson RHL, editors: Conflict and creativity: control of the mind, New York, 1963, McGraw-Hill, Inc.

Rutter M: The treatment of autistic children, J Child Psychol Psychiatry 28:193, 1985.

Rutter M, Tuma A, and Lann I: Assessments and diagnosis in child psychopathology, New York, 1988, The Guilford Press.

Sills R: Failure to thrive: the role of clinical and laboratory evaluation, Am J Disabled Child 32:967, 1978.

Skinner B: Walden two, New York, 1948, Macmillan Publishing Co.

Spitz R: The first year of life, New York, 1965, International Universities Press.

Townsend M: Nursing diagnoses in psychiatric nursing: pocket guide for care plan construction, ed 2, Philadelphia, 1988, FA Davis Co.

Watson J and Rayner R: Conditioned emotional reactions, J Exp Psychol 3:1, 1920.

Whaley LF and Wong DL: Nursing care of infants and children, ed 3, St Louis, 1987, The CV Mosby Co.

Chapter 8

Personality Disorders and the Latency Years

During the early years of infancy and toddlerhood, personality is fluid and undefined, gradually maturing and taking form as children age. Once established, personality traits and temperament are remarkably stable over the life span, and the mechanisms that contribute to the tenacity of these traits and the relationship of traits to the processes and mechanisms of coping are being studied by life-span developmental psychologists (Costa and McCrae, 1980). Their findings emphasize that the use of early and aggressive interventions when dysfunctional personality symptoms first appear—most often during the latency period—could prevent many lifelong debilitating personality problems and ineffectual coping patterns.

Definitions and Concepts

PERSONALITY DEVELOPMENT DURING LATENCY

Latency has not been studied as extensively as infancy and the preschool years because of the Freudian view of latency as "silent" years, characterized by diminished drive activity. There has been a shift from this historic perspective in recent years, and latency is now viewed as a significant time of development. The development tasks include ego consolidation, the development of a sense of industry, consolidation of values and social norms, and the development of a peer group. Reparative mastery during the latency period works through prelatency fantasies and distortions and facilitates normality in adolescent and adult life (Sarnoff, 1976).

Most psychoanalytic literature divides latency into two phases. The *early phase,* from 6 to 8 years of age, is marked by children's preoccupation with self, usually with an excessively strong superego that is strict and rigid. The second phase, from 8 to 12 years of age, is referred to as the *later phase.* Distinctions are also made between the age and state of latency.

Cognitive maturation and changes during latency are profound. During the early phase of latency, concrete operational thinking, abstract memory organization, and shifts in fantasy content from fantasy objects to reality objects occur. Fantasy is the primary means of adjusting to emotional stresses and becomes a defense mechanism (Sarnoff, 1976).

In the later preadolescent years, a shift to realistic knowledge of the world and the ability to find a concrete object for the expression of drives occurs. Physical changes culminate in the emergence of secondary sex characteristics, and parents are less often the center of attention relating to the discharge of drives. The superego reorganizes toward children's ethical individuation of their own motives derived from their parents' demands. Conflicts with parents over freedom prevail, and peers become the criteria for behavior. Once children's judgment improves, social leniency increases and greater freedom results. This shift from parents to peers and the gradual increase in freedom was called the *process of removal* by early experts in the area (Katan, 1937).

Normal latency-aged children have many transient symptoms such as obsessive compulsions and persecution fantasies, which are attributed to guilt feelings resulting from rebellion. Some experts believe that within this fluid, ego-emerging developmental context of latency, well-defined behavior patterns are lacking and the personality structures of most children are too unformed for many psychiatric diagnoses to apply (Sarnoff, 1976).

Clinical studies and practice experience, however, verify that many children have the beginning behaviors and symptoms of personality disorders during the years of toddlerhood. The incidence of the behaviors increases, and the symptoms are well defined once children reach the age of 10 or 11 (Adams and Fras, 1988). These children experience considerable psychologic pain and distress, and their symptoms cause frustration and problems for their peers, age mates, and the adults responsible for their care, necessitating diagnostic attention and interventions.

THE CONCEPT OF PERSONALITY

The study of personality disorders is one of the most fascinating areas of psychiatric nursing because it concerns the most human aspect of people. Everyone has personality traits and characteristics that make them unique human beings.

Despite this fascination, personality disorders are elusive mental health problems and lack the systematic explanations found for other psychiatric disorders. Definitions of personality, distinctions between healthy and disordered personalities, and methods that help adults and children with personality disorders are continuing mysteries. Research and clinical experience in personality disorders have been "least effective in modifying or extending the intuitive insights of the arts, literature and common sense" (Harvard Medical School Mental Health Letter, 1987).

Descriptions of children with unusual personalities can be traced back to the earliest records of mankind. Before scientists, artists and writers portrayed people with different personalities in character writings (Million, 1981). Today, children with different personalities receive considerable media coverage because the public believes that personality traits and child rearing experiences cause deviations. A decade ago, the film *The Bad Seed* shocked audiences and was followed by many articles and news columns commenting on the nature-nurture controversy and personality trait theories. Recently, the child star of *ET* appeared on *Good Morning America* to tell of her experiences in a drug rehabilitation program and reported that she had tried pot at the age of 10 and cocaine by the age of 12 and was drinking alcohol at the age of 9. Her life story differed remarkably from the social expectations for preteens, and her disclosures were followed by social consciousness raising by the media and the search for personality traits and experiences that set her apart. Although most professional health care workers have encountered children in their middle childhood years who engage in these practices, the American public was shocked to learn the extent of these behaviors among children and the peer pressures involved. Surveys show that 41% of fifth graders had been pressured by their peers to drink alcohol. The news media and popular dialogues that focused on this issue have coined a new meaning for the term *bottle babies* (Policoff, 1989). In many instances, children with addictive problems are diagnosed as having conduct disorders and/or dependent, borderline, or compulsive personality disorders, depending on the duration and extent of other signs and symptoms.

Although the words *personality, character,* and *temperament* are used interchangeably in the literature, character and temperament have definite meanings that distinguish them from personality. Character refers to those personal qualities that represent people's adherence to the values and customs of society; temperament refers to those biologically based dispositions that underlie energy level and moods (Million, 1981).

Definitions of personality imply that people's attitudes and behavior differ in ways that persist across changing situations. Traits are enduring "patterns of perceiving, relating and thinking about the environment and oneself, exhibited in a wide range of social and personal contexts" (American Psychiatric Association, 1987). Personality traits influence unconscious approaches to the world and are expressed in thoughts, emotions, and actions. When personality traits become inflexible and maladaptive and impair social or occupational functioning, they become personality disorders.

There are three major distinctions between normal children and those with personality disorders: (1) adaptive inflexibility in which children are rigid and lack alternative ways of relating, achieving goals, and coping with stress; (2) vicious cycles in which habitual perceptions and behaviors perpetuate and intensify difficulties; and (3) tenuous abilities in which children are fragile and lack resilience under stress (Million, 1981).

Personality Disorders

In the past, people with behaviors that conflicted with social norms were discounted and viewed as eccentric, perverse, and untreatable. Because of their disclusion and the lack of clear diagnostic criteria, the accuracy of the estimates of children with personality disorders in the population is limited. It is estimated that between 5% and 15% of the adult population have personality disorders, and ⅓ to ½ of psychiatric patients have personality disorders (Million, 1981).

Epidemiologic surveys indicated a higher incidence of personality disorders in socially impaired environments, and poor employment, marital adjustments, and difficulties with alcohol, drugs, and the law are also related to a higher rate. Some research has shown that with strong social support systems the incidence of personality disorders decreased, suggesting that personality disorders are not as incurable or as static as they have been viewed in the past (Vaillant and Perry, 1985).

Social psychologists have expressed considerable concern over recent statistics indicating that the number of people diagnosed with antisocial disorders has increased at an alarming rate, especially rates of persons with antisocial disorders involving aggression. Concerned at the increase in violence and stranger and serial murders, some experts advocate that the research and theoretic focus of psychiatry shift from narcissistic psychopathology to developing better understanding of and treatment regimes for personality disorders in which acting out is characteristic (Meloy, 1988). Others voice concern for the impact of contemporary child-rearing patterns on the next generation, warning that children raised in a "predominantly image-based, nonlinear, multimedia, briefly attentive society may not develop the deeper, unconscious levels of identity and meaning," resulting in lower empathy levels and higher anxiety levels (Gardner and Momarita, 1986).

DSM-III-R CRITERIA FOR PERSONALITY DISORDERS

A personality trait or character type may not hinder children's developmental progression, but a personality disorder will if it is undiagnosed and untreated. The mixed personality disorder NOS (not otherwise specified) diagnosis in the DSM-III-R is often used with children because their personalities usually fit into one or more diagnostic categories simultaneously.

The Group for the Advancement of Psychiatry (GAP) committee on child psychiatry first published categories for childhood personality disorders in 1966, and this system was widely used in child psychiatric care settings and stimulated extensive research (Goldstein, 1987; Rutter, 1987). The subsequent refinement and clarification of this criteria for childhood personality disorders contributed to the understanding of the origins of personality disorders in adolescents and adults.

Although the GAP categories used psychodynamic language and concepts, the DSM-III and DSM-III-R use a behaviorally oriented, atheoretic framework in the nomenclature. The DSM-III-R criteria specify that the diagnosis of antisocial personality disorders requires adolescents and adults to have a history of antisocial behavior including conduct disorders of childhood. After children reach the age of 18, continuing personality disorders of the pediatric age group that have been attributed to temperament should be reassigned to adult classifications.

The major changes in the DSM-III-R published in 1987 were the deletion and limiting of the overlapping behavioral criteria that were found in the 1980 edition of the DSM-III (Widiger and others, 1987). These diagnoses were found to be the least reliable and valid in clinical tests.

Most personality disorder categories used in the DSM-III-R are prototypal; that is, the characteristics are not necessarily shared by all persons with the specific personality disorder. Some criteria are optional, and all are presented in descriptive terms to avoid supporting a particular theory of personality development and

Table 8-1   DSM-III Classification of Personality Disorders

Cluster	Classification number	Disorder	Defenses
Eccentric	301.20	Schizoid personality	Isolation
Dramatic-erratic	301.50	Histrionic personality	Dissociation, acting-out, splitting, denial
	301.81	Narcissistic personality	Manipulation
	301.83	Borderline personality	Anger, crisis
Anxious	301.82	Avoidant personality	Isolation, passive-aggressive and fearful behavior
	301.60	Dependent personality	Overdependency
	301.40	Obsessive-compulsive personality	Rituals
	301.84	Passive-aggressive personality	Defiance

deviation. The prominent symptoms of personality disorders in childhood involve the areas of thought, developmental delays, and derangements.

Personality disorders have been grouped into three clusters by their characteristic adult defenses and have been adapted to children (Table 8-1). Antisocial, schizotypal, and paranoid personality disorders are not discussed in detail in this chapter because the symptoms described in the DSM-III-R rarely apply to children.

HISTRIONIC PERSONALITY DISORDERS

Egotism is a natural developmental stage in infancy and toddlers, and it fades when children become preschoolers. The diagnosis of histrionic personality disorders is seldom applied to children under the age of 7 but is usually reserved for latency-aged children, adolescents, and adults who cannot maintain lasting relationships, overreact to minor events, and lack genuineness. These disorders reportedly occur twice as often in females than in males, but some experts attribute the predominance in females as a historical sex bias because the clinical description of the disorders use terms that have also been applied in caricatures of women.

Clinical description.   Children with a histrionic personality clinically present as highly emotional, dramatic, expressive attention seekers, with behaviors that cause peers, parents, and teachers to reject and ignore them. These children crave an audience and the center of attention, acting out roles as if they were on a stage. They assume values, thoughts, and feelings that they believe are experienced by the people they are imitating (Rutter, 1987).

The conversation of histrionic children is exaggerated, with affect-laden anecdotes and the expression of vivid fantasies. These children manipulate others, have shallow, self-serving relationships and a low frustration tolerance, and overreact to minor stresses such as being ignored with irrational emotional outbursts, self-harming efforts, and tantrums. They lack consideration for others, yet rejection in social relationships often causes them intense distress. They demonstrate aggression, emotionalism, exhibitionism, oral-aggression, egocentricity, sexual provocativeness, and rejection of others. Their ineffective coping behaviors and impulsiveness put them at a high risk for self-injury (Nyman, 1988). Repression, denial, and dissociation are their major defenses (Ross, 1967), and they also exhibit an exaggeration of eye contact that may contribute to female stereotyping.

Their cognition is normal; however, they may lack the concentration abilities needed for problem solving and scholastic tasks. Their lack of self-discipline and perseverance may limit their learning performance, and physical preoccupations divert them from sustained intellectual focus or academic activities. They are more interested in creative and imaginative pursuits than in analytic or academic achievements. These children are impressionable, look to authority figures for magical solutions to their problems, evade external responsibilities, and lack goals and a life direction. The case example illustrates a child with the characteristic clinical presentation of histrionic personality disorder.

Case Example

Linda, a 9-year-old girl, was seen in the child mental health clinic with her father, who had received custody after a divorce when Linda was 7 years old. She was an attractive child and appeared much older than her years. Her father described her as "9 going on 29." She wore exaggerated eye makeup and a bright pink bodysuit and had a small, somewhat underdeveloped body.

Her teacher had suggested the visit because of Linda's inability to keep up with her classmates academically and her disruptive, attention-seeking behaviors at school. She had frequent tantrums in the classroom, fought with her peers, and was disliked for her manipulations. In a recent incident on the playground, Linda was not chosen to play on a softball team and responded by throwing a tantrum during which she scratched her own face in rage. Concerned at this new self-injuring behavior, the teacher conferred with Linda's father and suggested mental health consultation.

Linda said that she hated the "silly girls" in her class and that her teacher disliked her and picked on her constantly. She had no time for school work but spent hours in front of her mirror trying on makeup or exercising. She had uncontrollable crying spells at home and school and frequently asked her father why the other children did not like her.

Linda was happy when her father's friends visited. She would claim the center of attention and act somewhat provocatively. Her father reported that she had recently modeled her wardrobe for two of his friends and had banged her head with her hands in an uncontrollable tantrum when they showed a lack of interest. Linda clung to her father and talked of running away after the incident.

During the interview, Linda posed and emoted while she flipped the pages of a fashion magazine with casual disinterest, using exaggerated superlatives to describe the fashions displayed that caught her glance. Several times she interrupted the conversation by grabbing the clinician and pointing to a picture, saying, "It's me."

DSM-III-R criteria.   Criteria presented in the DSM-III-R are tentative because research in this area has been inconclusive and the diagnosis is relatively new. DSM-III-R definitions require that four of the following characteristics be present for diagnosis in an adult (Adams and Fras, 1988):
1. Speech content consisting of overstatement and hyperbole
2. Constant search for praise and approval
3. Inappropriate sexual seductiveness*
4. Overconcern with physical appearance*
5. Exaggerated emotional expression
6. Discomfort if not the center of attention
7. Perception of shallowness by others*
8. Egocentric and self-indulgent

Nursing management.   Children with histrionic personality disorder are especially dependent on the cooperation and assistance of their parents for recovery. It is unclear if these problems are episodic or characterologic; however, changes in children's behavior depend on changes in parents, their interactions with the child, and parenting behavior. Clinicians need to work with both generations, as well as teachers and other adults involved in children's daily life.

Most histrionic children demonstrate developmental delays by persisting in behaviors that they were encouraged to demonstrate at 3 or 4 years of age. They are unable to progress beyond the time when they were the natural center of attention. The parents often lack understanding of child development and change and continue with age-inappropriate discipline and rewards.

Behavior therapy and life experience peer groups are helpful treatment approaches. In some cases, group therapists will need to assist children in mastering earlier developmental tasks that were not negotiated, such as sharing and caring about peers. Parental guidance should focus on educating parents about normal behaviors and expectations and should provide skills in child discipline that will foster self-control.

When treated early, children with histrionic personality disorders can overcome the many crises that normally occur in life in less painful ways. However, the residual traits remain, and according to psychoanalytic theory, persons will be vulnerable to the more severe conversions, phobias, and dissociative disorders in subsequent stressful life experiences. Some authorities disagree, believing that neurotic symptoms originating during latency usually do not persist in adult life (Sarnoff, 1976).

NARCISSISTIC PERSONALITY DISORDER

The term *narcissism* was derived from the name of Narcissus, a vain young man in Greek mythology. It signifies extreme vanity and immature self-preoccupation in every day language and a Freudian description of a stage in identity development in psychiatric nomenclature. Healthy development in object relationships is accompanied by an increase in narcissism during late latency. Confusing changes in body

---

* Criterion seldom seen in children.

image draw self-attention and heighten the need for a strong ego (Sarnoff, 1976). Although the extent of the problem in the general population has not been confirmed by epidemiologic studies, the disorder appears to be more common in males than in females (Vaillant and Perry, 1985).

Clinical description.   Children with narcissistic personality disorders progress to latency indifferent to others and devoid of empathy and relatedness. These children present a clinical picture similar to that of histrionic children but also demonstrate *entitlement* behaving as if they possess special gifts and are entitled to special favors without reciprocity. They exceed histrionic children in their need for attention and manipulation of others (Mahler and Kaplan, 1977). They are greedy, demanding, and extroverted personality types who become angry when the actions of others do not meet their expectations. Narcissistic children lack sensitivity and manipulate others to achieve self-aggrandizement and to gain admiration and respect (Kohut, 1971).

This manipulation includes melodramatic behaviors such as smiling superfluously, weeping unsparingly, and acting bewildered, disarmed, or confused. Narcissistic children may demonstrate fastidiousness, forgetfulness, disparagement, and guileful adulation. The manipulation may be in the form of flattery, harassment, or intimidation, and it may include mimicking, pantomiming, and confrontation in the presence of others. Dishonest and devious behaviors may also occur as a means of manipulation, exemplified by acting out, which can range from back stabbing to anger, rage, and tantrums.

Parents, teachers, and peers usually believe that the manipulation is a conscious action, and will retaliate by medicating, isolating, punishing, or threatening the child. This reaction ignores the child's anxiety and pain and reinforces the narcissistic traits.

Some narcissistic children unconsciously use intellectualization as a defense against feelings of inferiority. It is a form of resistance that impedes the interpersonal process and discourages or blocks therapeutic change. They separate feelings from ideas and focus on the intellectual aspects of situations to avoid emotional awareness and to defend against experiencing pain and emotional reactions.

The families of narcissistic children have been extensively studied, and the identified patterns suggest areas that clinicians should address. Some family environments fostering narcissistic traits lack parental empathy, warmth, and support; others feature abuse and neglect. Parents often idealize a positive characteristic that they believe their child possesses. As a result, the child develops a superficial sense of omnipotence, fostering denial of any feelings of weakness, helplessness, or inferiority. Shared parent-child fantasies and magical thinking result in many neurotic problems as the child matures (Serban, 1982).

DSM-III-R criteria.   Narcissistic personality disorders first appeared in the 1980 edition of the DSM-III; however, narcissism has a long clinical and theoretic history (Satinover, 1986; Svarkic, 1985). The overlapping of narcissistic disorder criteria and the symptoms for other personality disorders creates difficulty in assigning the diagnosis to children. The DSM-III-R lists the following nine criteria for the disorders, and five must be present for the diagnosis (Adams and Fras, 1988):

1. Reaction to criticism consisting of feelings of rage and humiliation*
2. Grandiose sense of self-importance*
3. Alternation between extremes of overidealism and devaluation of others in personal transactions*
4. Belief that problems are exceptional and that a specially gifted person is needed*
5. Preoccupation with fantasies of unlimited success, power, brilliance, beauty, or ideal love†
6. Exhibitionism†
7. Disturbances in interpersonal relationships from entitlement†
8. Interpersonal exploitation†
9. Inability to recognize and appreciate the feelings of others†

Nursing management.   Different theoretic explanations for narcissism result in several perspectives on the management of narcissistic children. The long-range goals include assisting children in developing a stronger self-esteem, regulating outbursts of anger and hostility, and moving toward more age-appropriate relationships and regard for others. Long-term treatment is more involved than the interventions required for children with histrionic personality disorders. Family therapy, group experiences with peers, teacher collaboration, and individual psychotherapy provide a multiple approach that includes cognitive, behavioral, and social skill enhancement. Individual psychotherapy requires the knowledge and skills of a specialist if positive and lasting changes are to occur.

Because narcissistic children use manipulation for self-aggrandizement, specific intervention strategies are indicated. They include contracts with the child, parents, and teachers. The following guidelines for clinicians have been suggested (Chitty and Maynard, 1986):

1. Provide clear, consistent, and firm expectations that emphasize therapeutic concern.
2. If children test the limits of behavior, responses from everyone should be strong and consistent.
3. Responses to efforts to manipulate nurse-patient relationships should focus on the interaction process and not on the content of the attempts.
4. Provide explanations that are brief, clear, and limit setting.
5. Address rather than avoid children and their behaviors.
6. Avoid colluding with others to meet children's needs or to plan retaliatory actions.

With patient and supportive injunctions from clinicians and parents, children can recall repressed dissociated material and are usually surprised to learn of their own feelings. Helping them to become aware of their real feelings, abilities, and limitations and to accept the same in others is a major part of the therapeutic process with older children (Woosley, 1980).

Detachment is characterized by the refusal to acknowledge personal displeasure, painful sensations, or facts by acting aloof and unaware. By blocking

---

* Criterion seldom seen in children.
† Criterion seldom seen in adults.

out painful experiences, they cannot be worked through in the therapeutic sessions. Detachment needs to be differentiated from superficiality, which features shallowness, lack of attention to details, and disparagement of situations to reduce the intensity of emotions. Interventions in detachment depend on children's ability to assimilate and benefit from clarification and include the following:

1. Identification of the methods used by the child to remain detached from feelings
2. Identification by the child of the ego serving and self-defeating aspects of manipulation
3. Exploration of the fears and fantasies that inhibit the child from experiencing and integrating behavior, feelings, and thoughts
4. Emphasis on the emotive content of situations to prevent fear of emotions from continuing

It is difficult for parents and group activity peers not to react with frustration and annoyance at narcissistic children's forgetfulness of rules governing behaviors (Schacter, 1986). When confronted, these children dissociate using detachment and superficiality or have irrational tantrums and angry outbursts.

BORDERLINE PERSONALITY DISORDERS

Traditionally, the term *borderline* referred to psychopathology that fell between neurotic and psychotic and was seen as bordering on psychosis. Descriptions of borderline conditions have appeared in the literature since the 1900s and have included writings by Freud, Bleuler, Reich, and Deutsch. The theory of the separation-individuation process (Mahler, 1971) provides the basis for understanding the multiple defects affecting the borderline disorder (see Chapter 3). The particular deficiencies are related to the developmental subphase of rapproachement in which a conflict or crisis results from children's strong wishes for reunion with their mother and their intense fear of engulfment.

Discrepancies in clinical descriptions of borderlines are attributed to the variation in identity disturbances characterizing this disorder. Borderline personalities are devoid of constant features and present different deficits and pathologic signs.

Some experts claim that the diagnosis of borderline personality disorder does not apply to children during the latency years because of rapid shifts in their use of defenses. These children are referred to as *vulnerable* because of weaknesses in the latency ego structure and inadequate symbol formation (Sarnoff, 1976).

The similarity of narcissistic and borderline traits have led some experts to suggest that the two disorders are related and that borderline children mature to become adults with narcissistic personality disorders (Goldstein, 1987; Siever and Gunderson, 1979). Clinicians can easily overdiagnose borderline conditions by limiting the evaluation to a history and clinical examination.

Clinical description.   Children diagnosed as borderline manifest ego weakness (such as the inability to tolerate anxiety and frustration), poor impulse control, and underdeveloped sublimating channels. They demonstrate a typical pathology of internalized object relationships and fail to integrate images of self and others (Kernberg, 1975). They usually have superficial social skills, and their interpersonal relationships continue only as long as they meet their needs. Borderline children express entitlement and are overly sensitive to rejection, distrusting others in ways that sometimes approximate paranoia (Kaffman, 1981). Their adaptation is minimal, and they often complain of emptiness, boredom, and depression.

Despite early deficits, some children with borderline disorders have stable ego deficits and the ability to maintain reality testing except under extreme cases of stress, which result in transient psychotic episodes. They may perform adequately in school if a highly structured learning environment is provided. Although they lack consistent feelings, anger is the one emotion they can express without pretending.

Consistent patterns have been identified in studies of the families of borderlines, including neglect relating to the emotional unavailability of parents during critical developmental periods and overinvolvement featuring symbiotic control and withholding of emotional needs by children and mothers. Other dynamics noted in the literature include parents' projection of marital hostilities and conflicts onto the child and inadequate same-sex role modeling (Gunderson and Englishwoman, 1981; Gunderson, Kerr, and Eglund, 1980).

DSM-III-R criteria.   Clinicians must differentiate between borderline personality disorders, histrionic disorders, conduct disorders, and psychosis. In some cases, children have both histrionic and borderline personality disorders, but histrionic children are more unaware of their feelings and the responses of others and do not report feelings of emptiness. Children with conduct and histrionic disorders do not exhibit identity diffusion or brief psychotic episodes that are characteristic of borderline personality disorders. In regressed states, borderline children may seem psychotic, but this state is stress related with ego alien qualities; psychotic regression is unsystematized.

The DSM-III-R gives considerable attention to adult and adolescent borderline personality disorders, but there is little information regarding the childhood aspects. However, the theoretic explanations and diagnostic criteria can be applied to children. The following symptoms are characteristic features in children with borderline personality disorders (Adams and Fras, 1988):

1. Transient deficits in cognition, including minipsychotic episodes that involve bizarre ideation and concrete thinking as a response to interpersonal stress
2. Intense and unstable relationships with others that fluctuate and shift from valuation to devaluation
3. Poor impulse control demonstrated by inappropriate temper outbursts and behavioral difficulties with marked shifting of attitudes
4. Occurrence of depressed affect and terror and panic attacks when left alone or experiencing anxiety because of inadequate defense mechanisms
5. Poor self-concept and identity because of indiscriminate modeling of adults
6. Related symptoms of uneven development in other areas, including neurologic soft signs, hyperactivity attention deficits, and motor, language, and learning disorders and delays

Nursing management.   The treatment modality of choice for most borderline children is long-term hospitalization and intensive work with the parents and children after discharge. Their need for hospitalization results from their unstable interpersonal relationships, identity diffusion, affective liability, and feelings of emptiness and aloneness. Their intense and uncontrollable anger and physical fights usually precipitate the crises that bring them to the clinic or inpatient setting.

Viewpoints on managing borderline clients differ, and interventions have been adjusted to school-aged latency children in various treatment settings. Some experts claim that interpretation is essential with support systems and prolonged hospitalization (Kernberg, 1975). Others recommend a supportive, reality-oriented behavioral approach or a limit-setting holding environment to achieve gradual social adjustment. Most perspectives combine elements of conflict resolution and social learning with a minimal amount of regression (Sederer and Thorbeck, 1984; Vaillant and Perry, 1985).

Nurse clinicians need therapeutic treatment plans based on children's developmental stage. Initial treatment efforts should focus on assisting children in the resolution of the immediate crisis and should educate them about verbal expressions of anger that can be used in lieu of acting out (Sederer and Thorbeck, 1984). Short-term goals involve setting firm limits before individual treatment begins and enhancing support systems with other clients and the nursing staff.

Long-range goals are for children to delay immediate gratification, to redirect their impulses to socially acceptable behaviors, and to learn more emotionally rewarding social skills.

Some borderline children engage staff members in their magical expectations and demands, precipitating struggles among them (Duldt, 1981). Clinicians should avoid overinvolvement and be alert to transference phenomena. It is essential not to release children's inhibitions or acting out behaviors. Acting out usually occurs in the hospital milieu because of children's disappointments, dissatisfactions, and envy of sicker children who seem (to them) to get more attention. The relationships of staff members with other children are undermined, and hospital personnel often become the evil or persecuting persons in the eyes of borderline children (Mark, 1980).

A special problem in the management of borderline children is their alternating behavior in therapeutic relationships. Responses to the nurses and therapeutic process vary from highly valuing the relationship, reflecting their ego hunger, to rejecting and devaluing the treatment, demonstrating their ineffectual object relation. Retaliation to this defense mechanism is usually counterproductive (Adler, 1974; Coltranne and Pugh, 1979).

Treatment approaches require clinicians to do the following:
1. Contract with the child to achieve goals when appropriate.
2. Use role modeling, reinforcement techniques, and peer pressure.
3. Provide group therapy.
4. Avoid bargaining.
5. Calmly confront the child when behaviors are inappropriate.
6. Control the treatment regime.
7. Monitor interactions with less organized children.
8. Remain calm, providing a holding environment.
9. Montior for signs of regression.
10. Identify alternatives to tantrums and destructive behaviors.
11. Assist the child with self-responsibilty.

12. Identify needs that require immediate attention and those that can be delayed.
13. Reduce the child's boredom.
14. Assist the child to tolerate being alone for short periods of time.

Milieu management principles include the following:

1. Staff exchange information and follow similar, rigidly structured management strategies.
2. The nurse or therapist acts as case administrator, and team assignments are monitored.
3. The milieu provides an opportunity for children to use primitive defenses, and the staff's goal is to gratify positive strengths and protect clients from destructive behaviors.
4. The case administrator monitors the milieu for signs of interstaff friction (Bandura, Underwood and Fromson, 1975).

DEPENDENT PERSONALITY DISORDERS

Diagnosis of dependent personality disorders involves assessing overdependence and failure to develop autonomy as compared to the age-appropriate developmental sequence. Dependency disorders relate to children's expanding capacity for human relationships (see Chapter 3). In psychoanalytic theory the traits of dependence is related to the oral stage of psychosexual development. Adults with the residuals of oral-dependent problems demonstrate excessive concern with oral satisfaction, dependency, pessimism, passivity, and self-doubt. These oral traits are also found in older children who have been deprived and in most patients with psychiatric diagnoses. Dependent personality diagnoses are more commonly assigned to females than to males; a disparity that may exist because of the perception of the disorder's characteristics as feminine attributes.

Clinical description.   Children with dependent personalities establish relationships with others who will take care of them. They tolerate abuse from others and allow people to make decisions for them. They have not mastered autonomy and do not have a strong sense of self. Dependent children experience considerable discomfort when alone for even brief periods. Although they maneuver others into accommodating their strong attachment needs, they lack the demanding qualities of histrionic children.

DSM-III-R criteria.   The DSM-III-R defines dependent personality disorders in adult terms and requires that the following criteria characterize long-term functioning:

1. Passive allowance of others assuming responsibility for major areas of life
2. Subordination of needs to those of others
3. Lack of self-confidence.

Most of these criteria describe dependency in normal children. Most children have little choice in making major life decisions, must remain in relationships with people who mistreat them because of the fear of being alone, and experience hurt feelings from adult criticism and disapproval. Adams and Fras (1988) suggest that more appropriate criteria for diagnosing older children include: (1) agreeing with people even when they do not concur to avoid disturbing the relationship, (2) offering to do something unpleasant or demeaning to earn the favor of other people, (3) being preoccupied with the fear of being abandoned, and (4) feeling powerless or uneasy about being alone.

Nursing management.   Dependent personality traits involve learned helplessness. Feelings of helplessness are learned early in life and are a normal state for small infants and children and have also been observed in the phenomenon of job burnout. Response dependence is observed when people respond to situations with behaviors that have no relationship to the results. These people believe that outcomes will occur regardless of their action or inaction and that they are not in control of their life. The problem is usually identified in middle and late childhood when autonomy has not emerged and children show no motivation to gain control over any situation, which often occurs if the family process is inadequate. As a result, children become overly dependent on people that they believe have the ultimate power, such as authority figures (Schneider, 1980). If dependent children have an age mate who can teach them interdependence, the problem may disappear.

Children often cast nurses in the mother role, and clinicians unfamiliar with child development and normal dependency and autonomy unwittingly accept the role. Nursing interventions should focus on assisting children in learning the mutual benefits of peer relationships and include the following:
1. Setting age-appropriate and consistent limits and involving the family and significant others in the treatment plan
2. Avoiding retaliatory actions and emphasizing children's accountability for thoughts, actions, and feelings
3. Providing opportunities for children to control their life and assume responsibility for their actions
4. Fostering children's acceptance of their decision making
5. Keeping children informed of treatment activities
6. Directing children's thoughts and plans toward the future

Staff, parents, and children with dependent personality traits respond well to assertiveness training. Some clinicians have also found that group-training sessions for staff and latency-aged children in inpatient settings are effective.

COMPULSIVE PERSONALITY DISORDERS

Compulsions are commonplace traits in children and adults, and some experts believe that everyone has some compulsiveness in their personality armor (Vaillant, 1975). Compulsive personality disorders are among the most studied and described maladaptations, first appearing in the psychoanalytic literature in 1894 when Freud identified the relationships of isolation, displacement obsessions, and related compulsions to the anal stage of psychosexual personality development. Freud originally identified the three traits composing the anal character as orderliness, obstinacy, and parsiomony, traits that have consistently been emphasized in the professional literature.

Factor analyses studies of hospitalized and normal persons (Lazare, Klerman, and Armor, 1966) showed that these three traits were clustered with emotional constriction, perseverance, rigidity, strict superego, indecisiveness, and lack of provocativeness. The cognitive style of compulsive people demonstrates that the control functions of scanning and sharpening are highly developed.

Compulsions are unwanted actions associated with obsessions, and older children usually recognize them as silly and unnecessary. Other compulsions provide younger children with security and continuity. Some compulsions are productive, for example, checking for traffic before crossing streets, but others, such as the need to always be right, limit spontaneity, openness with friends, completing school assignment, and decision making. Children's compulsive behaviors are often used by them to resolve anxiety. In play therapy interventions, children project their concerns onto objects and toys, imagining scenes repetitively until problems are settled.

Even with early therapeutic interventions and resolution, the roots of compulsive habits are found in childhood. Children learn to displace anger and anxiety onto neutral objects, often to please parents who are harsh disciplinarians (Vaillant and Perry, 1985). Because compulsives are highly attracted to other compulsives, the parents usually have stable marriages in which work and occupational success are valued over relationships and friends.

Historically, more men than women have been diagnosed as compulsive, and the behaviors occur more frequently in the oldest child of a family. When diagnosed in childhood, compulsive personality disorders rarely become structured and develop into symptom neuroses. However, children may develop other neuroses such as phobias and anxiety disorders. The point at which compulsive personality traits become compulsive personality disorders is not yet known.

Clinical description.   Children with compulsive personality disorders demonstrate an inability to be warm and responsive and usually have few friends or social relationships. They are preoccupied with rules and rights and often discourage spontaneity and creativity. They are serious and formal children who seem unable to relax, laugh, or cry. They will describe but not display their feelings, and their voices are often strangely monotonous. These children often use the defenses of isolation, intellectualization, and displacement, and their lifestyle makes their days long and tiring. The case example illustrates the typical behavior of a compulsive child.

Case Example

Janet, a 10-year-old girl, was brought to the mental health clinic for her depression and fatigue. Janet was neatly dressed and presented an expressionless face. Janet's mother began the interview by saying that she was not certain she had come to the right clinic and that she feared Janet has a serious disease such as anemia or hepatitis. According to her mother, Janet never had the time or energy to play.

Janet said her schoolwork was so taxing that she had no time for anything or anyone else. She could hardly keep up and often had to stay awake long beyond her scheduled bedtime to complete her homework. Janet said writing took up most of her time because she did all her work in neat blocked printing, which she proudly displayed to the clinician for approval. Janet explained in detail that she needed at least five sharp pencils to complete her work each night. Although she earned high grades and her teachers said she was a model student, Janet feared she might not be the best student in the class. She did feel certain that she was the teacher's pet, accounting for the reason other children did not like her.

Janet had saved her schoolwork since first grade, neatly filing it on bookshelves. Janet's mother said that Janet was going to be an excellent secretary some day and had already mastered the word processor and spreadsheets on the family's computer.

Janet's chief complaint was her inability to make decisions and to "get through the day." With her mother's encouragement, she would lay out her clothes for the next day before going to bed. However, each morning Janet found that the clothes she had selected were not the right ones and had to try on her entire wardrobe before finding an outfit to wear. She showered immediately after school, after dinner, and again in the morning and expressed considerable concern about germs at school and at home. Janet said that after studying late, she was often tired and irritable and that her mother seemed indifferent to her exhaustion. Thus, Janet had crying scenes every night and resented her mother's efforts to help her organize her responsibilities.

Mornings were equally difficult for Janet. She would not leave for school until she had cleaned her room in a certain way, put fresh sheets on her bed, washed the ones she had slept on, and wrapped her school work in brown paper. She sometimes missed the bus because of trying to complete the morning tasks. Once on the bus, she needed to sit directly behind the bus driver, and other children would take her place. She usually had to argue with them and often arrived at school crying.

When describing her bedroom (her favorite place), Janet droned on about where each object went. She did not have many toys and did not like to play with them because she did not want them to become dirty. Janet's mother proudly stated that Janet carefully displayed these toys on the bookshelves in her room and would not allow visiting children to play with them. Janet and her father had carefully labeled each shelf so that when visiting friends wanted to hold the toys, Janet could quickly return her playthings to their proper place.

DSM-III-R criteria.   The DSM-III-R criteria for compulsive personality disorders have the highest degree of professional consensus of all personality disorders. Distinctions are made between obsessions and compulsions: obsessional people have an uptight, rigid lifestyle but no stark obsessions and compulsions and no personality disorder. People with an obsessive compulsive personality disorder show "perfectionism and inflexibility" to a degree that causes distress in the affected person and interferes with social functioning. Five of the following features must be present for diagnosis in children (Adams and Fras, 1988):
   1. Restricted expression of warm emotions and feelings
   2. Display of stinginess with time, money, and gifts even when personal gain is likely to result
   3. Perfectionism that hinders completion of a task
   4. Preoccupation with details, mechanics, or schedules at the expense of the major point of an activity
   5. Stubborn insistence that others submit to their manner of doing things
   6. Devotion to work to the exclusion of leisure and friendships
   7. Avoidance, postponement, or extension of decision making

8. Accumulation of worn or useless objects without sentimental value
9. Overly conscientious, scrupulous,and inflexible perspective of morality without a cultural or religious basis

Nursing management.   Unlike clients with other personality disorders, most adults and older children with compulsive personality traits are aware of their problems and seek treatment when their compulsions become restrictive. They respond well to nondirective techniques, and children particularly benefit from group therapies. Compulsive behavior that has been consistently rewarded from infancy is the most difficult to unlearn or modify.

Treatment using expressive psychotherapy is most effective if children are 10 or 11 years of age. Therapists must confront, advise, stress affects instead of thoughts, and discuss affects in present terms. They should prevent vagueness by stressing the need for concrete examples and should encourage risk taking and naturalness (Adams and Fras, 1988). Behavioral and cognitive strategies are useful, and because compulsive children usually have compulsive parents, family group therapies are often successful.

Some clinicians and health care professionals are highly self-disciplined and have developed compulsive traits. In child treatment settings these professionals may struggle for control with children and other staff. It is important to avoid child-therapist trait matching because a nontherapeutic replication of child-parent patterns may follow.

AVOIDANT PERSONALITY DISORDERS

When under additional stress and conflict, children with avoidant personality disorders (Axis II) may show symptoms of a phobic and/or panic disorder. Avoidant personalities have a trait disorder that can be placed on a continuum with a state disorder, and under adverse conditions a personality disorder becomes a neurosis. Some experts claim that these children desire closeness with other people, but others suggest that an avoidant disorder of childhood is a continuation of early fears of strangers (Vaillant and Perry, 1985).

Clinical description.   Children with avoidant disorders are hypersensitive to rejection and usually have few peer and social relationships. These children are not antisocial or shy but require strong guarantees of uncritical and unconditional acceptance before they will venture into relationships. They often devalue themselves and their achievements and appear nervous and hesitant when talking with others, as if they were waiting for approval. They often have waiflike, pathetic qualities. Children with avoidant disorders are also compliant and ingratiating with adults.

DSM-III-R criteria.   There is a lack of consensus on the DSM-III-R location of the avoidant personality disorders and the suitability of this diagnosis for children. Some experts claim that this diagnosis is more aptly formulated within the Freudian framework of the phobic character. They also believe that the DSM-III-R criteria are not indicative of a clear mental disorder.

For children to be assigned a diagnosis of avoidant personality disorder, four of the following signs need to be present (Adams and Fras, 1988):

1. Absence of close friends or confidants outside of home
2. Easily hurt feelings from disapproval and criticism

3. Reluctance to interact with people that may not like them
4. Avoidance of activities that require more interaction
5. Fear of new experiences and of looking foolish
6. Fear of losing control of emotions or impulses
7. Exaggeration of the risks inherent in everyday activites

Nursing management.   The treatment of children with avoidant personality disorders is the same as the process for children with mild phobias. Interventions and planning include behavior and cognitive therapies focusing on reducing displacement symptoms.

PASSIVE-AGGRESSIVE PERSONALITY DISORDER

Children with passive-aggressive personality disorders express their interpersonal conflicts through retrogressive anger. The diagnostic term was first used by military psychiatrists during World War II to describe soldiers who were passive and indirect in their anger toward authority. Passive-aggressive personality traits are learned during early childhood and are most frequently found in adults and children who are placed in subordinate positions and view themselves as powerless to express themselves. Child-rearing patterns contribute significantly to the disorder. Although similar to dependent personality disorders, passive-aggressive disorders occur more often in females than in males.

Clinical description.   These children express indirect resistance to the demands of those in authority. They procrastinate, are stubborn, make promises they fail to keep, and are intentionally inefficient and forgetful. They may turn their anger inward and use the mechanisms of denial and rationalization.

The parents are typically assertive and aggressive. They punish and block their child's normal expression of assertiveness, causing the child to become outwardly polite and respectful. The child learns to punish their authoritarian parents with inefficient habits.

DSM-III-R criteria.   The DSM-III-R lists the following criteria for the diagnosis of passive-aggressive disorders in adults:
1. Resistance to demands for adequate performance in both occupational and social functioning
2. Resistance that is expressed indirectly through at least two of the following characteristics:
   a. Procrastination
   b. Dawdling actions
   c. Stubbornness
   d. Intentional inefficiency
   e. Forgetfulness
3. Pervasive and long-standing social and occupational ineffectiveness
4. Persistence of the behavior pattern even when more self-assertive and effective behavior is possible
5. Absence of criteria for other personality disorders and, if under the age of 18, absence of criteria for oppositional disorder

Five of the following criteria are needed to diagnose passive-aggressive personality disorders in children (Adams and Fras,. 1988):

1. Procrastination or dawdling actions so that deadlines remain unmet
2. Deliberately slow and incorrect work to avoid an unwanted task
3. Unjustifiable protestations that others make unreasonable demands on them
4. Avoidance of duties and responsibilities by claiming forgetfulness
5. Display of sulkiness and protestation with unwanted tasks
6. Overvaluation of their job performance
7. Resentment of cogent suggestions from others
8. Failure to do proper share of work to block the efforts of others
9. Display of unreasonable scornfulness toward authority

Nursing management. Because passive-aggressive children can manipulate unseasoned clinicians and often react with scorn to persons in authority, they require treatment with experienced staff. Strict limit setting using behavior modification techniques have been found useful. These children need additional help with learning constructive methods of expressing their feelings, and assertiveness training is of value. Because they have difficulties with interpersonal relationships, structured group experiences focusing on the development of social skills are indicated. Family therapy interventions reduce family members' reinforcement of these children's subversive response patterns.

SCHIZOID PERSONALITY DISORDERS

Schizoid personalities demonstrate isolating behaviors. Longitudinal studies of children show that their behavior traits are stable throughout life and not the precursors of psychotic disorders (Kety, 1985).

Clinical description. Children with schizoid personalities are indifferent to praise, criticism, or responses of others. Some run away from home at an early age because they find family ties uncomfortable. They are reserved, aloof, and solitary by preference. They express little affection or anger and seem absent-minded and intellectually limited. They are detached from their environment and avoid eye contact and spontaneous conversation. As these children approach puberty, they show little interest in the opposite sex. They may be highly effective and creative in work requiring little human contact and may have perceptual illusions, paranoid thoughts, magical thinking, and communication problems.

DSM-III-R criteria. The DSM-III-R specified that children or adults can be diagnosed as having both schizoid and schizotypal personality disorders. The behaviors listed by the DSM-III-R are similar to those the GAP (1966) used to describe the behaviors of the *isolated personality disorder:*

1. Little desire for or enjoyment of close relationships, including family ties
2. Preference for solitary activities
3. Lack of experience with anger or other deep emotions
4. Little if any desire to have sexual experiences
5. Indifferent to praise or criticism
6. Absense of or few friends or confidants other than household members
7. Constricted affect

Nursing management. The isolating and isolated behaviors of these children are the major areas of management concern. Treatment usually does not include antipsychotic drugs, and hospitalization is unnecessary and to be avoided if possible because institutional life may make them even more isolated and incompetent.

SCHIZOTYPAL DISORDERS

Schizotypal personalities are particularly mystifying. The usual history includes inherited limitations in brain functioning and child rearing in a family or environment that is cold, severe, and uncommunicative. Schizotypal children are often avoided by others, and because of few opportunities to develop social skills, they turn to fantasy and solitude.

Schizotypal personality disorder is a diagnosis rarely made for children, and the DSM-III-R criteria apply only to adults. Signs include bizarre behaviors and deficits in interpersonal relatedness, appearance, speech, behavior, and thinking. Children presenting these symptoms are usually diagnosed as having borderline disorders, schizophrenia, or autism.

The signs of schizotypal disorders often overlap with the symptoms of paranoid personality disorders. Both are thought to be genetically related to schizophrenia and are regarded as part of the schizophrenic spectrum. Few schizotypal children, however, develop schizophrenia.

Transference and Countertransference

Issues of transference and countertransference that develop during therapeutic work are especially difficult when the children involved have personality disorders. If transference and countertransference are ignored, they may restrict clinicians' efforts and limit or negate therapeutic process and progress.

Countertransference occurs when clinicians act out feelings toward clients that are unresolved characterologic or cultural conflicts or biases within themselves. These responses may or may not be induced by corresponding feelings in clients (Gorkin, 1987) but are often reactions to clients' efforts to sabotage relationships. They usually occur outside clinicians' conscious awareness.

The following suggestions and definitions are based on clinical work and the literature. They are a small sample of recent contributions to the clinical management of transference and countertransference issues found in the treatment of children with personality disorders (Basch-Kahre, 1984; Clegg, 1984; Lakovics, 1983; Robertiello and Schoenewold, 1987; Vaillant and Perry, 1985; Witherspoon, 1985):

1. A constructive approach to understanding the biologic bases of personality traits does not mean accepting the traits as solely genetic or denying the possibility of change and developments. Interventions need to be individually designed so that children can work within the parameters of their developmental stage, temperament, and the traits of the disorder. Provision of different opportunities, adjustment of limits, and frequent review facilitates reconditioning and relearning.
2. Clinicians should provide a model of mature behavior for children and parents and develop positive relationships without intellectually analyzing them. They need to convey concern, consideration, and respect.

3. Nurses should adopt a collaborative, sharing attitude about children's problems to improve communication.

4. Clinicians should encourage children to participate in group activities. When functioning as the group leader, they need to focus on alleviating children's feelings of isolation through use of the group process.

5. Children with some personality disorders have rigid personality structures, severe emotional deprivations, and lack of the motivation and social support systems that facilitate good treatment responses. The therapeutic milieu provides a corrective experience, and the skillful use of group process and peer pressures help alleviate these features.

6. Children with some personality disorders unconsciously attract others who reinforce their pathology. In the therapeutic milieu, peer associations need to be monitored and explored so that negative transference issues do not emerge among clients' peers.

7. The verbal and nonverbal messages of clinicians should not conflict.

8. Clinicians should focus on problem behavior and not ask for explanations for actions.

9. Clinicians should emphasize teaching and problem-solving skills and not interpretation or the development of insight. In some cases, confrontations and interpretations aggravate children's fears of abandonment or anger them.

10. Supportive interventions are essential for children to develop self-awareness, self-esteem, and accountability.

11. Instead of ignoring children's repetitious complaints, nurses need to convey that their behavior is not productive communication and explain ways in which others respond.

12. Contracts may be self-defeating because the expectations are often beyond children's capabilities at the time of treatment.

13. Because children with histrionic, narcissistic, and borderline personality disorders have traits that may result in self-destructive behaviors and aggressive acting out, clinicians should be nonrejecting and directly address their behavior. If aggressive actions occur, children need to be removed from the environment immediately and helped to regain self-control.

14. Acting out behaviors should be replaced by problem-solving strategies. Verbal communication assists children in depending less on nonverbal actions to express themselves and their needs.

15. Unless nurses identify unhealthy client maneuvers and design deliberate plans of intervention, they may become burned out from the emotional drain of reacting to behavior as if it were normal. Symptoms of countertransference in clinicians include being preoccupied with clients during leisure time, being late for meetings with them, and experiencing uneasy feelings during and after meetings.

16. Clinicians should not feel shame or discomfort when they are fooled by manipulative children. Unless they view the behaviors associated with personality disorders as pathologic, they will be unprepared for some children's actions.

17. In negative transference, children usually express their hostility verbally and nonverbally. Milieu and group experiences moderate the intensity of relationship work and lessen the possibility of transference.
18. Outpatient treatment of children with personality disorders may be complicated by their dependency on food or drugs or by the social and legal implications of their disorders.
19. Parents respond better to their child's treatment when they participate concurrently in a peer-group therapy designed for adults with related parenting issues, for example, Weight Watchers, Compulsives Anonymous, Gamblers Anonymous, and Parent Abuser.
20. Personality disorders may coexist with other psychopathology and may decompensate to psychosis. Personality states are also noted on Axis IV as adjustment disorders linked to life stress, occurring within 3 months of the life event. When children have an intermittent episode in which their personality traits become inflexible, rigid, and maladaptive, they are considered to have a personality disorder.
21. The DSM-III-R multiaxial system provides clinicians with concise information on the mutual influence and interactions of personality traits and mental disorders. Axis II guides the planning of care specific to personality traits, tracks developmental progress and changes, and uses characteristic behavior styles to accomplish goals.

REFERENCES

Adams PL and Fras I: Beginning child psychiatry, New York, 1988, Brunner/Mazel, Inc.

Adler G: Valuing and devaluing in the psychotherapeutic process, Arch Gen Psychiatry 22:454, 1974.

American Psychiatric Association: Diagnostic and statistical manual of mental disorders, ed 3, rev, Washington, DC, 1987, American Psychiatric Association.

Bandura A, Underwood B, and Fromson ME: Disinhibition of aggression through diffusion of responsibility and dehumanization of victims, J Res Pers 9:253, 1975.

Basch-Kahre E: On difficulties arising in transference and countertransference when analyst and analysand have different sociocultural backgrounds, Int Rev Psychoanal 11:61, 1984.

Chitty KK and Maynard CK: Managing manipulation, J Psychosoc Nurs Ment Health Serv 24:8, 1986.

Clegg HG: The reparative motif in child and adult therapy, Northvale, NJ, 1984, Jason Aronson, Inc.

Coltranne F and Pugh C: Danger signals in staff/patient relationships in a therapeutic milieu, J Psychosoc Nurs Ment Health Serv 16:34, 1979.

Costa PT and McCrae RR: Still stable after all these years: personality as a key to some issues in adulthood and old age. In Baltes PB and Brim OG, editors: Life-span development and behavior, vol 3, New York, 1980, Academic Press, Inc.

Duldt BW: Anger: an occupational hazard for nurses, Nurs Outlook 29:510, 1981.

Gardner RW and Momarita A: Personality development at preadolescence, Seattle, 1986, University of Washington Press.

Goldstein W: Current dynamic thinking regarding the diagnoses of the borderline patient, Am J Psychother 61:4, 1987.

Gorkin M: The uses of countertransference, Northvale, NJ, 1987, Jason Aronson, Inc.

Group for the Advancement of Psychiatry: Psychopathological disorders in childhood: theoretical considerations and a proposed classification, Rep No 62, New York, 1965, Brunner/Mazel, Inc.

Gunderson JG and Englishwoman DW: Characterizing the families of borderlines, Psychiatr Clin North Am 4:159, 1981.

Gunderson JG, Kerr J, and Eglund DW: The families of borderlines: a comparative study, Arch Gen Psychiatry 37:27, 1980.

Harvard Medical School Mental Health Letter: Personality and personality disorders, part I, Harvard Medical School Mental Health Letter 4:1, 1987.

Kaffman M: Paranoid disorders: the core of truth behind the delusional system, Int J Fam Ther 3:29, 1981.

Kaplan B and Sadock J, editors: Comprehensive textbook on psychiatry IV, vol 1, Baltimore, 1985, Williams & Wilkins.

Katan A: The role of displacement in agoraphobia, Int J Psychoanal 32:41, 1937.

Kernberg O: Borderline conditions and pathological narcissism, Northvale, NJ, 1975, Jason Aronson, Inc.

Kety S: Schizotypal personality disorders: an operational definition of Bleuler's latent schizophrenia? Schizophr Bull 11:590, 1985.

Kohut H: The analysis of self: a systematic approach to the treatment of narcissistic personality disorders, New York, 1971, International Universities Press, Inc.

Lakovics M: Classification of countertransference for utilization in supervision, Am J Psychother 37:245, 1983.

Lazare A, Klernman G, and Armor D: Oral, obsession and hysterical personality patterns: an investigation of psychoanalytic concepts by means of factor analysis, Arch Gen Psychiatry 14:624, 1966.

Mahler MA: Study of the separation-individuation process and its possible application to borderline phenomena in the psychoanalytic situation, Psychoanal Study Child 26:404, 1971.

Mahler MS and Kaplan L: Developmental aspects in the assessment of narcissistic and so-called borderline personalities. In Hartocollis P, editor: Borderline personality disorder: the concept, the syndrome, the patient, New York, 1977, International Universities Press, Inc.

Mark B: Hospital treatment of borderline patients: toward a better understanding of problematic issues, J Psychosoc Nurs Ment Health Serv 18:25, 1980.

Meloy JR: The psychopathic mind: origins, dynamics and treatment, Northvale, NJ, 1988, Jason Aronson, Inc.

Million T: Disorders of personality, New York, 1981, John Wiley & Sons, Inc.

Nyman G: Infant temperament, childhood accidents and hospitalization. In Chess S, Thomas A, and Hertzig ME, editors: Annual progress in child psychiatry and child development, New York, 1988, Brunner/Mazel, Inc.

Policoff SP: Bottle babies, Ladies Home Journal, p 183, May 1989.

Robertiello RC and Schoenewold G: 101 common therapeutic blunders: countertransference and counterresistance in psychotherapy, Northvale, NJ, 1987, Jason Aronson, Inc.

Ross N: The "as if" personality, J Am Psychoanal Assoc 12:59, 1967.

Rutter M: Temperament, personality and personality disorders, Br J Psychiatry 18:46, 1987.

Sarnoff C: Latency, New York, 1976, Jason Aronson, Inc.

Satinover J: Jung's lost contribution to the dilemma of narcissism, J Am Psychoanal Assoc 34:4014, 1986.

Schacter D: On the relationship between genuine and simulated amnesia, Behav Sci Law 4:47, 1986.

Schneider J: Hopelessness and helplessness, J Psychosoc Nurs Ment Health Serv 18:12, 1980.

Sederer LI and Thorbeck J: First do no harm: short term inpatient psychotherapy of the borderline patient, Hosp Community Psychiatry 37:692, 1984.

Serban G: The tyranny of magical thinking: the child's world of belief and adult neurosis, New York, 1982, EP Dutton.

Siever LJ and Gunderson JG: Genetic determinants of borderline conditions, Schizophr Bull 5:59, 1979.

Svrakic D: Emotional features of narcissistic personality disorder, Am J Psychiatry 142:720, 1985.

Vaillant GE: Sociopathy as a human process, Arch Gen Psychiatry 32:178, 1975.

Vaillant GE and Perry JC: Personality disorders. In Kaplan H and Sadock B, editors: Comprehensive textbook of psychiatry, ed 4, vol 1, Baltimore, 1985, Williams & Wilkins.

Widiger TA and others: The DSM-III-R personality disorders: an overview, Am J Psychiatry 145:786, 1987.

Witherspoon V: Using Lakovic's system: countertransference classifications, J Psychosoc Nurs Ment Health Serv 23:30, 1985.

Woosley D: A working concept of intellectualization, J Psychosoc Nurs Ment Health Serv 18:36, 1980.

Chapter 9

Disruptive Behavior Disorders of Early Childhood

Oppositional defiant, conduct, and attention-deficit hyperactivity disorders are categorized under disruptive behavior disorders in the DSM-III-R. Children with these disorders exhibit socially disruptive behaviors that are usually more distressing to others than to them. In contrast to parents' and teachers' reports and concerns, most of these children see themselves as victims of circumstances and do not view their behavior as oppositional, defiant, or noncompliant. Some authorities stress that disruptive behavior disorders are influenced by social and political factors because the appraisals and diagnoses of these children are usually based on moral evaluations by parents and teachers (Adams and Fras, 1988).

Statistics indicate that as many as 75% of children with attention-deficit hyperactivity disorders also have conduct disorder problems (Safer and Allen, 1976). The shared symptoms and concurrent incidence of these disorders led some experts to suggest that hyperactivity is the necessary ingredient for children to display severe conduct disorders (McMahon and Forehand, 1988).

Children with disruptive behavior problems are referred to mental health and child guidance centers more frequently than children with any other psychiatric diagnosis. Estimates are that over 50% of the children seen in mental health care settings have disruptive behavior disorders, reflecting the predominance of literature addressing the disease.

Disruptive children are usually referred because their behaviors cannot be controlled by parents or significant others. The chief complaints include: (1) aggressiveness toward others, for example, hitting, kicking, and fighting; physical destructiveness; disobedience; and temper tantrums; (2) a high rate of annoying behaviors, such as yelling, whining, and being verbally threatening; and (3) violations of community rules, for example, stealing and fire setting. Behaviors seldom occur in isolation but form patterns that have been labeled as *oppositional, noncompliant, defiant, aggressive, delinquent,* and, most recently, *conduct disordered* activities.

The problems are seen more often in boys than in girls, with ratios ranging from 4 to 1 to 12 to 1 (American Psychiatric Association, 1987). Developmental studies comparing children with nonproblematic behaviors with children referred because of their disruptive behaviors show that almost all children, referred and nonreferred, exhibit disruptive behavior at some point during their early childhood years (Patterson, 1982).

Referral usually occurs when children who have argued, demanded attention, teased, and been impulsive during the early home years enter kindergarten or preschool programs requiring a structured, sustained attention span and impulse control. Although parents have coped with the behaviors, teachers or other adults in the community perceive a problem and urge the parents to seek professional counseling.

The usual age of onset of the disorders is between 4 and 6 years of age, the time when children enter school. The number of children presenting disruptive behavior problems declines in older age groups. If untreated, children often exhibit similar patterns of behavior into adolescence, and the likelihood of delinquent and criminal behaviors also increases. As adults, they are at increased risk for psychiatric impairments, such as antisocial personality disorders, poor occupational adjustment, low educational attainment, marital disruptions, and poor physical health (Kazdin, 1985).

The severity of adult outcomes, the frequency of conduct disorders occurring with other childhood mental and physical health problems, and the many referrals for young conduct-disordered children emphasize the need for nurse clinicians to become highly proficient in this area. Nurses need to evaluate the degree of severity of the behavior and the appropriate interventions, instruct and enlist parents and teachers in planning and management, therapeutically intervene in the direct care of children when appropriate, and recognize the indications for more sophisticated interventions and medications. The short-term goal of care is to alleviate children's immediate difficulties, and preventing juvenile and adolescent delinquency and adjustment problems is the long-range aim of treatment.

Conduct Disorders

DEFINITIONS AND CONCEPTS

Historically, classification systems for childhood conduct disorders organized problem behaviors into patterns or distinctive clusters and were combined with childhood problems of crime and antisocial behaviors, resulting in diverse explanations and management techniques that have been disputed in juvenile delinquency and child psychology literature. Despite these disagreements, there is a strong consensus among all disciplines that conduct disorders during childhood are the precursors to later delinquency.

The developmental progression from minor antisocial behavior to the more serious antisocial behaviors is unknown. Scientists also do not know which childhood disruptive behavior patterns have the most serious prognosis. These unresolved issues are similar to the gray areas among the legal and psychiatric systems affecting adults whose antisocial behaviors violate community rules (Lewis and others, 1985).

The GAP committee on child psychiatry published a series of historically significant monographs addressing diagnostic and treatment issues with conduct-disordered children (1957, 1966, and 1982). Of these monographs, the 1966 GAP classification system was most strongly criticized for its use of psychoanalytic concepts and terms and its exclusion of concepts and terms from the behavioral and social sciences. Critics also noted its failure to reflect the traditionally held social expectations of values for children. For example, childhood oppositional defiant disorders were compared with the passive-aggressive personality syndrome seen in adults even though society expects children to obey their parents.

Drawing on the previous GAP monographs, the DSM-III (American Psychiatric Association, 1980) included two categories of childhood behavior disorders: conduct and oppositional. Conduct disorders involved aggressive-nonaggressive and socialized-undersocialized dimensions. The aggressive aspect was labeled by some researchers as *overt antisocial behaviors* and included children's actions that violated the rights of others, such as physical violence against people or property. The nonaggressive dimension included behaviors labeled *covert antisocial behaviors* and included actions that did not involve confrontations with others and were nonviolent, such as truancy, lying, stealing, and, in older children, substance abuse (Loeber and Schmaling, 1985).

The socialized dimension indicated children's degree of social attachment to others; the undersocialized dimension expressed children's failure to establish empathy or affection with others. According to the DSM-III, oppositional children were disobedient and stubborn and violated minor rules, displayed tantrums, and showed insolence. These dimensions were found unsatisfactory when clinically tested. The low reliability and validity found in clinical studies led some critics to stress that the DSM-III dimensions had little basis or support in clinical practice.

To address these concerns, the DSM-III-R replaced the subtypes based on aggressive-nonaggressive and socialized-undersocialized dimensions with three different dimensions: (1) solitary aggressive, which corresponds to the DSM-III subtype of undersocialized aggressive; (2) group, which approximates the DSM-III socialized nonaggressive conduct problems occurring mainly as a group activity with peers; and (3) undifferentiated, a diagnosis of conduct disorders for children whose pattern of behavior does not fit into either of the other two subtypes.

The DSM-III definition and classification of oppositional disorders has been subsumed by the conduct disorder diagnoses in the DSM-III-R. The essential features of oppositional defiant disorders is a "pattern of negativistic, hostile and defiant behavior without the more serious violations of basic rights of others that are seen in conduct disorders" (American Psychiatric Association, 1987). Definitions of conduct and oppositional defiant disorders are based on the severity and number of different behaviors displayed. The category of pervasive developmental disorders is a broad classification of severe disorders that affect children's social skills, language, attention, perception, reality testing, and motor activity.

Some behavioral psychologists object to the DSM-III-R system because of insufficient clinical or research evidence for separating oppositional and conduct disorders (Wells and Forehand, 1985). Reviews of the extensive empirical behavioral science studies performed on children with conduct disorders and statistical findings using factor and path analyses procedures demonstrate differences between research findings and clinical practice experiences. Clinicians need to be alert to methodologic flaws in many studies (Adams and Fras, 1988). Kaplan and Sadock (1985) give more credence to clinical findings than to most organized studies.

Antisocial Behaviors

1. Fights	6. Uncooperative	11. Irritable
2. Temper tantrums	7. Disruptive	12. Attention seeking
3. Disobedient	8. Negative	13. Dominates others
4. Destructive	9. Restless	14. Lies
5. Impertinent	10. Boisterous	15. Steals

Recent findings suggest that the dimensions of behavior are relatively independent of one another and that within each dimension, behaviors are highly related. Researchers believe that oppositional and conduct disorders represent end points of a single dimension of antisocial behaviors. Covert behaviors, such as truancy and stealing, are at one pole, and overt behaviors, such as temper tantrums, screaming, and demanding and impulsive actions, fall at the other end. It has been suggested that noncompliance should be the midpoint on this dimension conceptualization because it is seen as the keystone behavior that links covert and overt behaviors. Clinical studies show that noncompliance differs between the two end points.

Fifteen behaviors were statistically identified and placed on a continuum (see box). They involve direct confrontation or disruption of the environment and are similar to the overt and covert antisocial behaviors found in earlier editions of the DSM (Quay and Petterson, 1983).

THEORETIC EXPLANATIONS

During the 1970s many people claimed that the psychiatric diagnoses of conduct disorders and hyperactivity were artificial models constructed by inadequate parents, teachers who were intolerant of normal child exuberance, and professionals unable to find scientific evidence for these problems. This myth gained considerable acceptance through lay publications that attributed conduct disorders and hyperactivity to factors ranging from food dyes to stimulating colors in children's environments. Adult intolerance, however, cannot account for the physical, behavioral, and social differences demonstrated between conduct-disordered and normal children.

When referred children do not present the necessary behavior for a conduct disordered diagnosis, parental misperceptions of the problem are usually due to their own anxiety, distress, or depression. For example, maternal depression and child noncompliance have been found to be highly correlated. In these cases, clinicians need to help parents accept the need for counseling for their depression and emotional distress.

More frequently, parents underestimate the severity of their child's behavior and the need for professional help. They deny the precariousness of the behavior and wait for the child to "grow out of it." Children are brought for help when their behavior has caused a crisis with peers or the community.

The first signs of oppositional behaviors appear between the ages of 18 and 36 months. According to most theories of psychosexual development, they are part of normal development for this stage and phase. Children are expected to demonstrate and experience considerable parental conflicts and difficulties as autonomy emerges and power struggles predominate.

Most authorities agree that biologic and genetic influences in the form of temperament predispose children to many behavior problems (Chess and Thomas, 1984, 1986). Of special interest are the children who exhibit intense, irregular, negative, and nonadaptive temperaments from birth, often leading to maladaptive parent-child interactions. The parents usually provide negative reinforcement, which escalates and maintains the coercive behaviors.

Psychoanalytic theories emphasize separation-individuation, trait, and temperament theories. Social bonding theories reinforce this perspective by claiming that the ability to form intimate, mutually enjoyable, and enduring relationships with others is established during early infant-mother interactions (Reid, Hinojosa-Rivera, and Lorber, 1981). Failure to establish affection, empathy, and bonding is a criteria for conduct disorders. The positive signs of bonding include the following:

1. Existence of one or more peer group friendships with a duration of at least 6 months
2. Extension of self to others when no immediate advantage is likely
3. Feelings of guilt or remorse if a reaction is inappropriate
4. Avoidance of blaming or informing on companions
5. Concern for the welfare for friends

Achenback and Edelbrock (1983) have proposed a developmental model based on the empirically derived conduct-disorder dimension (Table 9-1). This model identifies a hierarchical progression of conduct disorders through oppositional, offensive, aggressive, and delinquent developmental stages. The sequence progresses from overt to covert actions, minor to more serious disruptive behaviors, and parents and home to school and community. Earlier behaviors do not disappear but continue as the hierarchy of more complex patterns develop.

Family characteristics and parenting behaviors are frequently cited as etiologic factors. Epidemiologic studies show that parents of children with conduct disorders have more marital and personal problems, antisocial personalities, and alcohol dependency than the general population.

Parenting behaviors, especially those of the mother, have been studied extensively and are considered as the basis for many conduct disorders by experts. Longitudinal, comparative behavioral studies of nonreferred and referred conduct-disordered children and parents were conducted using parent, peer, and teacher interviews; parent and child self-reports; and sociometric studies and observations of children in various settings (Patterson and Blank, 1984; Patterson and Stouthamer-Loeber, 1984). Researchers added two constructs describing parenting behaviors to their model that supplemented previous research: inept parental discipline and monitoring. Inept discipline occurs when parents fail to carry out discipline, nag their child about trivial and significant deviant behaviors, and use extreme forms of physical punishment. Monitoring refers to parents' failure to be aware of or to believe reports of their child's conduct-disordered behaviors.

Some parental behaviors may reinforce noncompliance in conduct-disordered children. Studies have shown that these parents are more commanding and critical, use poor disciplinary measures, and inadequately monitor their school-age child's

Table 9-1   Developmental Progression of Conduct-Disordered Behaviors

Stage	Behavior
Oppositional	Presence of arguments; boastful speech; attention-seeking behavior; disobedience at home; impulsiveness; temper tantrums; stubbornness; teasing actions; loudness
Offensive	Presence of cruelty; disobedience at school; screams; poor peer relationships; fights; sulkiness; obscenity; dishonesty
Aggressive	Presence of destructiveness; threats; attacks; maladaptive friends; larceny at home
Delinquent	Presence of arson; larceny outside the home; alcohol/drug use; truancy; running away; vandalism

Modified from Achenback TM and Edelbrock CS: Manual for the child behavior checklist and revised child behavior profile, Burlington, Vt, 1983, University of Vermont.

activities (Patterson and Blank, 1984). They monitor their younger children with less concern than they supervise their adolescent children. Parents in these families also manage the children differently. Fathers usually take a secondary role and manage the children less than fathers of nonreferred children (Patterson and Stouthamer-Loeber, 1984).

The parents experience more depression anxiety, marital conflict, and stressful events than parents of children without conduct-disordered behaviors. Marital distress often leads to rejecting the children, which is more frequently directed at boys than at girls (Rutter, 1970). They are isolated from and dissatisfied with friends, neighbors, and the community. Family interactions with relatives and helping agencies are negatively perceived, and the level of positively perceived support from friends is low. Their depression and anxieties are associated with misperceptions of their child's behavior.

CLINICAL DESCRIPTION

Some clinical distinctions between normal and conduct-disordered children include the following:
1. Family interactions: Children with disordered conduct behaviors have more adverse behaviors in family interaction contexts.
2. Peer interactions: Children with disordered conduct behaviors demonstrate adverse behaviors with their peers. They were less socially competent than other children and more likely to be rejected.
3. Cognitive distortions: Children with conduct disorders misread hostile intentions in others. Aggressive children distort social cues in interactions and perceive others (including family members) to have hostile intentions for them.

4. Social problem-solving skills: Aggressive children are deficient in social problem-solving skills and value aggressive interpersonal styles. They are also less empathetic than nonaggressive children (Lamb, 1982).
5. Depression: The relationship of depressions and conduct disorders is much higher in boys than in girls (McMahon and Forehand, 1988).
6. Academic achievement: Children with conduct disorders have poorer academic achievement than their counterparts starting from the elementary grades. Low academic performance and repeating a grade occurred three times as often in children with behavior disorders than in matched control groups. Reading disabilities are highly associated with conduct disorders.

DSM-III-R CRITERIA

Suggestions for unifying oppositional defiant and conduct disorders into a single diagnosis illustrate the need for extreme care in diagnostic formulations. The revised DSM-III-R category for conduct disorders represents a major effort to correct the past problem of clinicians using conduct disorders as a blanket diagnosis. The new criteria and descriptions isolate the more serious juvenile delinquent behaviors from behaviors that are more socially acceptable and useful.

Random acts of conduct disorder are not sufficient for the application of the diagnosis and should be coded as antisocial behavior. The DSM-III-R definition stresses that repetitive, persistent patterns of behavior are to be of at least 6-months duration. The basic rights of others and major age-appropriate societal rules are violated.

Two elements combine the components of aggression and socialization and are found in all conduct disorders: lack of empathy, varying in amount or degree, and the inability to comply with society and its demands for inner values and outward conduct. Indicators of the absence (undersocialization) of adequate social empathy, bonding, and attachment include superficial peer relations, ego centricism, manipulation, lack of concern for others, and lack of guilt and remorse. Attachment bonds are judged on peer group friendships, the ability to extend self for others, degree of guilt feelings, loyalty for companions, and concern for other's welfare. If only one of these characteristics is present, the undersocialized subtype diagnosis is appropriate.

Conduct disorders are present in 9% of males and 2% of females in the general population (American Psychiatric Association, 1987). The age of onset varies but usually occurs at prepuberty in girls with the solitary aggressive group type. Early onset is a poor prognostic indicator. Although milder forms of these disorders may resolve with maturity, the more severe forms often become chronic when children are untreated. The group type of disorder has the best prognostic outcome; however, children's antisocial behaviors usually persist into adulthood and take the form of illegal activity. Conduct disorders in children somewhat correspond to antisocial and borderline disorders in adults.

OPPOSITIONAL DEFIANT DISORDERS

The important distinction between oppositional defiant disorders and conduct disorders is that although both feature disobedience and opposition to authority figures, children with conduct disorders violate the rights of others and children with oppositional defiant disorders do not. These children are disobedient, defiant, negativistic, angry, and aggressive in their opposition to adults (Adams and Fras, 1988). The case example illustrates the typical behavior of an oppositional defiant disorder.

Case Example

For the past year the client, a 12-year-old boy, has been irritable and vindictive and seems to deliberately annoy others. For example, he taunts his siblings and classmates even when parents or teachers are present. He argues, often hotly, with his parents and teachers and has such an unreasonable temper that he has been thrown off the baseball team (a favorite activity) for fighting and talking back to the coach. Everyone agrees that his behavior is well outside the range of adolescent turmoil and annoyance seen in other boys of his age and development.

He seems uncomfortable at times but does not meet the criteria for a mood disorder. His school performance is good when he applies himself, and there are no prodromal signs of a psychotic disorder. He is not particularly cruel (except verbally) and has not run away from home; broken into, stolen, or destroyed property; or used weapons in any of his several fights.

Modified from Spitzer RL and others: A psychiatrist's casebook: the DSM–III casebook, Washington, DC, 1986, American Psychiatric Press.

The usual age of onset is approximately 8 years of age. The course of the disorder is unknown. If it appears before puberty, it is usually more common in males than in females.

Irritability, hypomania, and antisocial behaviors are also seen in bipolar disorders of children and may be early signs of schizophrenia and/or the major depressive disorders. Attention deficit hyperactivity and specific developmental disorders are other problems commonly associated with an oppositional defiant disorder, which may progress to a conduct disorder (axis I) of childhood or to a passive-aggressive or antisocial disorder (axis II) of adulthood. For the diagnosis of oppositional defiant disorder the DSM-III-R requires that at least five of the following behaviors be present (Adams and Fras, 1988).
1. Frequent loss of temper
2. Frequent arguments with adults
3. Active defiance or refusal of adult requests or rules
4. Frequent deliberately annoying actions
5. Frequent displays of blaming others for own mistakes
6. Frequent irritability
7. Anger and resentfulness
8. Spitefulness or vindictiveness
9. Frequent use of obscene language

The severity of an oppositional defiant disorder depends on the number of symptoms present and the amount of poor functioning. The mild classification is applied when the minimum or slightly more than minimum number of symptoms are present, and there is little or no impairment in school and social functioning. Children are diagnosed as moderate when the symptom or functional impairment is intermediate between the mild and severe categories, in which many more criteria than are necessary to make the diagnosis are present, and significant and pervasive impairment in functioning at home and school and with other adults and peers occurs (American Psychiatric Association, 1987).

Nursing management.   Treatment planning is based on children's symptoms and predominating behaviors. Most interventions include a combination of behavioral, emotional cognitive, and family group therapies, and it is essential to involve the family, teachers, and other significant adults in treatment plans.

Because problem behaviors appear predominantly in interactions with well-known adults and peers, nurses may not observe many disruptive behaviors during the initial screening. Several assessment interviews need to be conducted, and psychologic and behavioral scales need to be used.

When working with children with conduct disorders, clinicians should not inadvertently reinforce noncompliant behaviors by giving attention to negative actions during behavior therapy. When emotive-cognitive interventions are used, clinicians need to focus on parenting, comforting, attachment, teaching, and advocacy.

Discipline and consistent external controls are the most important aspects of working with children with conduct disorders, and parents' collaboration is essential. Fostering children's self-control is also important, and changes and growth can be measured against the context of responses to adult/parental authority.

Children with undersocialized and aggressive conduct disorders have the poorest prognosis as compared to clients with other conduct disorders. They respond best to long-term, high-quality residential treatment settings that provide structure, support, and identification by an interdisciplinary team. Unfortunately, residential care is expensive, and children from families that cannot afford long-term treatment are often channeled into correctional settings or are cared for in outpatient community mental health agencies.

When children are treated in outpatient settings, including parents and teachers in the planned interventions is essential. Parents need to be taught ways in which their child can learn more effective self-management behaviors. Because preventing difficult behavior is easier than punishing it, the most effective discipline training includes preventive techniques. Clinicians' relationship with children should be based on identification with their healthier ego, and traditional analyzing techniques should be avoided because they often cause acting out and may worsen the disorder.

Children with undersocialized and nonaggressive conduct disorders often present devious behaviors that may frustrate unseasoned therapists. They are often exploitive of others; thus their family and peer relationships need to be carefully monitored. As a group, they have been found to be less physically robust, which may explain the reason they handle their anger by devious revenge (Adams and Fras, 1988). These children usually respond well to reality therapy, behavior modification, and family therapies. Experienced clinicians with special training are best qualified to work with these children, especially if clients and their family are outpatients.

Children with socialized nonaggressive diagnoses are more socially aware and responsive and thus have better prognoses than children with aggressive conduct disorders. They are less self-centered, and their ability to relate to others results in a high rehabilitation potential. With long-term psychotherapy, they can learn to outgrow antisocial relationships and replace them with different, constructive interactions.

Clinical specialists who are imaginative and patient are best suited to working with children with conduct disorders. However, fears that children will continue in their nonfunctional patterns are common, and mentor and peer supervisory support is highly recommended.

Attention Deficit Disorder with Hyperactivity

DEFINITIONS AND CONCEPTS

Research has provided remarkable insights into the understanding and treatment of hyperactive children. The associated disorder is referred to as *attention deficit disorder with hyperactivity* (ADHD), and it is one of the most studied and most frequently seen childhood disorders.

The main features of ADHD are distractibility and the inability to contain stimuli, resulting in children's excessive and random movements and short attention span (Adams and Fras, 1988). Developmentally inappropriate degrees of inattention, increased gross motor activity, impulsive, careless performance, excessive running or climbing, low self-esteem, mood lability, low frustration tolerance, and temper outbursts are also common characteristics. Most definitions of the disorder emphasize the triad of developmentally inappropriate behaviors: inattention, impulsiveness, and hyperactivity. Symptoms cannot be uncovered in laboratory tests, and diagnoses must be made from the reports of parents and teachers. ADHD is not a uniform concept but requires the same care and multiple assessment measures used for screening conduct-disordered children.

ADHD was first described in 1902 as *volitional inhibition,* that is, defects in moral control. During the past 90 years, hyperactivity has been renamed more than 20 times (Barkley, 1981). The most recent DSM-III-R term reflects the general consensus of scientists that the major deficiency in hyperactive children is their attention problems. Descriptive terms such as *hyperactive, hyperkinesis syndrome,* and *minimal brain damage* found in the past literature are confusing and imprecise; however, hyperactivity, hyperkinesis, and attention deficit disorder continue to be used interchangeably in most contemporary writings. Some scientists use *hyperactivity* to describe activity level problems and the latter two terms to characterize associated symptoms.

THEORETIC EXPLANATIONS

Since the first writings describing hyperactivity in the 1900s, neurologic factors have been postulated as a cause for hyperactivity. The similarity between the behaviors of children with ADHD and children suffering from brain injuries have been attributed to the same organic factors. Children who were overactive, distractible, inattentive, and impulsive were diagnosed as having brain injury, even in the absence of laboratory evidence or history of brain injury. The popular diagnoses of minimal brain damage (MBD) and minimal brain dysfunction implied an underlying brain impairment that was based on evaluations of children's behaviors by parents and teachers.

The neurophysiologic mechanisms responsible for MBD could not be found, and the theory was discarded. Statistics indicated that less than 5% of children with ADHD have identifiable organic changes (Rutter, 1984).

Research seeking organic explanations for childhood overactivity continued. During the 1960s the focus shifted to measuring the motor degree, level, and frequency of activity levels. Cumulative findings indicated that other behavior problems such as attention deficits and poor impulse control coexisted with overactivity, broadening the concept to a syndrome.

The primary behavior symptoms appearing in the literature during the 1970s and the diagnostic term of *hyperkinetic reaction of childhood* from the DSM-III were changed to the label of *attention deficit disorders*. Genetic theories of hyperactivity were popular explanations that replaced the earlier notion of undefinable yet present MBD. For example, research on the personality or temperament traits of parents of hyperactive children showed impulsiveness, poor judgment, and sociopathy were more common than in the parents of normal children. On-going twin and adoption studies strongly support these genotype factor influences.

Maturation or developmental lags have also been studied as etiologic factors contributing to hyperactivity. *Lag* refers to children's nervous system not developing according to the expected norm. This biologic dysmaturation is not global and affects some areas more than others. For example, gross motor development may be normal while fine motor coordination and perception are not. When these children are tested, there is a "scattering" of results, identifying areas of delay.

Other biologic factors are associated with the prenatal period. These intrauterine damages include congenital anomalies, intrauterine subclinical lead poisoning, cigarette smoking, and maternal alcoholism and drug abuse. Allergies, intolerance of dyes, and sugar tolerances are other physical responses that have been viewed as causative factors for hyperactivity. To date, no systematic studies have definitively supported these various biologic hypotheses.

Two contrasting physiologic theories with strong research evidence have changed thinking about hyperactivity during the last 40 years. In the 1950s, Laufer, Denhoff, and Solomons (1957) suggested the following biochemical explanation: The center of the brain stem (the reticular activating system) is the central controller of all sensory input. In hyperactive children, excitatory and inhibitory neurons are biochemically inadequate to function, and overactivity is a result of deficient quantities of these neural transmitters that lower stimuli thresholds. Although no general agreement as to which neural transmitter is most instrumental has been reached, dopamine has been implicated most often. According to this model, amphetamines increase the synaptic conduction time, which raises the stimulus barrier and calms hyperactive children. Psychostimulants also increase cortical control over the highly disorganized brain stem activity, improving purposeful behavior and the attention span. This theory gains additional support because of the reactions of ADHD children to phenobarbital, a drug that suppresses cortical activity and, instead of sedating them, makes them more hyperactive (see Chapter 16).

Scatterfield, Satterfield, and Cantwell (1981) presented a contrasting model, hypothesizing that a lowered excitability in the midbrain reticular activating system is present, requiring more stimulation. Hyperactivity results from *stimulus hunger,* and an impressive body of research supports their theory.

Biologic explanations are currently the most widely accepted explanations for hyperactivity. The following factors may contribute to the diagnosis of ADHD:

1. Prematurity
2. Signs of fetal distress
3. Precipitated or prolonged labor
4. Perinatal asphyxia and low Apgar scores
5. Feeding and sleeping difficulties during the first few weeks of life
6. Presence of colic at 3 months of age
7. History of brain damage or injury to the central nervous system from trauma or infections, cerebral palsy, or neurologic disorders
8. Family history demonstrating alcoholism, hysteria, and sociopathy; parental history of hyperactivity; learning disabilities, and developmental learning disorders and/or impulse control problems.

Other theorists claim that hyperactivity evolves from the neurophysiologic substrate and is reinforced by the reciprocal interaction of children with their social environment. According to this substratum theory, behavior symptoms are secondary and are due to immature, primitive, erratic behaviors. Conflicts with peers and adults result from children's distractibility and poor interpretation of their interpersonal world.

Most psychologic explanations for hyperactivity focus on a social-learning framework. Some attribute hyperactivity of childhood to *conditioned lifestyle hyperactivity,* a theory positing that children's interaction patterns with significant adults produce the signs of the disorder. Children's direct imitation of parental actions and reactions and parental conditioning are contributing factors. Children's attributes of introspection and delayed gratification are suppressed by selective inattention. Quick action is rewarded and becomes necessary for emotional survival.

CLINICAL DESCRIPTION

ADHD involves all the symptoms of oppositional defiant disorder, conduct disorder, and other specific developmental disorders. Nonlocalized neurologic soft signs and motor perceptual dysfunctions, such as poor eye-hand coordination, may be present.

According to the current DSM-III-R criteria, hyperactivity is found in approximately 3% of children in the general population and occurs 6 to 9 times more often in males than in females. The age of onset is before the age of 7, usually at 3 or 4 years of age when children enter kindergarten or preschool. The behaviors must be present for at least 6 months for the diagnosis, and symptoms include distractibility, inability to contain stimuli, random movements, short attention span, developmentally inappropriate inattention, impulsiveness, hyperactivity, and immaturity.

Children's impulsiveness and angry outbursts usually interfere with interpersonal relationships and may result in guilt, self-hate, helplessness, feelings of inadequacy, and low self-esteem. Antisocial acts that defy authority are frequent. Hyperactive children are easily led to membership in gangs, where they find the structure they need, as well as acceptance and spirit of adventure. Stealing, fighting, truancy, and drug and alcohol abuse are found more often in ADHD child than in children in the general population.

If untreated, their traits of immaturity continue into adolescence, manifesting as superficiality, poor judgment based on concreteness, need for immediate gratification, and poor impulse control. As adults, females are prone to hysteria and males to antisocial personality; both sexes are at greater risk for alcoholism and drug abuse. The prognosis depends on psychosocial conditions, such as the family and school providing the appropriate structure, support, and motivation. Children from stressful environments have poorer prognoses. Physical violence, repeated arson, and cruelty to animals are often reported.

There is considerable controversy about whether the incidence of hyperactivity is increasing. Some writers claim that the higher rate results from improved detection in contemporary society, due to more comprehensive preschool screening programs, greater dissemination of information about hyperactivity to professionals and parents, and an increased awareness in the general population about developmental and psychiatric conditions. Sophisticated medical neonatal technology and more effective life-saving techniques for endangered infants who develop disorders from residual deficits has also increased the rate. Others claim that the incidence has actually increased because of the greater number of dysfunctional families, increased environmental pollutants, permissive child-rearing practices, and poor nutritional habits.

In contrast, the life histories of many highly successful and creative people demonstrate hyperactivity problems during their youth. Maintaining childlike inquisitiveness, activity, and involvement throughout life contributes to their achievements.

Risk factors of children likely to become hyperactive have been studied thoroughly. Longitudinal research of children born with minor physical anomalies shows a higher predisposition to developing hyperactivity (Rutter, 1984). Infant studies suggest that children born with difficult temperaments, that is, displaying high activity levels, being colicky, having irregular eating patterns, and showing fussiness when held, are at high risk for developing ADHD (Barkley, 1981).

Hyperactivity presents differently at developmental stages, and there are characteristic signs alerting clinicians to the problem when assimilating a developmental history from parents. As infants, these children show higher activity levels than other children, reject the usual comforting measures, and need extraordinary measures to restrain them in their cribs and ensure their safety. As they begin to crawl and climb, they seem fearless, and parents become preoccupied with safety. For example, parents may report nailing furniture to the wall or removing bureau drawers to prevent the furniture from being used as a makeshift ladder, or placing a restrictive top on the crib to keep their child from climbing out and falling.

Most parents become aware of their child's hyperactivity when the child is between 2 and 3 years of age. The child is described as noncompliant, restless, and constantly active. Because of clumsiness and poor coordination, these children are accident prone, and parents must use extraordinary measures to childproof the home. They are noisy and demanding and cry more than other children, exhausting their mother or caretakers. These children are difficult to settle into a routine, seldom nap, and are sporadic eaters. Developmental milestones, such as weaning, drinking from cups, and toilet training, are more difficult than with normal children. Adequate nutrition is a major concern because ADHD children are fussy and uninterested in chewing and taking the time needed to eat. Because many of them have food allergies plus colds, respiratory infections, and injuries, frequent visits to the hospital are necessary. Their lack of attention to environmental changes and safety appears as a lack of concern for self.

Between the ages of 3 and 5, the major problem these children present is noncompliance. Sleeping and toilet training problems may continue, and they seem to have less of a conscience than expected. They also begin to show difficulties with *rule-governed behavior,* that is, the ability to use language to guide their behavior instead of responding impulsively to circumstances. Seasoned parents find themselves increasingly frustrated because disciplinary measures are not effective. ADHD children display rage and aggression toward their parents and caretakers, as well as toward their peers and playmates. They destroy toys and property when others do not accommodate them. They have violent, uncontrollable temper tantrums, causing their parents to isolate them from public places and crowds. These constraints reduce the parents' social experiences and add to their feelings of isolation and frustration. Because of the veiled suggestions from teachers and friends that they have failed to discipline their child properly, parents begin to feel guilt ridden.

By the time the child is 5 years or older, parents have been the recipients of complaints and have been judged by teachers, their child's peers and playmates, and neighbors. Parents are often quite defensive when the behaviors are reviewed during the initial contact with clinicians. ADHD children usually repeat kindergarten or first grade, and because they are often unaware of others' concerns about their behaviors, they react with feelings of rejection and failure. By the time they are in second grade, their learning disabilities are evident, and they may be placed in special classes. The parents' frustration with the pattern of school failure continues. These children are usually rejected by their peers and become loners or members of gangs of children who also have ADHD or other conduct disorders. They may steal, lie, and demonstrate other defiant and aggressive behaviors to gain acceptance. Their actions further alienate them and anger their teachers, peers, and parents. The case example illustrates the typical behaviors of a child with ADHD at this age.

Case Example

The school referred Jim, a 6-year-old boy, because "he requires constant supervision to keep him from disrupting classroom activities." He is also described as "stubborn, defiant, and quarrelsome," and as having a very short attention span. Every school he has attended has had the same complaints about his behavior: he is overactive, uncontrollable, disruptive, and impulsive.

His mother states that at home Jim never keeps still for any length of time; he is always running, jumping, rocking, or fiddling with something. She describes him as doing three or four things at a time without completing anything. He has poor judgment and goes off anywhere by himself and does whatever he wants to do. He is extremely intrusive and disrupts any activity in which others are attempting to engage. His mother feels that he demands her undivided attention. Furthermore, she says, he is always provoking his older brother, and has a wild temper, which erupts very dramatically and suddenly and disappears in the same fashion.

As an infant, Jim was constantly climbing out of his crib and highchair, and could not be contained. As a toddler, he was into everything, and his parents made many visits to the emergency room because of his minor accidents. He climbed, jumped on the furniture, and refused to stay in his playpen.

During the evaluation, Jim spent most of the time walking around the office or tilting a chair, leaning on its back, and rocking back and forth. He jumped from subject to subject and talked incessantly. He acknowledged having some difficulty in school, but felt it was strictly because the other children picked on him.

Modified from Spitzer RL and others: A psychiatrist's casebook: the DSM-III casebook, Washington, DC, 1986, American Psychiatric Press.

During later childhood, hyperactive children usually show signs of depression and low self-esteem. Success at school, at home, and in social relations is rare, and acting-out behavior increases as they try anything to be accepted. During these years, truancy begins and they may run away from home when tensions peek. Many hyperactive children have their first contact with juvenile authorities during this time.

DSM-III-R CRITERIA

Changes made in the DSM-III-R were based on studies showing that the clinical diagnosis without hyperactivity was seldom assigned. In the rare cases when a diagnosis of ADHD without hyperactivity is made, it is placed in the DSM-III-R category of specific developmental disorders, NOS. The case example describes the behavior of a child with ADHD without hyperactivity.

Case Example

An 8-year-old boy was referred to a mental health clinic because of increasing difficulty at school. His teacher reported that he often seemed to be in a world of his own in which he appeared "not to be listening." He did not finish classroom assignments unless the teacher continuously supervised his performance. When she succeeded in gaining his attention, he was able to deal with academic tasks easily, which was not surprising since he had learned to read at the age of 4 in a Montessori nursery school. His writing was usually illegible. He spent a good deal of time drawing spaceships. The child was somewhat obese and awkward (appearing to be the size of an 11- or 12-year-old), and his physical awkwardness resulted in his being chosen last in baseball or volleyball. He tended to be bossy with his peers and often abruptly quit games because he could not tolerate waiting for his turn.

The client was the product of a difficult breech delivery at term. His mother reported that he had been an irritable baby and that she had had a difficult time establishing sleeping and eating routines. She stated that as a toddler he was "always into everything" and was difficult to control. For example, at age 2 she told him a dozen or more times not to go into the street, yet he often did; this situation was finally controlled by putting him in a fenced backyard. As he grew older, he had a proclivity for getting into other dangerous situations. He often ran off to play without telling his parents. At times they had found him walking the railroad tracks or playing on the thin ice of a not-quite-frozen reservoir.

Even now the client requires fairly consistent parental supervision. He does not like to watch television, but enjoys being read to and knows many books by heart. His play patterns have been relatively immature, and his room is generally cluttered. When requested to clean his room or perform chores, he is often noncompliant. He seems incapable of organizing his activities and, as a result, approaches them in a haphazard manner, leaving much undone. At home he is a friendly, cuddly child who is absentminded and sometimes disobedient.

On a Wechsler Intelligence Scale for Children the client's performance IQ was 110 and his verbal IQ was 140. A screening neurologic examination revealed impaired balance and impaired fine-motor coordination. Eye contact was good, and his thought content was typical for an 8-year-old boy.

Modified from Spitzer RL and others: A psychiatrist's casebook: the DSM-III casebook, Washington, DC, 1986, American Psychiatric Press.

The diagnosis of ADHD is based on a complete longitudinal history from parents and teachers. No special neurologic examinations or laboratory tests presently support the diagnosis. Behaviors must be present for at least 6 months, and the severity of the disorder is rated according to the number of symptoms demonstrated.

Nursing management.   At the first encounter, clinicians need to be sensitive to the distress and guilt most parents are experiencing and focus on seeking solutions. Most clinicians will also encounter parents whose expectations of children's behaviors are too demanding or who are naive about normal child development.

In most cases the history from the mother is the most reliable. However, she may report defensively in response to others' criticisms. The extent of distractibility, attention deficit, overall life style, and characteristic way of reacting are important information for initial screening and assessment.

When taking a history from the parents, clinicians should do the following:
1. Explore the parents' report of their child's attention span in detail to determine symptoms of a stimulus barrier deficit.
2. Elucidate information about the child's activity level.
3. Discuss the child's impulsiveness, watching for signs of a serious defect, such as killing of animals.

In unstructured playroom settings the attention span of ADHD children deteriorates after approximately 15 minutes, and they display many extraneous movements of restlessness. These are usually signs that the child needs sensory input and is searching for distractions.

Nurse clinicians need to become familiar with behavior checklists and rating scales that are essential tools for the evaluation and management of children with ADHD. The hyperactive child's low self-esteem and short attention span are major areas for clinicians to focus on during individual psychotherapy.

The major principle in counseling all adults with ADHD children is to communicate the child's need for structure. Interventions need consensus among all participants in the child's life, which is difficult because the behavior challenges adults' self-esteem. Disagreements among parents of hyperactive children are more frequent than parents of normal and/or children with other psychopathology, and the stress on the family system is often the reason for divorce. Clinicians need to assist with other weakened family interactions and focus on parents' perceptions of their child. Descriptions of the child's daily activities are addressed initially, including play behavior (alone or with other children), self-responsibility (such as eating and sleeping behaviors), and responses to visitors and people in public places.

For each situation the parents should be asked the following (Barkley, 1981):

1. Is this a problem area?
2. What does the child do in this situation that bothers you?
3. What is your response?
4. What will the child do next?
5. If the problem continues, what will you do next?
6. What is the usual outcome of this interaction?
7. How often do problems occur in this situation?
8. How do you feel about the problem?
9. On a scale of 0 to 10 (not a problem to a severe problem), how severe is this problem for you?

Behavioral modification interventions using operant conditioning that rewards self-control and delay of gratification are among the most widely and successfully used treatments. Behavior techniques assess parental training interventions, drug effects, and self-control training. Most experts suggest using behavior tools that are statistically reliable, such as the Conner's parent rating scales. These excellent adjuncts assist in gathering baseline data and track treatment progress (Adams and Fras, 1988). They are widely used for children with conduct disorders or ADHD by school counselors, psychologists, special educators, and other members of the interdisciplinary teams and are detailed in Table 9-2. Nurse clinicians' special skills in family therapy, psychopharmacologic management, and behavior modification techniques qualifies them to work with these children, their teachers, and their families.

Parental guidance and educational and psychopharmacology measures are useful interventions. Parental counseling and guidance should provide parents with a framework for understanding their child and ADHD. Only the aspects of parenting that contribute to or interfere with their adaptation to the child should be addressed and not their general parenting skills. Preventive measures are emphasized to minimize disruption and overstimulation. Parents and teachers focusing on accomplishing age-appropriate tasks raises parents' and the child's self-esteem.

Parents and teachers need to learn ways to screen the child's peer relationships, and the child should be gradually taught ways to select social contacts. Interventions should be adapted to the short-term perspective of the child by consisting of shorter sessions and longer intervals, and restructuring the child's defenses is inappropriate. The successful use of psychopharmacologic measures does not exclude children's need for individual therapy or the parents' need for guidance. Psychopharmacology is most successful when given concurrently with supportive, educative therapy.

Table 9-2   Evaluation Instruments Used to Assess Noncompliance

Rating scale	Description
Child behavior checklist (CBCL)	Consists of 20 social competency and 118 behavior problem items; scale used for ages 2 to 3, 4 to 5, 6 to 11, and 12 to 16 for both sexes; addresses developmental changes and sex strength; verifies schizoid, depressed, uncommunicative, somatic complaints; obsessive, social withdrawal; hyperactive, aggressive, delinquent behaviors
Conners Parent Rating	Consists of 48 items involving conduct, learning, psychosomatic signs, impulsive-hyperactive behavior, anxiety; used to evaluate hyperactive children and response to treatment; separate hyperactive scale for children 4 to 5 years of age; briefer than CBCL; sensitive to medication and parent training interventions; used for baseline pretreatment measures
Home Questionnaire Situations	Evaluates problem areas using 16 situations as guidelines; discriminates ADHD from normal children; sensitive to drug and parent training intervention changes
Werry-Weiss-Peters Activity Rating Scale	Consists of 31 items addressing activity levels in 7 settings: play, mealtimes, sleep, television, homework, public places, school
Self-Report rating scales for children	Used for children ages 11 to 18; uses first person wording; validity norms not established but useful for comparisons of perception differences of child, parents, teachers
Behavior problem checklist (BPC)	Consists of 89 items completed by parents and teachers; measures conduct problems, personality problems, inadequacy-immaturity, social-delinquency; addresses conduct disorders, socialized aggression, attention problems, anxiety, withdrawal, psychotic behavior, motor excess; used for screening, evaluating dimensions of deviant behavior and treatment outcomes
Eyberg Child Behavior Inventory	Consists of 36 items completed by parents; used for children 2 to 15 years of age; normative data for children 2 to 12 years of age available; used for screening and treatment outcome measure
New York London Survey	Addresses temperament activity level, rhythmicity, approach to or withdrawal from new stimuli, adaptability to new situations, intensity of reactions, threshold of responses, quality of mood, distractibility, attention span; evaluates parents within developmental framework; infant, middle childhood temperament baselines available; reliability not confirmed
Self-Control Rating Scale (SCRC)	Consists of 33 items focusing on ability to inhibit behavior, follow rules, control impulsive behavior; useful for clinicians, parents, teachers in evaluating ADHD deficits; sensitive to treatment effects and self-control training

Parents often treat their hyperactive child with special diets before seeking professional help. The Finegold diet is a popular diet that has sometimes been successful. It excludes all foods with the natural salicylate radical tartrazine and with artificial colors. The low sugar diet is not effective and often causes greater hyperkinesis. Clinicians need to learn if any restrictive diets methods have been used. The danger in the popularity of these diets is that parents are more accepting of the disorder when they can label the cause and will avoid seeking professional care.

The coexistence of ADHD and developmental learning disabilities is frequent; therefore nurses should offer support and counseling to teachers. They may also need to mediate between parents and the school because parents and teachers often displace blame on each other for the behavior. Evenhandedness, patience, and a structured classroom in which learning is interesting but not overstimulating for the child should be emphasized. More frequent repetition of instructions is required, and complex tasks should be divided into segments. On-going interactions with teachers, school psychologists, and the school social worker, as well as use of all available resources, are necessary. In many inpatient settings, nursing staff accompany the child to school and participate in the child's learning process, reinforcing the knowledge and applying it to other areas of the child's life.

REFERENCES

Achenback TM and Edelbrock CS: Manual for the child behavior checklist and revised child behavior profile, Burlington, Vt, 1983, University of Vermont.

Adams PL and Fras I: Beginning child psychiatry, New York, 1988, Brunner/Mazel, Inc.

American Psychiatric Association: Diagnostic and statistical manual of mental disorders, ed 3, Washington, DC, 1980, American Psychiatric Association.

American Psychiatric Association: Diagnostic and statistical manual of mental disorders, ed 3, rev, Washington, DC, 1987, American Psychiatric Association.

Barkley RA: Hyperactive children: a handbook for diagnosis and treatment, New York, 1981, The Guilford Press.

Chess S and Thomas A: Origins and evolution of behavior disorders: infancy to early adult life, New York, 1984, Brunner/Mazel, Inc.

Chess S and Thomas A: Temperament in clinical practice, New York, 1986, The Guilford Press.

Edelbrock E: Conduct problems in childhood and adolescence: developmental patterns and progressions, Unpublished manuscript, 1985.

Group for the Advancement of Psychiatry: The diagnostic process in child psychiatry, New York, 1957, Group for the Advancement of Psychiatry.

Group for the Advancement of Psychiatry: Psychopathological disorders in childhood: theoretical considerations and a proposed classification, New York, 1966, Group for the Advancement of Psychiatry.

Group for the Advancement of Psychiatry: The process of child therapy, New York, 1982, Brunner/Mazel, Inc.

Kazdin AE: Treatment of antisocial behavior in children and adolescents, Homewood, Ill, 1985, The Dorsey Press.

Lamb ME: Parental influences on early socioemotional development, J Child Psychol Psychiatry 23:189, 1982.

Laufer MW, Denhoff E, and Solomons G: Hyperkinetic impulse disorder in children's behavior problems, Psychosom Med 19:38, 1957.

Lewis D and others: Conduct disorder and its synonyms: diagnosis of dubious validity and useful. In Chess S and Thomas A: Annual progress in child psychiatry and child development, New York, 1985, New York University Press.

Loeber R and Schmaling KB: Empirical evidence for overt and covert patterns of antisocial conduct problems: a meta-analysis, J Abnorm Child Psychol 13:337, 1985.

McMahon RJ and Forehand R: Conduct disorders. In Mesh J and Terdal LG, editors: Behavioral assessment of childhood disorders, ed 2, New York, 1988, The Guilford Press.

Patterson GB: Coercive family process, Eugene, Ore, 1982, Castalina.

Patterson GB and Blank L: Bootstrapping your way in the nomological thicket, Behav Assess 8:49, 1984.

Patterson GB and Stouthamer-Loeber M: The correlation of family management practices and delinquency, Child Dev 55:1299, 1984.

Quay HC and Peterson DR: Interim manual for the revised behavior problem checklist, Unpublished manuscript, 1983.

Reid JB, Hinojosa-Rivera G, and Lorber R: A social learning approach to the outpatient treatment of children who steal, Unpublished manuscript, 1981.

Rutter M: Sex differences in children's responses to family stress. In Anthony EJ and Koupernick C, editors: International yearbook for child psychiatry and allied disciplines, vol 1, New York, 1970, John Wiley & Sons, Inc.

Rutter M: Prevention of children's psychosocial disorders: myth and substance. In Chess S and Thomas A, editors: Annual progress in child psychiatry and child development, 1983, New York, 1984, Brunner/Mazel, Inc.

Safer JD and Allen RP: Hyperactive children: diagnosis and management, Baltimore, 1976, University Park Press.

Scatterfield JH, Satterfield B, and Cantwell D: Three-year multimodality treatment study of hyperactive boys, J Pediatr 98:650, 1981.

Spitzer RL and others: A psychiatrist's casebook: the DSM-III casebook, Washington, DC, 1986, American Psychiatric Press.

Wells KC and Forehand R: Conduct and oppositional disorders. In Bŏrnstein PH and Kazdin AE, editors: Handbook of clinical behavior therapy with children, Homewood, Ill, 1985, The Dorsey Press.

Chapter 10

Specific Developmental Disorders

Linda Whisonant-Haberman

Specific developmental disorders affect academic development and are not caused by physiologic or psychologic conditions. They are subclassified according to the predominant area of cognitive functioning involved and include reading, arithmetic, language, and mixed or atypical developmental disorders.

Mastery of academic skills provides the social and emotional context for many developmental issues of childhood such as the process of separation, adjustment to a new environment, adaptation to social contacts, competition, and assertion. There are reciprocal interactions between children's success with these issues, level of school performance, and developmental progress. According to systems and transactional models, mastering academic skills is a component of the student role. Children whose academic achievement is positive find that school provides them a satisfying, productive student role; children with specific developmental disorders usually find that school requirements and their student role are fraught with frustrating, stressful experiences.

This chapter discusses two interrelated perspectives: the DSM-III-R classification and criteria of specific developmental disorders and educational practices and perspectives on Public Law (PL) 94-142 and PL 99-457. PL 94-142 is the Education for All Handicapped Children Act (1977), and it provides legal guarantees for special services for handicapped school-aged children in the Unites States and supplements and redefines the requirement of compulsory school attendance. It is an essential consideration of treatment plans for all children with psychiatric and specific developmental disorders. In 1986, PL 99-457 was passed as a preventive legislation to minimize the need for special education and related services after handicapped infants and toddlers reach school age.

Nurse clinicians working with children diagnosed with specific developmental disorders need to be aware that the idea of teaching these children is a relatively new concept. In the past, children with specific developmental disorders usually did not attend school, and if they did, subject contents were often unrelated to their learning and academic progress. It was thought that many of these children were incapable of learning.

Definitions and Concepts

PREVALENCE

Statistical estimates on the prevalence of learning disabilities differ among settings and geographic areas. Gaddes (1987) estimated that in countries such as the United States, Canada, and parts of Europe, the incidence of underachievers is about 15% and approximately 7% are children with cerebral dysfunctions who display perceptual, cognitive, and/or motor impairments. Learning disabilities continue to be recognized more often in males than in females, with ratios varying from 2 to 1 to 5 to 1.

Some professionals and parents claim that school settings during the early years discriminate against boys and contribute to the preponderance of learning disorders and behavioral problems a number of young males experience. These critics believe that the effects of higher hormonal levels causing more aggression, restlessness, and impatience lead to the disparity in the rate. Others note that young boys have more rugged bone structures, display greater muscular reactivity, and have a strong tendency toward restlessness and vigorous covert activity. Differences in the basal metabolic rates (BMR) of young boys and girls have also been hypothesized as the reason for higher rates in males. Boys are estimated to be nine times more hyperactive than girls, and research indicates young males 5 to 8 years of age are more aggressive and negative, have poorer relationships with teachers, and have twice as many classroom disturbances as girls (Humphrey, 1986). These critics of school environment advocate that more action-oriented curriculums be implemented to meet school-aged boys' basic needs for motor activity. Incidents of male students being mismatched with female teachers are also cited in the literature, causing some experts to advocate male and female first grade teachers.

Achievement-related anxiety is the major source of academic problems in school-aged girls. It has been posited that girls may avoid being successful in academic areas because of fear of social rejection or a loss of femininity, especially when academic success and accomplishments require aggression and competition with boys.

Although the available epidemiologic data addressing age prevalence is limited, learning disabilities are thought to become more frequent and severe as children progress in elementary school (Taylor, 1989).

Academic difficulties are the major reasons young children are referred to mental health professionals. Estimates are that as many as 30% of the 12 million school-aged children in the United States have adjustment problems related to mastering academic skills and peer relationships and that approximately 20% require mental health counseling or psychiatric interventions (Opie and Slater, 1988).

ETIOLOGIC FACTORS

Five models have been identified as useful in understanding etiologic factors in learning disability and developmental disabilities during infancy and early childhood. The explanatory models are not mutually exclusive because the origins of learning disabilities and delays are multidimensional (Aman and Singh, 1983):

1. Difference model: Individual differences in cognitive ability are normally distributed throughout a population, and learning difficulties result from the natural occurrence of poorly developed learning skills.
2. Deficit model: Learning difficulties are associated with organic conditions that interfere with learning. These conditions may include mixed cerebral dominance, maldevelopment or disease of the brain, and vestibule and ocular difficulties.
3. Delay model: Learning difficulties are associated with immaturity in development. Eventually, adequate achievement in skills will probably develop.
4. Disruption model: Extraneous factors such as severe anxiety or depression disrupt the learning process.
5. Personal-historical model: The basic skills needed for learning are not acquired because of environmental factors such as failure in the teaching or learning process.

DSM-III-R CRITERIA

The DSM-III-R categories of specific developmental disorders reflect the belief that academic/cognitive deficits and difficulties may be unrelated to diagnosable psychiatric disorders. The use of educational language does not infer that psychologic mechanisms are not operative—there are strong associations between emotional maladjustment and low academic achievement. However, mental disorders do not inevitably prevent adequate or superior school performance. For example, children with schizophrenic and borderline disorders often do well in academic areas, despite gross dysfunction in other areas.

Emotional conflicts are evident in most children with these disorders, but elements of depression, anxiety, and stress do not meet the requirements for a clinical diagnosis of a severe psychiatric disorder such as psychosis or depression. In contrast, children with specific developmental disorders frequently have concurrent psychiatric diagnoses of the conduct disorders and/or ADHD (see Chapter 9). Specific developmental disorders may also be the result of congenital defects, chronic degenerative brain disorders, and acute brain assaults such as brain injuries due to trauma, infections, and disease.

The DSM-III-R criteria stress that the diagnosis of academic skills disorders is to be used when children with adequate intellectual capacity develop a pattern of failing grades or underachievement. Three circumstances are specified: (1) absence of evidence of a mental disorder that accounts for academic problems (determined by a complete psychiatric evaluation and IQ test), (2) absence of evidence of a physical disorder that accounts for the academic problems, and (3) presence of a mental disorder that does not cause academic problems.

The definition of mental retardation in the DSM-III-R uses specific IQ score parameters and adaptive behavior levels. Some critics object to the use of IQ scores, suggesting *performance deficit* would be a more neutral label because the tests measure responses to questions and other demands (Corning, 1986). Others support the use of IQ test scores, stressing that many mental health professionals and the general public incorrectly believe that mental retardation correlates with a low IQ, and the DSM-III-R's precise definition is of critical clarifying importance (Adams and Fras, 1988).

The DSM-III-R uses the same definition as the American Association on Mental Deficiency (AAMD) for mental retardation. Two diagnostic areas are stressed: children must function on a retarded level both intellectually and in terms of adaptive functioning.

Subaverage intellectual functioning in the DSM-III-R refers to an IQ of 70 or below on an individually administered IQ test. Approximately 80% of all mentally retarded children fall into this educable category and have IQ levels between 50 and 70. These children are therefore eligible for and benefit from assistance mandated for special educational programs under PL 94-142.

Adaptive behavior refers to the effectiveness of children in meeting standards of personal independence and social responsibility expected for their chronologic age and cultural group (Adams and Fras, 1988). Good social and emotional adaptation can compensate for lower intelligence.

Axis V in the DSM-III-R is used to specify children's highest level of adaptive functioning during the past year. However, it is difficult to ascertain when a problem goes beyond a V-code severity to a mental disorder, and the V-code diagnosis is cursory at best (Bemporad and Schwab, 1986). If this functioning is evaluated as high, it can offset the potential diagnosis of mental retardation using the IQ score criteria (Adams and Fras, 1988). The DSM-III-R states that good adaptive functioning may be present in children whose IQ is near but not lower than 70, and children whose IQ falls between 70 and 85 with good adaptive functioning are referred to as having *borderline intellectual functioning*. These borderline cases are the most difficult level to diagnosis because there are no specific symptoms. However, borderline is a critical distinction for the DSM-III-R diagnosis and for the educational diagnosis of handicapped children with learning disabilities under PL 94-142. These deficits are usually first identified by teachers when children enter school and their adaptive functions present problems.

Children with moderate, severe, and profound mental retardation are usually detected before entering school by pediatric professionals during routine well-child screenings. These children have delayed or deficient developmental landmarks that are often detected using the Denver Developmental Screening. Additional psychologic tests such as the WISC-R and Vineland Social Maturity test confirm or rule out screening discrepancies. Professional services for many of these handicapped preschool aged children now fall under PL 98-457 (Part H), an amendment to PL 94-124.

Treatment of the emotional disorders in mentally retarded children is similar to treatment of children with normal intelligence. Child psychiatric nurse clinicians do need to adjust specific treatments to children's cognitive level.

The DSM-III-R does not use the term *learning disabilities* but refers to specific disorders in learning (see box). These disorders present when academic skills are below expectations of age-appropriate skills (American Psychiatric Association, 1987).

DSM-III-R Classification of Specific Developmental Disorders

Mental retardation

317.00 Mild mental retardation (educable: IQ 50-70)
318.00 Moderate mental retardation (trainable: IQ 35-49)
318.10 Severe mental retardation (IQ 20-34)
318.20 Profound mental retardation (IQ below 20)
319.00 Unspecified mental retardation

Specific developmental disorders

Language and speech disorders.

315.39 Articulation disorder
307.00 Cluttering
307.00 Stuttering
315.31 Expressive language disorder
315.31 Receptive language disorder

Academic skills disorders.

315.00 Reading disorder
315.80 Expressive language disorder
315.10 Arithmetic disorder

Motor skills disorders.

315.40 Coordination disorder
315.90 Specific developmental disorder NOS

Other developmental disorders.

315.90 Developmental disorder NOS

From American Psychiatric Association: Diagnostic and statistical manual of mental disorders, ed 3, rev, Washington, DC, 1987, American Psychiatric Association.

Some educators are concerned that the DSM-III-R's language has done little to clarify the diagnostic difficulties resulting from PL 94-142. Both resources fail to state specific methods or criteria to be used when assessing children with learning disabilities.

PL 94-142

DEFINITIONS AND CRITERIA FOR LEARNING DISABILITIES

During the 1960s, disagreement with the belief that the family and not the government or state was the key decision-maker for children occurred. Spirited public concern for preschool children at risk for learning difficulties, fostered partly by school desegregation and human rights advocates, resulted. Public pressures influenced the passage of federal legislature for two groups of children: children of the poor and handicapped children with physical and mental defects. Examples of federally funded programs initiated for these preschoolers

Table 10–1   Federal Programs Serving Young Children

Program	Authorization	Purpose
Medicaid	Title XIX; Social Security Act	Provide medical services for low-income families
Early Periodic Screening, Diagnosis and Treatment (EPSDT)	Title XIX; Social Security Act	Provide comprehensive and preventive health services for diagnosis and treatment of physical and mental defects
Child Welfare State Grants	Title IV, Part B; Social Security Act	Strengthen child welfare services—enable child to remain in-home
Head Start	Title V; Social Security Act	Provide health, education, and social services for preschoolers of low-income families
Maternal and Child and Health-Block Grant	Title V; Social Security Act	Provide health care for mothers and children
Social Services Block Grant	Title XX; Social Security Act	Prevent, reduce, or eliminate dependency, neglect, and abuse
Education of all Handicapped Children	Title VI, Part B; Education of the Handicapped Act	Assist states in providing a free, appropriate public education
Infants and Toddlers with Handicaps	Education of the Handicapped Act Amendments of 1986 (Part H)	Help states plan and develop comprehensive services for infants and toddlers with handicaps

Modified from Smith B: A comparative analysis of selected federal programs serving young children, Chapel Hill, NC, 1986, University of North Carolina Press.

include Head Start and the Early Periodic Screening Diagnosis and Treatment (EPSTD) programs (Gallagher, 1989) and are summarized on Table 10-1. The passage of PL 94-142 represented an effort to elicit major structural changes in the public educational system through mandatory requirements.

The concept of learning disabilities included in PL 94-142 was first proposed by Kirk, who suggested scientists concerned with perceptual handicaps shift their focus from seeking the causes of these problems to research and clinical studies that identify and treat learning problems. Scientists had used the term *learning disabilities* to refer to the group of symptoms related to minimal brain dysfunction (MBD). The paradigmatic change that resulted initiated the establishment of the field of learning disabilities (Taylor, 1989).

Since then, the learning disabilities educational field has shifted from serving only children with neurologic difficulties to those with other problems, including difficulty in the school setting (Torgensen, 1986).

Psychoneurologic perspectives during the late 1960s concentrated on unifying factions of special educators addressing learning disabilities and MBD. For example, Johnson and Myklebust (1967) paired sensation, perception, imagery, symbolization, and conceptualization processes with visual, auditory, and motor channels. Kirk and Kirk (1971) posited a psycholinguistic model consisting of three types of overlapping learning disabilities: (1) academic disorders, including deficits in reading, writing, and arithmetic; (2) nonsymbolic disorders, encompassing the ability to recognize, integrate, and use sense impressions; and (3) symbolic disorders, pertaining to children's ability to understand and/or express visual and auditory symbols meaningfully.

The National Advisory Committee on Handicapped Children's definition of special learning disabilities contributed to the development of PL 94-142 and the DSM-III-R:

... a disorder in one or more of the basic psychological processes involved in understanding or using spoken or written language. These may be manifested in disorders of listening, thinking, talking, reading, writing, spelling or arithmetic. They include conditions which have been referred to as perceptual handicaps, brain injury, minimal brain dysfunction, dyslexia, developmental asphasia, etc. (US Office of Education, 1968).

The definition used in the 1977 U.S. PL 94-142 was similar. Differentiating learning disabilities from problems not primarily due to visual, hearing, motor handicaps, mental retardation, emotional disturbances, and environmental disadvantages were major concerns and later became the *exclusion factor* in the law.

PL 94-142 statute served as a legal guarantee of special education assistance for learning disabled school-aged children in the United States. The intent of PL 94-142 was to guarantee the following (Gallagher, 1989):

... (1) services available for all handicapped children; (2) fairness in diagnosis and treatment, particularly for minority children and families; (3) a clear set of educational objectives for the handicapped child to ensure that the child was not merely being put aside by the educational community; and (4) an opportunity for parents to have some say in their child's educational planning.

Six principles formed the foundation for the law (Gallagher, 1989):
1. Zero reject: No child would be denied special services
2. Nondiscriminatory evaluation: No child would be given tests that might discriminate ethnically or racially
3. Individualized educational programs: Each child would have a written program with clear objectives and records of performance toward those objectives
4. Least restrictive environment: The child could experience as normal as possible classroom setting
5. Due process: Parents could protest if they believed that the school was treating the child unfairly
6. Parent participation: Parents would be ensured a role in the development of their child's program

Despite efforts toward clarification, the statue's language and intent were vague, and its passage caused considerable dispute because of difficulties in implementation. Many mental health professionals, educators, parents, and politicians equated learning disabilities, mental retardation, and behavior disorders. One congressman noted that research had identified 53 learning disabilities and labeled 99 MBD and that "No one really knows what a learning disability is" (Congressional Record, 1975). Because the statute did not specify disorders, such as listening, thinking, talking, and reading, educators who had emphasized these areas were disconcerted (Taylor, 1988). Critics also claimed that the definitions and terminology do not consider external variables such as educational opportunities, expectations, and motivational and social influences on learning.

It is generally accepted in educational circles that the definition of learning disability in the statute is not one disorder but a collection of distinct disorders with numerous manifestations. Anderson (1979) described children with learning disabilities as having hidden handicaps, which hinder children's progress in the typical school setting.

In 1981, the National Joint Committee for Learning Disabilities (NJCLD) redefined the term and stated (1) learning disabilities was a generic term and not a specific diagnosis, (2) learning problems are heterogenous, and (3) learning disabilities may present with other handicapping conditions (Hamill, 1978).

The US Department of Education's sixth annual report to Congress in 1984 indicated that the prevalence of learning disabilities had doubled since 1974 and that more than 40% of children in special education programs were classified as learning disabled, representing 4% of all school children nationally. The government estimated that only 2% of the American school-aged population could be classified as seriously learning disabled. Many states report the prevalence of learning disabilities ranged from 26% to 64%, indicating the diversity of procedural criteria to identify these children (Chalfant, 1989).

DEFINITIONS AND CRITERIA FOR BEHAVIOR DISORDERS

There is no single, universally accepted definition of behavior disorder, and inconsistencies in the placement of children are also seen. Some districts differentiate by recommending placements into emotionally handicapped or severely emotionally handicapped programs, but other districts refer to these students as behaviorally disordered.

Although they have not been universally embraced in the field (Morgan and Jensen, 1988), current federal definitions of seriously emotionally disturbed children describe a condition in which one or more of the following characteristics exist over a long period of time and adversely affect educational performance:

1. Inability to learn that cannot be explained by intellectual, sensory, or other health factors
2. Inability to build or maintain satisfactory interpersonal relationships with peers and teachers
3. Presence of inappropriate types of behavior or feelings under normal circumstances
4. Display of general, pervasive mood of unhappiness or depression

5. Tendency to develop physical symptoms or fears associated with personal or school problems

The federal definition includes children who are schizophrenic but not those who are socially maladjusted, unless it is determined that they are seriously emotionally disturbed. Other factors must be present for an educational diagnosis of emotional handicaps to be assigned. Primarily, discrepancy between expected and actual performance of children according to chronologic and mental age must be seen.

Although limitations in PL 94-142 have been noted in the literature, there are many advantages to the current concepts of learning disabilities and emotional handicaps. The law has necessitated that scientists reexamine the traditional theoretic explanations for cognitive skills required for learning. Cognitive processing factors such as self-concept, locus of control, temperament, and behavior problems have also been reevaluated (Bender, 1987a).

Theoretic Explanations

Cognition plays a major role in both child development and child psychiatry, and current perspectives view it under the headings of cognitive processing and cognitive deficits (Rutter, 1989). Recent theories posit that people's cognitive processing of ways in which others view them and the biases resulting from this are related to many social and psychologic disorders. These biases are thought to be caused by early experiences, temperamental styles, and cognitive deficits.

PSYCHOLOGIC PROCESS MODELS

Psychologic process models have been developed by educational specialists, and they vary according to the definition and psychologic processes emphasized. Chalfant and King (1976) recommended the following operational definition for psychologic processes:

1. Attention: The ability to focus on appropriate stimuli selectively
2. Discrimination: The detection of differences of given stimuli
3. Memory: The ability to recognize or recall what has been learned
4. Sensory integration: The ability of two or more sensory channels to function simultaneously (for example, visual-motor integration)
5. Concept formation: The ability to understand and provide a specific response based on the type of stimuli
6. Problem solving: The ability to use prior knowledge and reorganize the information to produce a solution and achieve a desired outcome

There is no generally accepted theoretic basis for the diagnosis of psychologic processes and limited educator consensus on the processes and syndromes to be considered. Because of the dearth of valid instruments for measuring psychologic processes, inferences about abilities and disabilities can best be made from observations.

Dysfunction in psychologic process is one of the criteria for the diagnosis of learning disabled in PL 94-124. The others are task failure, achievement potential discrepancy, etiologic conditions, and exclusionary conditions. The federal statute did not identify the psychologic process that should be dysfunctional, resulting in many differences between states in selection and emphasis and in debatable estimates of the prevalence of learning disabilities.

For example, some states classify perceptually handicapped children with children with learning disabilities, and some districts include perceptual-motor skill training in their programs. Critics stress the study findings that strongly suggest this training has little effect on academic achievement. Some researchers have found that training children in perceptual deficit areas does not produce better school performance or perceptual motor growth (Hamill, 1978; Wallace and McLaughlin, 1979). Despite difficulties in classifications, 18 states have reported that the psychologic process criteria are helpful and have included them in their state guidelines (Chalfant, 1989).

Because of the alarming increase in school-aged children being assigned the educational diagnosis of learning disabled, public funds for implementing PL 94-142 are limited, and the field of learning disabilities is facing policy adjustments and probable cutbacks. Possible solutions include eliminating the category of learning disabilities and reverting to the initial format. Others suggest practitioners need to be more rigorous in the use of existing criteria to reduce the overidentification of learning disabled children and return to the initial 2% cap and categoric emphasis of the 1970s (Chalfant, 1989). Reversion to the original format may stimulate practioners to reevaluate their criteria, tighten decision making, and generate a sound data base, leading to more realistic models.

There is a consensus among researchers that psychologic processes do not function in isolation. Table 10-2 identifies common terms used in describing these processes.

Educational practices have shifted since the passage of the law, perhaps indicating that the law has resulted in improvements in the services for learning disabled children. During the last decade the traditional focus on the categoric nature of handicaps has shifted to an emphasis on ways in which children are taught. The assistant secretary for the office of Special Education and Rehabilitative Services stated: "At the heart of the categorical approach is the presumption that students with learning problems cannot be effectively taught in regular education programs, even with a variety of support." Noting that the present educational system is composed of many nonrelative parts that result in a flawed vision of education for children, she urged "appropriate professional and other resources for delivering effective, coordinated, comprehensive services for all students be based on individual education needs, rather than eligibility for categorical programs" (Will, 1987).

Educational assessment of children begins with observing their present level of functioning in the intellectual, academic, and social/behavioral areas. A diagnosis of learning disabled results from a complete testing battery including standardized tests, criterion-referenced tests, observations, task analysis, case histories, and interviews. The purpose is to find appropriate intervention and meet with and counsel parents to gain their collaboration in a special educational program promoting prescriptive teaching.

The concepts and practices used for diagnosing and treating children with academic skills disorders is a basic framework applicable to all children who are mildly handicapped. "Many mildly retarded, hearing impaired, emotionally

Table 10-2   Common Terms Used in the Diagnosis of Learning Disabilities

Visual perception	Ability to obtain information from visual stimuli; poor ability frequently associated with diagnostic assignment of learning disabilities
Visual memory	Ability to recall accurately prior visual experiences (Vallett, 1969); impaired ability often associated with reading difficulties (Kirk, 1976)
Visual figure ground discrimination	Ability to focus on objects without distraction from background or other stimuli; poor ability results in difficulties classifying objects by size or shape (Wallace and McLoughlin, 1979)
Spatial relationships	Ability to sequence objects; poor ability associated with difficulty with sentences in paragraph, letters within words, math problems; problems with simpler tasks also seen
Form perception	Ability to adjust to earlier perceptual generalizations; dysfunction associated with reading disabilities
Visual motor integration	Awareness of concrete areas and ability to structure environment; poor ability associated with unsynchronized movements, difficulty coordinating fine muscle movement, disorganization of response, distraction
Visual motor coordination	Ability to integrate body movements and visual skills; dysfunction associated with reading difficulty
Auditory perception	Ability to interpret, understand, and recognize sounds; impaired ability associated with difficulty learning phonics
Auditory memory	Ability to store and retrieve information when needed; dysfunction associated with difficulty following directions, organizing environment, completing simple tasks; disability also affects language skills, sequencing, comprehension, mathematic skills, social skills
Auditory discrimination	Ability to differentiate between phonemic sounds; impairment associated with reading and spelling difficulties
Sound blending	Ability to synthesize single phonic elements or phonemes into words; dysfunction associated with reading difficulties
Auditory figure ground	Ability to select relevant auditory stimuli; impairment associated with high distractability
Haptic perception deficits	Ability to understand object qualities, bodily movements, and ways in which they interrelate (Lerner, 1976)
Tactile perception	Ability to learn and obtain useful information through manipulation
Kinesthetic perception	Ability to sense bodily movements; deficits associated with problems of spatial orientation, body image, and coordination; handwriting affected

disturbed, and culturally different young people exhibit characteristics and symptoms that fit the learning disabilities concepts and respond to materials and methods designed for the learning disabled" (Lerner, 1976).

SELF-CONCEPT

The central idea of the self-system is that individuals develop a set of beliefs about themselves and their environment, influenced by the interaction of self-esteem, self-efficacy and locus of control (Harter, 1983).

Normally, most children encounter difficulties in school work at one time that range from failure to acquire beginning reading skills to memorizing spelling lists or mastering math facts. Children usually react to these transitory learning difficulties with frustration, anxiety, stress, and a sense of isolation. Parents and teachers often react with disapproval and annoyance, further limiting children's ability to cope (Taylor, 1989).

Some authorities claim conditions in the classroom add to or create *competitive stress,* a condition occuring when children perceive that they "will not be able to respond adequately to the performance demands of competition" (Humphrey, 1986). Perceived as personally threatening, competitive stress often threatens normal children's self-esteem and results in a transitory stress reaction. Learning disabled children experience discomfort and threats to self-esteem almost daily.

Social comparisons, that is ways in which people define themselves in relation to others, are fostered by the reflected appraisals of teachers and peers. In the school setting, comparisons of children's abilities with those of other children are made so that they can evaluate their position. They are rewarded for being right and punished for being wrong, usually by the grading system. The Society for Research in Child Development provided extensive longitudinal studies on test anxiety as it relates to school children and presented suggestions for reduction of test anxiety and performance stress (Hill and Sarasen, 1966). Text anxiety may begin in childhood and last throughout life.

Self-regard is vitally influenced by children's social surroundings. Primary education attempts to implant standards that may allow children to determine whether they are correct (valued) or incorrect (devalued). The more intensive the learning of these standards, the less susceptible children may be to reflected appraisals and comparisons in the immediate situation. Unfortunately, such early learning may also reduce their capacity to adapt to new and changing circumstances (Gergen, 1971).

In general, young children are not competitive, and when competition does exist, the extent varies with earlier home experiences, family composition, and self-system strengths. By middle school years, children become more competitive, with the intensity ranging from intense to mild to nonexistent.

Learning disabled children are frequently characterized in the literature as having negative or lower-than-normal self-concepts (Gardner, 1978; Wallace and Kaufman, 1978). Fear of failure may prevent them from completing or even attempting to complete an assignment or examination. They often exhibit extreme concern about what others think of them and lack self-confidence. Research findings suggest a strong association between self-concept and achievement. Children with positive self-concepts were not as easily threatened by difficult tasks and had steadier achievement than children with negative self-concepts (Purkley, 1970). However, several research studies indicate that this relationship does not necessarily continue through adolescence (Bender, 1987b). Discrepancies may occur because as children grow older, they often develop more positive and realistic self-concepts, which may be independent of school failures.

Continuity in self-esteem has been the focus of many clinical studies and observations. Some experts emphasize the importance of cognitive interpretation of experiences, which change as cognitive processing abilities mature. Some experts claim that for experiences to have long-term effects on the self-system, cognitive transduction must occur, explaining the reason many early infancy and childhood experiences do not have long-term psychologic outcomes. In contrast, Bowlby (1980) holds that trauma or loss during infancy and early childhood impairs the self-system permanently.

TEMPERAMENT

Some interacting aspects in task mastery have been partly attributed to children's innate temperamental disposition, that is, the way they characteristically behave when approaching a task or life experience. These factors include cognitive appraisal of the task or experience, mental reaction to the appraisal, and their resulting action (Rutter, 1989). In a longitudinal study of the association between temperament and IQ, these characteristics were measured in children at 4 and 8 months of age and again at 4.7 years of age. Two extremes of the temperament continuum were used: difficulty and easiness. Findings suggested that children who are difficult infants activated special family resources stimulating intellectual development (Maziade and others, 1969). Comparisons of learning disabled children with 35 nonhandicapped peers indicated that the nonlearning disabled group were more task oriented than the learning disabled children (Bender, 1987a).

LOCUS OF CONTROL

Children's self-perceived extent of control over their fate may have a direct relationship to their self-concept and learning disabilities. The methods used in clinical studies involve asking children what they believe contributes to their success or failure. They may attribute it either to their own internal personal characteristics or to external causes (Byran and Pearl, 1979). Research findings have not verified that children with learning disabilities ascribe their problems to one factor over the other as compared to their nonhandicapped peers. However, knowledge of children's locus of control orientation is clinically vital because it affects study habits and the selection of the most beneficial teaching methods (Bender, 1987b). It has also been found to be highly correlated with the effects of social skills training and delinquency (Henderson and Clive, 1983).

BEHAVIOR PROBLEMS

Learning disabled children and emotionally handicapped children have deficits that interfere with reading, writing, and mathematic skills. Their personal-social development and behavioral progress and control are also affected because they often become frustrated, depressed, and defensive regarding their lack of academic success. A casual relationship between social and emotional problems and learning disabilities has yet to be determined by research, but there appears to be a reciprocal relationship between learning problems and behavior problems (Morgan and Jenson, 1988). Behavioral characteristics associated with learning problems include non-completion of tasks and the inability to follow directions and classroom rules and to stay seated.

DSM-III-R Criteria

ACADEMIC SKILLS DISORDERS

Academic skills disorders are specific developmental disorders not caused by other psychologic disorders. Academic disabilities are seldom confined to just one area because problems have a ripple effect, influencing other learning skills. The older terms such as *specific learning disorder* or *LD* created confusion with other psychogenic learning disorders and are not used in the DSM-III-R. Other terms once used include *dyslexia, alexia, word blindness,* and *aphasia*.

Developmental lags that are caused by mental retardation, pervasive developmental disorders, and other physical impairments are not diagnosed as specific developmental disorder. For example, blind children are usually unable to read, but this developmental lag should not be diagnosed as developmental reading disorder (Webb and others, 1981). Nor are these diagnoses to be used for slow learners or underachievers. For a diagnosis to be made, a significant discrepancy between actual and expected levels of performance must occur. Determining what constitutes a significant delay demands clinical judgment and knowledge of normal development. The criteria for specific developmental disorders in the DSM-III-R are summarized in the box.

DEVELOPMENTAL READING DISORDERS

Reading is loaded with anxiety for many children. Estimates of the incidence of developmental reading disorders in American children is between 1% and 15% depending on the diagnostic criteria. The incidence is higher among socially disadvantaged children, and the male to female ratio ranges from 2 to 1 to 4 to 1. The incidence is lower in Oriental cultures in which writing is read from top to bottom and characters are read from right to left (Adams and Fras, 1988).

Although the etiology of developmental reading disorders is unknown, dysfunction of the left hemisphere of the brain combined with skewed dominance of the right hemisphere is a current theory. However, it remains unconfirmed, and the most commonly accepted etiology is developmental or maturation lag (Adams and Fras, 1988).

The essential feature of developmental reading disorder as defined by the DSM-III-R is "marked impairment in the development of the word recognition skills and reading comprehension." Children with this disorder often have poor comprehension because they focus on decoding the written symbols. Their oral readings tend to be slow and halting and contain substitutions of words, for example, *this* for *that, what* for *when,* and *who* for *how.* The omission of suffices and prefixes and entire words also distort their reading.

Diagnostic Criteria for Specific Developmental Disorders

Developmental arithmetic disorder

Arithmetic skills, as measured by a standardized, individually administered test, are markedly below the expected level, given the person's schooling and intellectual capacity (as determined by an individually administered IQ test). This disturbance significantly interferes with academic achievement or activities of daily living requiring arithmetic skills and is not due to a defect in visual or hearing acuity or a neurologic disorder.

Developmental expressive writing disorder

Writing skills, as measured by a standardized, individually administered test, are markedly below the expected level, given the person's schooling and intellectual capacity (as determined by an individually administered IQ test). This disturbance significantly interferes with academic achievement or activities of daily living requiring the composition of written texts (spelling words and expressing thoughts in grammatically correct sentences and organized paragraphs) and is not due to a defect in visual or hearing acuity or a neurologic disorder.

Developmental reading disorder

Reading achievement, as measured by a standardized, individually administered test, is markedly below the expected level, given the person's schooling and intellectual capacity (as determined by an individually administered IQ test). This disturbance significantly interferes with academic achievement or activities of daily living requiring reading skills and is not due to a defect in visual or hearing acuity or a neurologic disorder.

Developmental articulation disorder

Consistent failure to use developmentally expected speech sounds. For example, in a 3-year-old child, failure to articulate p, b, and t is seen, and in a 6-year-old child, failure to articulate t, sh, th, f, z, and l is observed. The difficulties are not due to a pervasive developmental disorder, mental retardation, defect in hearing acuity, disorders of the oral speech mechanism, or a neurologic disorder.

Developmental expressive language disorder

The score obtained from a standardized measure of expressive language is substantially below that obtained from a standardized measure of nonverbal intellectual capacity (as determined by an individually administered IQ test). This disturbance significantly interferes with academic achievement or activities of daily living requiring the expression of verbal (or sign) language. It may be evidenced in severe cases by use of a markedly limited vocabulary, by speaking only in simple sentences, or by speaking only in the present tense. In less severe cases, there may be hesitations or errors in recalling certain words, or errors in the production of long or complex sentences. The problems are not due to a pervasive developmental disorder, defect in hearing acuity, or a neurologic disorder (aphasia).

Deficits in expressive language and speech discrimination and writing ability are usually present. The most effective way to increase writing and language skills is to increase reading ability. However, this method may have little value for children with reading disorders.

Diagnostic Criteria for Specific Developmental Disorders — cont'd

Developmental receptive language disorder

The score obtained from a standardized measure of receptive language is substantially below that obtained from a standardized measure of nonverbal intellectual capacity (as determined by an individually administered IQ test). This disturbance significantly interferes with academic achievement or activities of daily living requiring the comprehension of verbal (or sign) language. This may be manifested in more severe cases by an inability to understand simple words or sentences. In less severe cases, there may be difficulty in understanding only certain types of words, such as spatial terms, or an inability to comprehend longer or more complex statements. The difficulties are not due to a pervasive developmental disorder, defect in hearing acuity, or a neurologic disorder (aphasia).

Developmental coordination disorder

The person's performance in daily activities requiring motor coordination is markedly below the expected level, given the person's chronological age and intellectual capacity. This may be manifested by marked delays in achieving motor milestones (walking, crawling, sitting), dropping things, clumsiness, poor performance in sports, or poor handwriting. This disturbance significantly interferes with academic achievement or activities of daily living and is not due to a know physical disorder, such as cerebral palsy, hemiplegia, or muscular dystrophy.

Modified from American Psychiatric Association: Diagnostic and statistical manual of mental disorders, ed 3, rev, Washington, DC, 1987, American Psychiatric Association.

Developmental reading disorders in the DSM-III-R have the same exclusion factors as PL 94-142: a deficit not explainable by mental retardation, inadequate schooling, or hearing or visual defects. The DSM-III-R definition and the PL educational definition stress that when considering appropriate identification of these children, the diagnosis is made only after determining that the impairment significantly interferes with academic achievement or life skills. The DSM-III-R also associates these impairments with other deficits including developmental receptive language disorder, developmental coordination disorder, and disruptive behavior disorders.

The disorder is usually apparent by the age of 7 when children are usually reading simple sentences and stories and have developed a basic *sight word* vocabulary. In severe cases, the evidence of reading difficulty may be apparent as early as the age of 6 when children have difficulty with left to right orientation, visual discrimination, sound blending, and other essential prereading skills.

Children are sometimes able to compensate if they have high intellectual functioning. In these cases the disorder may not be readily apparent and diagnosed until the child is 9 or 10 or even later. With specialized instruction, the disorder is mild, and the difficulties are minimal and may not interfere with typical functioning in adulthood. If the disorder is severe despite instructional interventions, difficulties and some signs will remain for life. Research has shown that the disorder is more common in the first degree biologic relatives than in the general population.

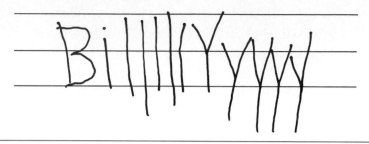

Figure 10-1   Perseveration.

How Is Your Visual Perception?

e ach ch ilb mitha le ar mimq bisadilith is am iubiubnal, het sowe qeueral cyaracteristics bo exist:

He or sye yas aver apr or adove aver ape iutellipeuce; sowe of tye wore qrevaleut shwqtows aqqear to de-- bis or bers of woter activith; bisorber sof ewotioualith; bisorbers of qerceq tiou; bisorber s of couceqtiou; dis orb ers o f weworh.

Difficulties in reading interfere with children's progress in other subjects. Alternative teaching methods are often needed to teach other areas in which their ability is not limited.

Visual perception deficits are seen in approximately 10% of the cases but can have far-reaching effects. The box shows an example of the way in which children with visual perception problems see words. Problems with visual motor integration result in perseveration in which children focus on a particular object and are distracted from the original task (Figure 10-1). In older children, disruptive behavior disorders may also be present and are usually due to academic frustrations and children's inability to succeed.

Disabilities are quantified by analyzing results of tests, checking for discrepancies between performance and ability, and identifying patterns that may be indicative of a learning problem. The Bannatyne method recategorizes the WISC subtests scores into spatial, conceptual, and sequential groups for more accurate diagnoses (Rugel, 1974).

ARITHMETIC DISORDERS

The prevalence of developmental arithmetic disorder is unknown, but it is less common than developmental reading disorders. According to the DSM-III-R, these disorders are apparent by the time children are 8 years old and perform- ing multiplication and division tasks with a basic understanding of mathema- tical concepts. In some children the disorder is apparent as early as 6 years of age when they are learning basic numerical concepts. In other children it may not occur until the age of 10 or later when more complex mathematical tasks are introduced. Research findings have not yet associated a familial pattern of

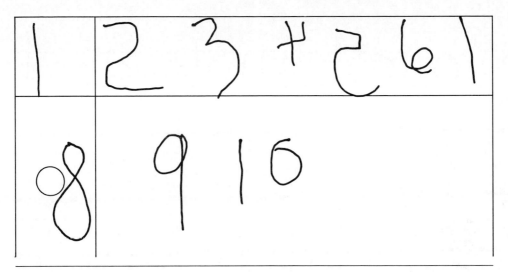

Figure 10-2   An example of what numbers resemble when written by a learning disabled child. Note that the numbers are not within the paper and margin borders.

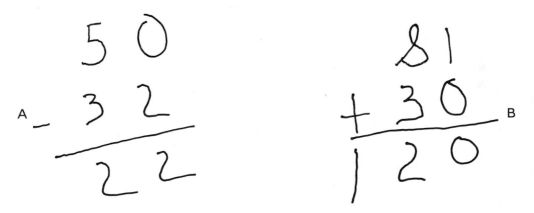

Figure 10-3   Common computational problems exhibited by skill-deficit children. **A,** Difficulty with regrouping. **B,** Difficulty with place value.

arithmetic disorders. Examples of common errors are shown in Figures 10-2 and 10-3.

DEVELOPMENTAL EXPRESSIVE WRITING DISORDERS

Developmental expressing writing disorder is defined in the DSM-III-R as the following: "The impairment in the ability to compose written texts may be marked by spelling errors, grammatical or punctuation errors within sentences, or poor paragraph organization." In severe cases, it is evident by the age of 7 when children are expected to write simple sentences correctly (Figure 10-4). In less severe cases,

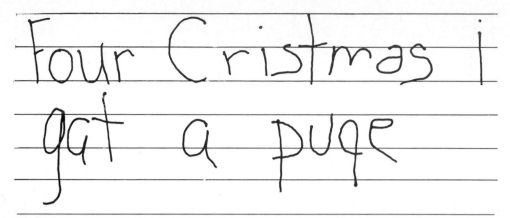

Figure 10-4   Common handwriting and spelling errors of learning disabled children.

the disorder may not be apparent until the age of 10 or later when children sequence and organize thoughts and follow basic syntax and semantic rules. First degree biologic relatives may also have developmental language disorders and academic skills disorders. Writing disorders have received little attention until recently, but it is estimated that they are as common as developmental reading disorders and have a similar course.

DEVELOPMENTAL COORDINATION DISORDERS

Motor deficiencies manifest in an impairment of the ability to use motor skills to enhance learning. Children may be deficient in gross motor skills including coordination, directionality, body image and body movement or in fine motor channels such as eye-hand coordination.

Motor skills disorders are categorized in the DSM-III-R as a developmental coordination disorder (315.40). The DSM-III-R states: "The manifestations of this disorder vary with age and development: young children exhibit clumsiness and delays in developmental motor milestones." The essential feature is a marked difficulty in the development of motor coordination, which may contribute to their low self-esteem. There is no information available on familial patterns. Commonly associated problems include difficulties in academic skills, particularly reading and writing, and in nonmotor areas such as articulation and receptive and expressive language problems.

Although the Dolman-Delcato theories are still considered extremely controversial, a 1985 article from the Oregon Hope and Help Center (a neurologic rehabilitative center) entitled "No Miracles" used these principles successfully. The case example summarizes one child's treatment.

Case Example

Randy, a 10-year-old boy, had hyperactivity and disabilities causing considerable strain on those who worked with him. Schools had been unable to cope with him. He was progressed through a rehabilitative patterning program involving passive movements imposed on his head, arms, and legs in a predetermined order and developmental exercises recapitulating movements from before birth to the walking stage. His therapy advanced to include cross-pattern walking and becoming totally right-handed. With special adaptations for scheduling and the continence of the patterning techniques, Randy became a successful student within 9 months and is a successful adult today both socially and academically.

Modified from Gold S and Kline J: No miracles, Acad Ther 21:2, 1985.

LANGUAGE AND SPEECH DISORDERS

Distinctions are made between speech and language in the communication disorders. Language disorders are peripheral speech or communicative disorders, for example, developmental articulation disorders.

Congenital, developmental, or specific language disorders are present from birth, but acquired language disorders can occur at any age and are usually treated by neurologic and pediatric specialists.

The DSM-III-R lists two subtypes of language disorders: developmental expressive language disorders and developmental receptive language disorders. The former involves impairment in encoding and producing language, and the latter includes understanding and producing language and is more serious. Both subtypes are given the same code number, and the specific subtype is to be noted. Speech therapy provided by specialists is the appropriate intervention.

The speech disorder of developmental articulation (dyslalia) is a disorder of mispronunciation. The most common speech disorder, it is found in approximately 6% of males and 3% of females.

Stuttering, the disturbance in rhythm of fluency of speech, is most pronounced when there is pressure to communicate. The psychodynamic explanation that stuttering represents aggressive acts against impatient listeners is generally discounted, with more accepted explanations linking stuttering to genetic and brain function theories. Specialized forms of behavior therapy are prominent methods of intervention.

Cluttering is a rare disorder, characterized by rapid speech that flows by fits and starts. Etiologic explanations for cluttering stress that it is a basic global linguistic-processing difficulty.

ELECTIVE MUTISM

Elective mutism occurs in children who have normal speech equipment, but choose not to speak. It is the only psychogenic communication disorder and is attributed to early emotional trauma, hospitalization in early life, rejection by ambivalent parents, and other family pathologic factors. *Symbiotic* mutism occurs when children excessively sides with their mother; *passive-aggressive* elective mutism presents in children assuming a controlling and manipulative role by selectively withholding speech, and *speech phobic* elective mutism is the displacement of extreme anxiety onto speech (Hayden, 1980).

When mutism occurs after a traumatic event, the condition is called *traumatic mutism* and is not the same as elective mutism. For example, children involved in auto accidents or witnessing violence may be scared speechless. In these instances, treatment is guided by posttraumatic shock theory and interventions.

Educators working with children with learning disabilities identify cognitive processes and linguistic functions as primarily verbal or nonverbal. Verbal speech-language functions include the following (Taylor, 1989):

1. Expressive language and listening comprehension
2. Accuracy and speed in naming and articulation (speech-motor control)
3. Ability to use phonologic (speech-sound) codes to remember verbal stimuli, produce rhymes and recognize phonemic similarities, and segment and blend phonemes into words
4. Ability to use verbal coding or rehearsal generally
5. Awareness of morphologic and syntactic structures in language

Deficient nonverbal areas include the following:

1. Visual perception and visual-motor skills
2. Ability to discriminate or remember the temporal order of nonverbal stimuli
3. Presence of neurologic soft signs, including motor steadiness, motor sequencing and agility, and somatosensory skills

Generalized cognitive dysfunctions appear in the following areas:

1. Cross-modal and intermodal matching abilities
2. Short-term memory for verbal and nonverbal stimuli
3. Vigilance and attentional capacity
4. Use of strategies that enhance task performance, including accuracy or comprehensive monitoring, stimulus encoding, rehearsal, clustering, and elaboration
5. Miscellaneous high-order cognitive abilities, such as the ability to shift mental sets, reason abstractly, solve problems, and conceptualize.

Nursing Management

INTERDISCIPLINARY PERSPECTIVES AND COLLABORATION

Children diagnosed with specific developmental disorders require the collaboration of professionals and specialists from different clinical and theoretic disciplines concerned with neurophysiologic and cognitive development and deviations. In some instances, child psychiatric nurses may serve as case manager, coordinating specialists in their primary interventions, and they often provide supportive psychotherapy. Children must receive instruction that is beneficial to them in both the academic and affective realms. For children with a psychiatric disorder and a learning disability, nurses implement the treatment goals in the affective realm, working in close collaboration with teachers and parents. They should also be aware of federal programs providing support.

Typically, four areas contribute to the care of children with specific developmental disorders: medicine, psychology, language, and education.

Psychiatrists, psychoanalysts, and psychiatric nurses are often more cause oriented in their approach than educators. This may be partly due to their belief that once an etiology is determined, a cure or specific caring measures can be emphasized and described. The use of psychopharmacology in interventions is frequent, especially when the academic disorder or learning disability presents concurrently with hyperactivity.

Psychologists observe, test, evaluate, and characterize outward behaviors. For over 50 years, they have attempted to detect presumed organic brain changes in children with specific developmental disorders. However, the complexity of brain-behavior relationships has been an obstacle.

Neuropsychologic evaluations assess the range of adaptive abilities that are controlled by the central nervous system. They include planning and abstract reasoning; receptive and expressive language; attention; memory, sensory, and perceptual and motor functioning; and perceptual motor problem solving. However, not all neuropsychologic measures examine children's emotional status or attempt to link organic and psychologic factors (Allen and others, 1987). Deficits that may be noticed in an adolescent are often not recognized as the delayed effects of an early childhood trauma. Because of limitations of developed screening measures, neuropsychologists are now focusing on developing tests that evaluate higher cognitive functions (Lewis and Sinnett, 1987). Problem-solving skills are a higher functioning cognitive skill that play an integral part in children's learning. For example, children with significant brain damage that are unable to use abstract reasoning may rely on the less successful methods such as trial and error.

Rehabilitative specialists have become interested in methods that enhance interpersonal skills deficits through social skills training programs using instruction, shaping, prompting, modeling, feedback, reinforcement, and behavior rehearsal. Self-monitoring feedback has been found to be effective in numerous clinical studies (Gajor and others, 1984).

The concerns of psycholinguistic specialists overlap with those of educational specialists in learning disabilities. The diagnosis of the *language-learning-disabled child* has appeared recently in both psycholinguistic and educational literature. Understanding ways in which normal children learn and develop language is essential for understanding children with specific developmental disorders (see Chapter 3). For educators, the cause of the dysfunction is often not their focus, and "education often begins where medicine stops" (Kirk, 1972).

PL 99-457, PART H

Because PL 94-142 did not include children under the age of 3, PL 99-457, Part H was developed. It enlarges the themes of interdisciplinary collaboration and family empowerment developed in PL 94-142 and ensures that no child is denied special services and that evaluation does not discriminate ethnically or racially. Some experts believe that this law is the predecessor of future legislation providing needed health, social services, and educational support to children and their families. The purposes of the law are the following (Gallagher, 1989):

1. To enhance the development of handicapped infants and toddlers and to minimize their potential for developmental delays
2. To reduce the educational costs to our society by minimizing the need for special education and related services after handicapped infants and toddlers reach school age
3. To minimize the likelihood of institutionalization of handicapped individuals and maximize the potential for their independent living in society

4. To enhance the capacity of families to meet the special needs of their infants and toddlers with handicaps

PL 99-457 was enacted for children experiencing developmental delays as measured by appropriate diagnostic instruments and procedures in cognitive development, physical development, language and speech development, psychosocial development, or self-help skills. It also affects children with a diagnosed physical or mental condition having a high probability of resulting in developmental delay. Under the terms of the law, individual states must define children who are *at risk* medically and environmentally and must provide the following:

1. Case manager: Each family must have a case manager assigned to it who is most appropriate for the situation. This person is responsible for the implementation of the plan and for coordination with other agencies and persons. The provision is designed to simplify the family's contact with the professional world.
2. Multidisciplinary assessment of the child and family: A comprehensive and multidisciplinary assessment of the functioning of each child and the needs and strengths of the families is essential, involving different professional disciplines in decisions affecting the family.
3. Interagency coordinating council: This council enlists the participation of parents and the public and advises and assists the lead agency in identifying sources of financial support and in promoting interagency agreements.

Professionals have recognized the difficulties in acquiring family involvement in a total treatment program. Diagnostic and reimbursement policies that are designed to focus on the individual, professional competitiveness, barriers between disciplines, and inconsistent training programs also contribute to uncoordinated assistance for these families.

Reforms requiring parents' participation enhance the capacity of families to cope with infants and toddlers who have handicapping conditions. Individualized Family Service Plans (IFSP) provide a statement of children's development, the family's strengths and needs, and the intervention services that will be used to deal with those needs and necessitate the involvement of the family.

Critics of the IFSP note the potential of intruding into the privacy of the family and lowering the family's sense of responsibility for the child. Numerous safeguards have been proposed to protect confidentiality by limiting the examination of records and requiring a written notice to parents when services by intervention agencies change.

EDUCATIONAL INTERVENTION TECHNIQUES

The purpose of remedial tutoring is to identify and support children's independence, reduce stress and anxiety, interpret difficult areas of both content and process, strengthen motivation, and address early signs of psychological issues. To be successful, it must accomplish the following:

1. Enlist students' interest so that they can attack the academic task (commitment)
2. Simplify the task through reduction of required acts
3. Maintain students' pursuit of objectives

4. Provide feedback about responses
5. Control frustration
6. Demonstrate the proper solution

Prescriptive teaching occurs once the level of functioning has been identified. Clinicians continually teach children based on their unique needs, and evaluate their performance. Through this process, the effectiveness of the teaching intervention can be determined.

In defining the *modality concept,* Wepman (1967) stated that to define children's learning type, their maximal modality or pathway of learning needs to be understood. When children show that their strength in learning is in a visual channel, a visual method of instruction is encouraged. Immediate auditory reinforcement and training to improve other capacities or channels are also suggested for this approach.

The skills-sequence approach analyzes the specific skill to be taught and breaks it into a series of explicit subskills. For example, for children to learn to write their name, they are taught the way to position the paper, to hold a pencil, to form the latters, and to avoid repetition of letters. Many educators recommend combining the modality-processing and skills-sequence approaches.

Direct instruction is a preferred practice method of teaching both learning disabled and behaviorally disordered children. The concept is based on three basic assumptions: (1) all children can be taught, (2) teachers and administrators are responsible for learning, and (3) learning depends on active participation.

The method involves introducing new materials, providing extensive practice opportunities, and associating the new material with previously learned information. High mastery standards are set and maintained, and it allows only one interpretation of the material. It maximizes active learning and available teaching time and often includes a behavioral management system in the implementation.

Precision teaching is another preferred practice in education. It involves procedures based on direct and daily measurement of observable behavior of students, monitoring that has been positively associated with student achievement. Evaluating intervention strategies and modifying them according to the needs of the student are also effective measures (Kerr and Nelson, 1983). Five principles guide precision teaching (White, 1988):

1. The learner knows best: If data suggest that satisfactory progress is being made, the instruction is appropriate.
2. Focus on direct observable behavior: Behaviors are observed and counted, have a beginning and an end, and are repeatable.
3. Frequency is the basic measure of performance: Behaviors are recorded according to their appropriateness.
4. The standard celeration chart is critical: Graphs on a semilogarithmic scale record, display, and analyze student performance, enabling equal dimensions of change to appear, some without regard to absolute frequency.
5. Analyze environmental conditions: Evaluating the impact events may have on the performance of a child is essential.

Clinicians should apply these educational approaches when teaching children with learning and emotional disabilities (see box).

Techniques for Working with Children

1. Eliminate distractions as much as possible for attention-deficit children. Clinicians need to be aware of visual distractions, such as mobiles, posters, and murals, and auditory distractions, such as humming noises and conversations of others.
2. Provide activities that children can master and that foster success.
3. Schedule courses that are based on children's learning style and that induce success.
4. Present material in small, sequential steps.
5. Reinforce basic concepts with supplementary materials.
6. Arrange seating to minimize distractions.
7. Provide a course syllabus to overcome problems of disorganization.
8. Furnish written records of homework assignments.
9. Provide a written copy of the work that is put on the board, to reduce copying errors and time required.
10. Segment learning experiences into shorter time blocks to accommodate the child's short attention span.
11. Use prerecorded "talking books" in lieu of reading assignments.
12. Use oral instead of written tests.
13. Remove time restrictions from tests or administer tests in two sessions.
14. Substitute oral reports, graphic displays, or other projects for written reports.
15. Replace selected reading assignments with audio-visual presentations.
16. Form a contract with children based on fulfilling mutual goals.
17. Arrange for peer tutoring.
18. Provide positive feedback consistently and frequently.
19. Recognize and use children's special talents to promote learning and feelings of self-worth.
20. Allow and encourage children to monitor their daily progress through the use of charts or graphs.
21. Maintain a structured program but remain flexible within it.
22. Build self-confidence in the students.
23. Begin on children's developmental level.
24. Teach remedial material, material that needs to be relearned, and new material.
25. Use physical proximity to refocus children on their task.
26. Include the use of cues and aids until children can perform alone.
27. Use methods of instruction needed by the child and vary the work tasks.
28. Allow time for group and individual work and plan activities requiring some physical movement and verbalization.

Summary

Academic problems are often the reason for children's first contact with mental health professionals. Clinicians should consider children's reaction as significant; they are in need of crisis or stress intervention and psychologic support. This first negative experience may signify a more serious psychiatric disorder in the early stages of development.

Nursery and elementary school nurses' therapeutic roles usually focus on the areas of poor motivation, poor self-concept, and underachievement. Resolution of immediate problems requires a definite plan of intervention dependent on the demands confronting the student and should include stress management techniques and remedial tutoring.

School nurses should also continually monitor children with academic problems. They are in a unique position to follow the progress of these children longitudinally during grade progression. Interdisciplinary collaboration between teachers focusing on the academic progress and nurses managing and providing the emotional components needed may avert or lessen more severe illnesses. When child psychiatric nurses are contracted to provide consultation services to teachers in their management of deviant children, they need to understand teachers' roles and goals and be aware of the educators' language, educational viewpoints, operational problems, teaching methodologies, and concepts.

School nurses and child psychiatric consultants may have a critical role in the required process for diagnosing children under PL 94-142 or 99-457. Parental consent must be given before children can be placed in a special program, and nurses' skill and experience in working with families renders them qualified for the successful negotiation of this process. Children are expected to attend school and progress academically with the help of the child psychiatric nursing staff.

REFERENCES

Adams P and Fras I: Beginning child psychiatry, New York, 1988, Brummer/Mazel, Inc.

Allen JA and others: Neuropsychological assessment in a psychiatric setting: the mind-body problem in linical practice, Bull Menninger Clin 50:5, 1987.

Aman MG and Singh NN: Specific reading disorders: concepts of etiology reconsidered. In Gadow KD and Bialer I, editors: Advances in learning and behavioral disabilities, vol 2, Greenwich, Conn, 1983, JAI Press, Inc.

American Psychiatric Association: Diagnostic and statistical manual of mental disorders, ed 3, rev, Washington, DC, 1987. American Psychiatric Association.

Anderson LE: Helping the adolescent with the hidden handicap. In Wallace G and McLoughlin AS: Learning disabilities: concepts and characteristics, ed 2, Los Angeles, 1979, Merrill Publishing Co.

Bemporad JR and Schwab ME: The DSM-III and clinical child psychiatry. In Million T and Klernman GL, editors: Contemporary directions in psychopathology: toward the DSM-IV, New York, 1986, The Guilford Press.

Bender WN: Behavioral correlates of temperament and personality in the inactive learner, J Learn Disabil 20:5, 1987a.

Bender WN: Secondary personality and behavior problems in adolescents with learning disabilities, J Learn Disabil 20:5, 1987b.

Bowlby J: Attachment and loss III: loss, sadness and depression, New York, 1980, Basic Books, Inc, Publishers.

Byran T and Pearl R: Self-concept and locus of control of learning disabled children, Clin Child Psychol 8:223, 1979.

Chalfant JC: Learning disabilities: policy issues and promising approaches, Psychol 44:392, 1989.

Chalfant JC and King FS: An approach to operationalizing the definition of learning disabilities, J Learning Disabilities 9:4, 1976.

Congressional Record: Washington, DC, 1975.

Corning WC: Bootstrapping toward a classification system. In Million T and Klernman GL, editors: Contemporary directions in psychopathology: toward the DSM-IV, New York, 1986, The Guilford Press.

Gaddes WH: Prevalence estimates and the need for definition of learning disabilities. In Obrzut HE and Hynd GW, editors: Cognitive dysfunction and psychoeducational assessment in individuals with acquired brain injury, J Learn Disabil 209:10, 1987.

Gajor A and others: Effects of feedback and self-monitoring on head trauma youth's conversation skills, J Appl Behav Anal 17:3, 1984.

Gallagher JJ: A new policy initiative: infants and toddlers with handicapping conditions, Psychol 44:387, 1989.

Gardner W: Children with learning and behavior problems, Boston, 1978, Allyn & Bacon, Inc.

Gergen KJ: The concept of self, New York, 1971, Holt, Rinehart & Winston, Inc.

Gold S, and Kline J: No miracles, Acad Ther 21:2, 1985.

Hamill DD: Assessing and training perceptual and motor skills. In Hamill DD and Bartel NR, editors: Teaching children with learning and behavior problems, ed 2, Boston, 1978, Allyn & Bacon, Inc.

Harter S: Developmental perspectives on the self-system. In Hetheringtron EM, editor: Socialization, personality and social development, vol 4, ed 4, New York, 1983, John Wiley & Sons, Inc.

Hayden TI: Classification of elective mutism, J Am Acad Child Adolesc Psychiatry 19:118, 1980.

Henderson M and Clive H: A critical review of social skills training with young offenders, Criminal Justice and Behavior 10:3, 1983.

Hill KT and Sarasen SB: The relation of test anxiety and defensiveness to test and school performance over the elementary school years, Society of Research in Child Development Monograph, 1966.

Humphrey JH: Profiles in stress, New York, 1986, AMS Press, Inc.

Johnson D and Myklebust H: Learning disabilities: education principles and practices, New York, 1967, Grune & Stratton, Inc.

Kerr MM and Nelson M: Strategies for managing behavior problems in the classroom, Columbus, Ohio, 1983, Merrill Publishing Co.

Kirk SA: Educating exceptional children, Boston, 1972, Houghton Mifflin Co.

Kirk SA: Teaching reading to slow and disabled learners. Boston, 1976, Houghton Mifflin & Co.

Kirk SA and Kirk WD: Psycholinguistic learning disabilities: diagnosis and remediation, Chicago, 1971, University of Illinois Press.

Lerner JW: Children with learning disabilities, ed 2, Boston, 1976, Houghton Mifflin Co.

Lewis L and Sinnett R: An introduction to neuropsychological assessment, J Counsel Dev 66:3, 1987.

Maziade M and others: Temperament and intellectual development: a longitudinal study from infancy to four years. In Myklebust HR and Boshes B: Final report: minimal brain damage in children, Washington DC, 1969, Department of Health, Education and Welfare.

Morgan DP and Jenson WR: Teaching behaviorally disordered students, Columbus, Ohio, 1988, Merrill Publishing Co.

Opie ND and Slater P: Mental health needs of children in school: role of the child psychiatric mental health nurse, J Child Adolescent Psychia Mental Health Nurs 1:31, 1988.

Purkley WW: Self-concept and school achievement, Englewood Cliffs, NJ, 1970, Prentice-Hall, Inc.

Rugel RP: WISC subtest scores of disabled readers: a review with respect to Bannatyne's recategorization, J Learning Disabilities 1:46, 1974.

Rutter M: The role of cognition in child development and disorder. Chess S, Thomas A, and Hertzig ME, editors: Annual progress in child psychiatry and child development, New York, 1989, Brunner/Mazel, Inc.

Smith B: A comparative analysis of selected federal programs serving young children, Chapel Hill, NC, 1986, University of North Carolina Press.

Taylor HG: Learning disabilities. In Mash EJ and Terdal LG, editors: Behavioral assessment of childhood disorders, ed 2, New York, 1989, The Guilford Press.

Torgensen JK: Learning disabilities theory: its current state and future prospects, J Learn disabilities, 19:399, 1986.

US Office of Education: First annual report, national advisory on handicapped children, Washington DC, 1968, Department of Health, Education and Welfare.

Vallett RE: Programming learning disability children, Belmont Calif, 1969, Fearson.

Wallace G and Kaufman JM: Teaching children with learning problems, ed 2, Columbus, Ohio, 1978, Merrill Publishing Co.

Wallace G and McLoughlin JA: Learning disabilities: concepts and characteristics, ed 2, Columbia, Ohio, 1979, Merrill Publishing Co.

Webb LJ and others: DSM-III training guide, New York, 1981, Brunner/Mazel, Inc.

Wepman JM: The perceptual basis for learning. In Frierson EC and Barbe WB, editors: Educating children with learning disabilities, selected readings, New York, 1967, Meredith Corp.

White OR: Precision teaching-precision learning, exceptional children. In Morgan DP and Jenson WR, editors: Teaching behaviorally disordered students: preferred practices, Columbus, Ohio, 1988, Merrill Publishing Co.

Will MC: Educating children with learning problems: a shared responsibility, J Learn Disabil 20:5, 1987.

Part III

Physical, Social, and Emotional Disorders

Chapter 11

Gender and Sexual Identity Disorders

Gender and sexual identity disorders involve problems in gender, sex drive, and sexual expression. Components include gender identity (the inner conviction of being male or female) and sexual preference (roles, sexual orientation, and the emotional and social qualities perceived as masculine or feminine). Gender identity also refers to people's capacity to experience themselves as female or male in social and sexual relationships and includes acceptance of gender, integration of genitalia, and body image sensations.

Social and cultural stereotypes influence gender and sexual concepts, and conflicts arise when expectations of gender and sexuality identity are not fulfilled. People often assume that their beliefs are universally held and view values as *good* or *bad* based on ethnocentric concepts. These traditional, rejecting attitudes cause stigmatization and discrimination against children with sexual and gender behaviors different from their culture's norms.

During the last decade a new psychology of sex roles has emerged in which sex role development is a dynamic, interactive process modified by social and biologic forces. The traditional psychology of sex roles held that the familiar division by sex of work and domestic responsibilities was essential for the development of healthy males and females. This chapter discusses the psychologic, emotional, and social interactions occurring during physical biologic development.

Definitions and Concepts

Major obstacles in identifying and treating childhood gender and sexual identity problems are the ambiguous use of the terms *gender* and *sex* and vague definitions of differences in masculine and feminine gender and sexual behaviors. Most dictionaries use three main definitions for sex: (1) gender, that is, the two divisions of males and females; (2) anything connected with sexual gratification or reproduction; and (3) the character of being male or female.

Although these definitions are outdated, they influence popular and professional perceptions. The first definition is based on anatomic and chromosome configuration at birth and fails to include contemporary psychologic aspects of behavior relating to gender. The second definition limits sex to reproduction and the sex act, and the third definition uses the word *character,* interpreted to refer to the quality of people's sexual behavior as compared to cultural expectations.

The terms *gender* and *sex* are also used ambiguously by professionals in the literature and clinical practice. In different contexts, they are used to describe the genetic composition, reproductive organs, secondary sex characteristics, and the intrapsychic characteristics associated with being male or female. Some define normal sexual identity as occurring when identity correlates with anatomy, despite considerable evidence that the definition is limited (Gadpaille, 1981).

In contrast to the older definition in which sex and gender are interdependent, Unger (1979) suggests partitioning the concept of sex on the basis of biologic and social functions. He advocates limiting the term *gender* to descriptions of nonphysiologic components of sex that are considered culturally appropriate. Applying these distinctions would provide more accurate data for specific assessment and interventions but is difficult because of limitations in separating the interactions, especially in the cognitive area (Shepherd-Look, 1982). Growing evidence also exists that the physiologic dichotomy between males and females is not as absolute as older theories assumed. Researchers found little correlation between chromosomal, hormonal, and morphologic indicators of sex in people (Money, 1988; Money and Ehrhardt, 1972).

The terms used contribute to the confusion because they are referred to in both outdated and new theories. *Cross-sexed* applies to people who have incorporated a sex-role standard opposite from their biologic sex; in the past, it was synonymous with *androgenized.* The inaccurate assumption was that masculinity and femininity fell at opposite poles of a single continuum.

Androgenization is not the same as *androgyny,* a concept developed by Bem (1974, 1975) in the 1970s. It views masculine and feminine traits as existing on two separate continua, with degrees of masculine and feminine behavior ranging from high to low and occurring in both sexes when measured independently. A major goal of interventions in gender and sexual disorders is to expand children's repertoire of androgynous behaviors to maximize their human potential. Androgynous individuals are less rigid, more adaptive, and more effective in situations that call for characteristics of both sexes.

DSM-III-R Diagnoses

Advances in scientific and clinical understandings have resulted in clearer definitions of these disorders, reflected in changes in the terminology and concepts of the DSM-II, DSM-III, and DSM-III-R. In the DSM-III-R, gender disorders were moved from the adult section to the childhood disorders section because they invariably begin in childhood (see box).

Current concepts hold that the predominant characteristics of gender identity disorders are an inconsistency between the sex assigned at birth and gender identity. They are early and fundamental disturbances in children's sense of self that may involve delusional thinking.

> ### *Gender Identity Disorders*
>
> 302.60 Gender identity disorder of childhood
> 302.50 Transsexualism; specify sexual history: asexual, homosexual, heterosexual, unspecified
> 302.85 Gender identity disorder of adolescence or adulthood, nontransexual type; specify sexual history: asexual, homosexual, heterosexual, unspecified
> 302.85 Gender identity disorder (NOS)
>
> From American Psychiatric Association: Diagnostic and statistical manual of mental disorders, ed 3, rev, Washington, DC, 1987, American Psychiatric Association.

Historically, female gender and sexual disorders were not given the same clinical attention and research as male disorders because of the double standard valuing future male adult roles over female roles. Gender problems are reported at least eight times more often in boys than in girls (American Psychiatric Association, 1987).

The GAP's Women's Task Force for consciousness raising of female issues petitioned for and elicited changes in the proposed criteria of gender disturbances for females in the DSM-III-R. These criteria were based on clinical and research studies on males conducted by male physicians, despite considerable research evidence that psychosexual development in males and females differs and that interventions used for males would not be appropriate for females (Kaplan, 1983; Kass, Spitzer, and Williams, 1983).

In the DSM-III-R diagnoses, gender identity disorders of childhood are characterized by persistent distress about assigned gender that presents before the age of puberty. These children overidentify with stereotypes of the opposite sex, rejecting the behaviors, activities, and interest of their sex. In acting out wish-fulfillment fantasies, they may injure themselves when attempting physical activities that conflict with their physical endowment. Transsexual disorders are characterized by persistent discomfort and the sense of inappropriateness about the assigned sex, with the preoccupation lasting at least 2 years. Children with the disorder express the desire to eliminate primary sex characteristics and assume those of the opposite sex. Cross-gender identity problems exist when children are convinced that they are a member of the opposite physical sex. A conflicted sexual identity is the state in which strong feelings of masculine and feminine identity coexist.

Gender identity disorders not otherwise specified include cross-dressing instances in children. Although a child that has met the criteria for gender identity disorder could be regarded as a child transsexual, the diagnosis is conventionally reserved for adults (Adams and Fras, 1988).

While gender role and identity relate to biologic sex, they are not shaped by biologic factors, distinctions provided for in the DSM-III-R multiaxis system. Gender disturbances do not refer to sexual activities, proclivities, or homosexuality, and physical abnormalities of sex organs are rarely associated with these disorders. If present, they are noted on Axis III.

Theoretic perspectives

SOCIAL AND CULTURAL ASPECTS

During the past 30 years, American culture has been undergoing remarkable cultural, social, economic, and political change concurrent with psychocultural shifts in sexual and gender role concepts and stereotypes. Although some adults have expanded their ideas of acceptable sexual and gender lifestyles, traditional notions still prevail within and between cultures. Public opinion surveys indicate that little change in traditional gender and sex role traits expectations has occurred (Mason, 1973; Mason, Czajka, and Arber, 1976). Most Americans expect men to demonstrate competence, independence, rationality, control, and assertion and women to exhibit warmth and expressiveness.

Some variations in culturally accepted sex-role stereotypes have been found, and these variations are important for nurse clinicians to identify when screening children and their parents presenting gender and sexual identity concerns. The change in family situations has greatly affected roles. Only 6% of American families fit the traditionally held image of the wife at home rearing the children and the male husband working (Klein, 1983). Statistics also show that 12.7 million children under the age of 18 live with their mother and 1.3 million children live with their father (US Bureau of Census, 1984). However, the changes that have occurred have not been adequately assimilated by many adults, who are ambiguous role models for children developing their sexual identities.

Many researchers are involved in studies concerning the modification of traditional assumptions. The proliferation of scientific publications in sex-role psychology since the mid-1960s reflects their professional concern. Some scientists hope to correct misconceptions about sex differences, believing that they are the reason for sex discrimination and sex stereotyping in contemporary society. Others focus on investigating social policy to determine the types of jobs members of the two sexes should or could hold and the life styles that would maximize potential and androgyny in both sexes.

Most scientists view the psychocultural shift in sex and gender as one of the greatest changes for maximizing human potential and are optimistic that less rigid stereotypes will evolve to less restrictive sex-role and gender definitions and a fully human view of both sexes. Block (1973, 1978, 1984) has stated that socialization changes will permit sex-role definitions transcending the limiting concepts of masculinity and femininity imposed in the past. Extensive research confirms that it is more accurate to speak of sex-related differences than of sex differences (Harris, 1982).

Understanding gender identity and sex roles requires awareness of the cultural perceptions shaping female and male sexual and gender behaviors. Standardized questionnaires and survey tools have been developed that measure sex-role attitudes and orientations, such as the Index of Sex Role Orientation (Dreyer, Woods, and James, 1981) and the National Fertility Survey Sex Role Attitude Inventory (Mason, Czajka, and Arber, 1976). Nurse clinicians can use them for value clarification interventions with families, students, and staff in inpatient clinical settings (Rieker and Carmen, 1983).

There are differences in attitudes held by subgroups in the population. Sex-role standards are more rigidly defined with less tolerance for deviation in men from lower social classes and in the less educated. Young educated men maintain more rigid sex-role standards than women. Women students and college-educated women perceive the feminine role as involving greater independence and achievement than older or less educated women. When compared with children of unemployed mothers, children whose mothers were employed held more educational aspirations and viewed males assuming housekeeping tasks as appropriate (Shepherd-Look, 1982).

Masculinity, femininity, androgyny, and preferred modes of sexuality are learned as children develop and involve a complicated and sequential process of interactions within multiple lines of development. Many concepts occur unconsciously, influenced by the on-going role modeling of significant adults. Either biologic sequences or child-rearing experiences may influence deviations from the normal developmental progression, producing psychosexual identity disorders. Therefore, the interaction of developmental components need to be considered concurrently:

The sexual instincts of man do not suddenly awaken between the thirteenth and fifteenth year, i.e., at puberty, but operate from the onset of the child's development, change gradually from one form to another, progress from one stage to another until at last adult sexual life is achieved as the final result from this long series of developments (Freud, 1946).

PSYCHOANALYTIC EXPLANATIONS

Early psychoanalytic theories attributed differences in gender to biologic factors and the presence or absence of a penis. Sigmund Freud established the most fully developed descriptions of the development of gender identity. He noted that maleness and masculinity were more natural states and considered femininity to be less valuable (Stoller, 1985). Anna Freud's descriptions of the complex development of defense mechanisms during childhood (1946) clarifies Sigmund Freud's theory of psychosexual development and psychoanalytic explanations for gender disorders (1959).

Pre-Oedipal children's ties to their mother are tenacious and intense and are necessary to master early development tasks. According to Anna Freud's theory the defense mechanisms of repression and identification mature as children enter the Oedipal stage, providing a defense against these past bonds and facilitating negotiation of Oedipal developmental tasks. The overuse of repression results in the massive denial noted in the absence of or limited memory of pre-Oedipal experiences.

Freud held that shifting identification was more difficult for girls than for boys and that as a result, girls developed less restrictive superegos and the feminine traits of softness, compassion, flexibility, and effectiveness were facilitated:

1. A boy has a loving relationship with his mother and sees his father as a rival and an object of envy and hostility because he stands in the way of the boy owning his mother. At the same time the boy fears his father will castrate him in retaliation for his sexual desire toward his mother (castration complex). For resolution of the Oedipal stage, the boy must transfer his identification with his

mother to his father. Freud's classical case of "Little Hans" (1955) described this transference process and the phobias children may develop as a defense against their sexual anxieties.

2. A girl observes that little boys have penises and infers she has been castrated and blames her mother. To compensate for this deficiency, the girl develops a desire for a penis (penis envy) and a wish to have a child by her father, who becomes her primary love object. Because the mother is his primary love object, she becomes the child's rival. To successfully resolve her Oedipal conflict, the girl must make a third transference (from mother to father then back to her mother).

With increased awareness of the impact of cultural expectations on female personality growth and development, the theory of defensive identification in girls is generally discounted and viewed as historically specific to the Victorian era. Some claim that the concept of penis envy is a symbolic representation of roles, rights, responsibilities, and out-dated cultural double standards that value males more than females (Block, 1984; Gilligan, 1983).

Others view the theory as clarifying trait differences and holding positive implications for females. Freud (1961) postulated that the special characteristics of the Oedipal complex and its resolution resulted in women developing a final superego structure that was less strict. If this assumption is correct, it may explain why females escape more psychosexual conflicts than males even though female development is more complex and sensitive than male psychologic development, (Nagera, 1981).

The Oedipal theory continues to be a source for explanation of psychosocial disorders. Psychoanalytic theory holds that before the Oedipal stage, sexual and aggressive drives are fused. Through defensive identification, two different and distinctly focused drives emerge (Kohut and Wolf, 1978). Some experts believe that when women fail to negotiate this task, they continue to exhibit aggressive behaviors our society values in men.

In contrast to the Freudian notion that the post–Oedipal latency years are a wasteland in which sexual drives are dormant, Sarnoff (1976) presents a psychoanalytic view of the latency years as rich in drives and developmental events and notes the occurrence of difficulties reflecting sexual and gender issues. Possible psychopathologies occurring during latency explain sexual and physical disorders in children, such as eating and sleep disturbances, which are related to biologic changes, sexual fantasies, and maturational difficulties.

1. Failure to enter the state of latency
   a. Failure of the development of cognitive precursors
      (1) Failure to develop the symbolizing function due to impaired displacement, delay, repression, or object relations
      (2) Failure in maturation of symbolizing functions and impairment in the development of behavioral and object constancy due to poor superego formation, poor models, or poor superego from failure of identification
   b. Overstimulation

2. Regressive deterioration of the ego structure of latency in children who have already reached the latency state from decompensation of the ego structure, resulting in acting on fantasies themselves and being driven by overstimulating events such as seduction and beatings
3. Regression to prelatency behavior due to loss of mechanisms of restraint and the structure of latency
4. Inadequate symbol formation due to an inadequate structure of latency
   a. Severe mourning reactions
   b. Patterns of good behavior in school coupled with poor behavior at home
5. Neurotic symptoms
   a. Hysteria
   b. Phobias
   c. Obsessions
6. Depression
   a. Persecutory states
   b. Unsuccessful attempts to adjust to new peer groups
   c. Psychosomatic responses
   d. Obsessional states
   e. Oral regressive states accompanied by overeating
7. Psychotic states

EGO PSYCHOLOGY

Ego psychologist Eric Erikson attributed distinctions in gender to social and cultural influences. Erikson contributed to the understanding of gender differences with his research on children's choice of play objects and play configurations (1964). The differences begin when children have independent opportunities to make choices, usually after walking is mastered and play materials are not provided and controlled by caretakers. Play materials and free play activities that normally occur at specific ages and stages provide important early sex and gender conflict screening data and can be employed by clinicians when play therapy and behavior modification are used as interventions in these disorders (Rekers, 1977a).

SOCIAL LEARNING THEORIES

In contrast to the psychoanalytic perspective, social learning theories emphasize the role of reward, punishment, generalization, and imitation in the development of gender identity, with imitation in observational learning critical. These theories also believe that identification is more difficult for boys because they must imitate the parent with whom they have the least contact, the father, who is absent from the home most of the day due to working conditions or divorce.

Social learning theorists stress that children's early and profound love for the primary model, their mother, establishes a powerful identification. However, they postulate that when small boys perceive anatomic sex-organ differences, they transfer their identification from their mother to their *father likeness,* a transference facilitated by social and peer interactions and prevailing male prescriptions (Bandura, 1977; Maccoby and Jacklin, 1974).

COGNITIVE-DEVELOPMENTAL THEORIES

Cognitive-developmental theorists draw on Piaget's theory to explain normal gender identification, positing that children's concept of their bodies and the bodies of others determine gender identity (Belenky and others, 1986; Kohlberg, 1966; Phillips, 1969). The schemata begin with the initial labeling by parents or significant others who inform and reassure children about being a boy or a girl. These injunctions are internalized and become a self-categorization, stabilizing as cognitive maturation continues. Children develop a *gender schemata* and place a positive value on clothing, toys, and activities that support and strengthen it to achieve cognitive consistency (Rosen and Teague, 1974). However, the behavioral repertoire of children with gender identity disorders is often more limited than members of the sex they emulate, and their fantasy life and problem solving are circumscribed.

Body image, core gender identity, and self-concept are established by 30 months of age and contribute to the gender schema. Children's ideas of masculine and feminine behavior are derived from universally perceived gender differences, and gender identity becomes stabilized at 5 or 6 years of age. Piaget's theory of conservation holds that children then learn to conserve, and gender concepts become concise and fixed.

SYMBOLIC INTERACTIONS THEORIES

Symbolic interactions theorists stress humans as symbol-using creatures who exist in a world with meaning created by their symbols of verbal and nonverbal language, signs, and objects (Blumer, 1969; Grecas and Libby, 1976). They describe gender and sexual activities in terms of religious, romantic, recreational, and utilitarian-predatory meaning. Children's use of opposite sex mannerisms may elicit rejection from their peers although they are unaware of the behaviors contributing to their painful rejection (Berkowitz, 1985; Rosen and Teague, 1974). These theories provide the rationale for using nonverbal communication indices in the assessment and intervention of gender identity problems in children.

COMMUNICATION THEORIES

Children learning to speak and use language to communicate in the areas of sex and gender are confronted with a confusing array of terms fraught with ambiguities. The language of sex and gender in most cultures is expressed through gestures and mannerisms Goffman (1977) refers to as *genderisms*. These nonverbal gestures, such as a certain smile, frowns, winks, body postures, and use of physical space, convey specific gender messages and are learned and relied on by children during these early years (Gilligan, 1982; Michael, 1968; Thorne, Kramarae, and Henley, 1983). Anthropologic evidence also exists that distinctions in male and female gender behaviors differ from culture to culture. Each society has a set of masculine and feminine gender mannerisms conveying both normal and deviant messages (Kessler and McKenna, 1978).

Developmental Ages and Stages

PRENATAL PERIOD AND INFANCY

For most people, few aspects of human behavior are as closely linked to biology as sexuality. Sex is viewed as a biologic endowment present at birth and possessed by all animals that have gender (Money, 1988). Biologic etiologic explanations for gender and sexual disorders consist of genetic, constitutional, gonadal, external sex-organ anatomic, internal accessory genital anatomic, and sex endocrinologic variables, producing male or female concepts.

Biologic development of sexual identity begins with the presence of specific sex chromosomes, which influences gonadal differentiation and prenatal hormonal secretions. These secretions are responsible for the morphology of the external genitalia and the patterns of organization in the brain that influence future temperament and cognition. The sex of the fetus can be identified months before birth with ultrasound, and the sex assignment influences prenatal expectations and child-rearing patterns for boys and girls after birth. Male infants are born with an erect penis and females with vaginal lubrication, denoting a sexual readiness that is a natural function of being human and a recurrent vital characteristic throughout the life cycle (Adams and Fras, 1988).

During the first 3 or 4 months of life, infants' major task is individuation-separation (Mahler, 1971). Freud (1946) viewed this phase as bisexual or asexual because both male and female infants separate from a (female) mother body image. The influence of an initial female body image is viewed by theorists as evidence for the greater difficulties males have in sexual and gender confirmation (Casper and others, 1978; Fraiberg, 1961; Mahler, 1971).

Intersex Conditions

Hermaphroditism and pseudohermaphroditism are rare occurrences in which ambiguous or anomalous genitalia are present in newborns. Although the causative factors for these congenital anomalies are unknown, a number of variables have been suggested, including errors in genetic coding, X chromosome alterations, hormonal and substance exposures occurring before and during pregnancy, and embryologic developmental deviations. Male infants may present with hypospadias and undescended testes, and females may demonstrate hypertrophied clitoris. When surgical or medical interventions are indicated, the decision-making process involves chromosomal, gonadal, hormonal, and anatomic factors. Decisions to correct ambiguous genitalia must be made immediately after birth to prevent later identity problems.

Nursing management. Intersex conditions require the services of many professionals, and primary care nurses often monitor and manage these children during and after corrective interventions. A continuing team approach is usually necessary, and primary clinicians need to ensure that communication is maintained between specialists and the family. Reinforcement, support, continuation of interventions, and on-going evaluation are critical.

Because of infants' limited communication ability, objective signs of sexual identity problems are rare at birth. The learning experiences that affect gender and sexual identity have also not occurred. Core gender identity appears at birth and almost always follows the sex assignment rather than the biologic state. In other rare instances the severe sexual identity dysfunction of transsexualism has been identified at birth (Stoller, 1985). Some child analysts claim that by the age of 8 months, children show signs of genital awareness and that by 15 to 18 months, they enter an early genital phase. Children at this age become flushed, perspire, and touch or grasp their genitalia when kissing or in close affectionate contact with a loved adult (Adams and Fras, 1988).

Once biologic sex is established, culturally defined cues greatly influence developing children. For example, when pseudohermaphroditism (biologic sex mistaken at birth) occurs and the incorrect sex is assigned, it is psychologically destructive to change this ascription by 2 years of age. Once children are 3 years old, most experts believe gender identity is well established and generally irreversible.

The presence of one or more of the symptoms in the physical areas of sex does not automatically imply a psychosexual disorder in infants. However, because these five variables produce male or female concepts, they are important initial screening criteria and indicate the necessity of a comprehensive clinical evaluation examining the frequency, setting, stage of emotional and social development, medical history, developmental progress, and general psychologic functioning.

An ambiguous or undifferentiated sexual identity presents during the developmental state in infancy or as a pathologic condition in later life in which a firm self-conviction of being male or female is lacking. Children developing transsexualism have the normal physical anatomy of one sex but identify with the opposite sex.

Parents of children with intersexual and genital anomalies that have been surgically corrected need on-going emotional support and specific educational help to cope with these conditions. Discussions with parents should minimize uncertainty about children's assigned sex, and concerted efforts should be made to prevent ambiguities in child rearing. The best approach is to emphasize that development is incomplete and requires medical management to assist nature. When questions arise, clinicians should be truthful and stress that no contradictory organs or elements exist in their child's body.

When parents or caretakers are overly concerned or are using ineffective coping mechanisms, adult role assessment formats such as the Fountaine Role Assessment tool clarify inconsistencies in adults' sex-role expectations of each other and of the child (Janosik and Davies, 1989). The goal is to provide consistent and unified gender and sexual child-rearing expectations to establish the most effective psychologic environment for the child. The basic principles for intersex management in infancy include the following (Gadpaille, 1981):

1. Most children develop healthy and unconfused sexual identity to their assigned and reared sex providing that this identity is unambiguously adhered to by parents and others aware of the initial dilemma, even when the sex assignment contradicts biologic determinants of sex (Money and Ehrhardt, 1972).
2. The assigned and child rearing sex is most effectively determined by the predicted anatomic ability for optimal adult sexual function.
3. When a functional penis is not expected to develop naturally in a genetic male, it is preferable to rear the child as a girl because surgical and medical methods

for creating a satisfactory female sexual appearance and function are more successful.

Advances in psychodiagnostics and treatment procedures make the goal of preventing the adult conditions of transsexualism, transvestitism, and other chronic sexual behavior disorders feasible. When biophysical conditions are present, nurse clinicians caring for these children can monitor early signs of distress and conduct long-term developmental tracing of sexual adjustment, facilitating detection of early psychologic signs that may warrant special interventions.

EARLY CHILDHOOD AND PRESCHOOL YEARS

The schemata of self-regard, body image, and core gender identity are established and accepted by children by the age of 30 months, and stereotypic masculine or feminine patterning at 4 or 4½ years of age. The effects of these major developmental milestones should be considered for children 1½ to 5 years of age. Most children become acutely aware of anatomic sex differences during this time period, and if congenital genital anomalies were present at birth, children's evolving body image concept should be monitored, especially when medical or surgical corrective measures are continuing.

Body Image Disturbances

As a major component of sexual identity, body image is the way children perceive their physical self as an object different from other objects. Combined with ego identity or social self, the perception of the physical self shapes ways in which children feel about themselves as a person and as a male or female sexual being.

Periods of rapid physical growth precipitate remarkable changes in body image. Most writings on body image discuss adolescent identity crises in which physical growth and sexual maturation coincide. However, the on-going subtle adaptations of body image that affect human sexuality are continuous. Concept distinctions basic to understanding gender identity problems include the following:

1. Neurologic body precept: This concept involves the postural image people have of their body as it functions outside central consciousness. It results from sensory impressions initiated during the embryonic stage and is organized during childhood as the result of tactile and kinesthetic perceptions.
2. Body concept: This psychologic image includes perceptions, thoughts, and feelings that the ego has in viewing the body and self. Failure of the ego to self-observe results in inappropriate words and actions.

Medical consultation is indicated if assessment findings indicate that children's behaviors deviate from the normal developmental range and if the symptom pattern has a history of more than 6 months. When symptoms of gender disturbance are obvious, evaluation should include a history, physical exam and examination of external genitalia, and chromosome analysis.

Treatment outcomes of children born with congenital genital anomalies are predominantly positive. Studies of hermaphroditic children suggest that interventions are highly successful when biologic misassignments at birth were corrected early with parental guidance starting in infancy and continuing during the early years. The interrelationship of biologic, psychologic, and identity factors that occurs during this time has the greatest potential in the formation of sexual identity of a child. Interventions should focus on fostering the following (Wolman and Money, 1980):

1. Identification with and role modeling of parent figure and peers of the same sex
2. Development of complementary role behaviors toward members of the opposite sex
3. Recognition of and identification with sexual anatomy and reproductive function

Nursing management. Nurses must carefully examine their own belief system with regard to psychosexual behaviors and guard against imposing their values on others, especially when working with young female inpatients in psychiatric settings. These girls have weak gender identities, body images, and body boundaries. Clinicians also need to understand the complexities and ambiguous meanings of sexual and gender language when communicating with children and ensure that the clients and their family assign the same meanings to terms.

An example of the confusion that inaccurate terminology creates is found in the sex education courses provided by schools and clinicians in clinical interventions. These programs are often limited to genital-centered content that fails to include the wholeness of man or woman or the meaningful fulfillment appropriate to people's needs and roles in contemporary society. Sex education must emphasize the gender and anatomic differences between the sexes and use the correct terms for body parts. These language problems can have grave implications when courses involve AIDS education.

Mannerisms, play behaviors, the use of toys, and other early signs of gender conflict that clinicians should evaluate include the following:

1. Cross-dressing (transvestitism)
2. Intense emotional expressions of the desire to be a member of the opposite sex
3. Overuse of effeminate or masculine gestures and gait
4. Feminine or masculine vocal tones and inflections
5. Speech content dominated by feminine or masculine words
6. Preference for playmates of the opposite sex
7. Preference for toys and activities socially ascribed as appropriate for the opposite sex.

EARLY SCHOOL YEARS

The period beginning at 6 years of age and extending through puberty was called *latency* in the psychoanalytic literature and was depicted as sexually dormant years. Numerous early psychologic theories overlooked the active sexuality that occurs during this period, resulting in many misconceptions concerning developing gender and sexuality identity during this time. Between 5 and 6 years of age, the Oedipal conflict is resolved and same sex identity becomes firmly established. This confirmation is followed by many years of intense emotional investment in the genitalia and sexual body image.

Children's interactions with their environment and culture expand remarkably during this time as they move from the protection of family, neighborhood, and friends to the wider world of peers and school. They also have an expanded awareness of the values society accords males and females and their role expectations. Children with atypical but normal genital developmental patterns may experience unpleasant peer responses. Because young children usually think dichotomously and hold rigid masculine and feminine body image stereotypes, body and genital comparisons in school showers and toilets can be painful experiences.

Children entering school are presented with a new and different set of sex stereotypes, those related to learning, academic performance, and sex-related cognitive abilities:

1. Verbal abilities: There is considerable evidence that girls acquire verbal skills earlier than boys, attributed to earlier left-hemisphere brain maturation (Money, 1988). Reinforced by cultural experiences, girls' early preference for verbal modes limits their need to develop nonverbal spatial modes of thought. In contrast, boys explore spatial aspects and develop nonverbal modes of cognition (Harris, 1982, Sherman, 1967).

2. Visual-spatial ability: Boys excel in their visual-spatial ability, mental understanding, and manipulation of 2- and 3-dimensional objects (Erikson, 1963). These differences have been related to a recessive X-linked gene expressed more frequently in males. Research indicates that 50% of males and 25% of females show the trait phenotypes (Harris, 1982; Sherman, 1967). Differences in cerebral specialization are also attributable to male dominance in this area. Early cerebral lateralization in girls occurs at a premature stage in the right hemisphere, with a greater degree of cortical commitment to language.

3. Mathematical ability: Although the evidence is less impressive than in other areas, it appears boys excel in mathematics ability. This sex difference is not apparent until 12 to 13 years of age when visual-spatial skills become more important to understand more advanced levels of math (Shafer and Gray, 1981; Tobias, 1978). Socialization experiences also reinforce these differences (Klein, 1983). During grade school years, girls are more willing to take risks and can withstand ambiguity more than after adolescence; thus they are more prone to math anxiety (Tobias, 1978).

4. Physical and verbal aggression: When children engage in free play, boys are more physically and verbally aggressive than girls. The biologic foundation for these sex differences appear universal; males have been found to be more aggressive than females in all human cultures and in primates. The findings are related to sex hormones, particularly testosterone, and are strengthened by social influences. There is evidence that boys are more biologically prepared to learn aggression and that females have more difficulty expressing aggression, often channeling it into less constructive, socially prescribed outlets.

Culturally presumed myths about sex differences and intellectual abilities influence the expectations of parents, teachers, and classmates. Girls are presumed to be more social, suggestible, and auditory; better at rote learning and repetitive tasks; more motivated by achievement; and affected more by heredity. They are also thought to have a lower self-esteem than boys. Boys are expected to be better at tasks requiring high-level cognition, more analytic in their thinking, more affected by their environment, and more visual. Although there is scientific consensus that sex differences exist, biologic and social determinants of behavior are difficult to separate and measure. Biologic factors are most strongly implicated in visual-spatial ability and aggression.

Effeminacy and Tomboyism

Effeminacy and tomboyism are the most common gender identity problems leading parents to seek professional attention. In many cases, the behaviors were present earlier, and children may have already experienced family contempt and humiliation (see case example). Fathers may react to their son's unmanly behavior as an affront, and the degree of parental rejection depends on the amount of fathers' ego investment, anxieties, and identification (Pillard and Weinrich, 1986). Many parents misread signs of gender identity conflict as symptoms of emerging homosexuality.

Case Example

Ronald was referred for therapy at age 12 because of a history of odd, immature behaviors and inability to make friends, as well as recent concerns of parents and teachers about his rather marked withdrawal. Ronald was placed in a group therapy situation with four other preadolescent boys. He was a slightly built boy with glasses who appeared and acted several years younger than his age. Background data indicated that Ronald lived with his parents and two younger brothers. Both parents conveyed genuine caring for Ronald and concern about his problems. Ronald's father, a large, muscular, handsome man, expressed particular worry about Ronald's lack of interest or ability in physical activities such as football and hunting. Ronald was not well liked by his two male teachers, who viewed him as "babyish" and inappropriate. For several years, Ronald had been ostracized by many of his peers and labeled as a "sissy" and subsequently as a "fag."

Ronald came to the group somewhat reluctantly at first but became an eager, active participant. He frequently functioned as a group leader because of his intellectual ability and sensitivity to others. However, he demonstrated marked discomfort whenever the group's conversation focused on issues related to girls, girlfriends, or dating. At these times, he would display immature giggling and try to refocus the conversation. If the topic of conversation continued, he would withdraw from the group and engage in some form of immature play, such as using puppets in another part of the room.

Ronald continued in the group for almost 2 years. He developed age-appropriate friendships with boys inside and outside the group. He also began to openly discuss his dislike for activities that many of his male peers considered essential such as competitive physical sports. Ronald began to tolerate discussions about girls and dating behaviors and to share his feelings of attraction to certain girls. His conversations, however, indicated that he still felt unable to approach girls his own age. He continued to struggle with the belief that he was seen by others as somewhat abnormal sexually because he did not participate in the activities expected of males. Through the group process, he received some support as peers pointed out that there are a variety of ways to demonstrate appropriate male behaviors, for example, group leadership and assistance to others. Ronald's sensitivity helped him become a confidant and friend, if not a "boyfriend" or "date," for several female peers.

Group work with Ronald emphasized helping him recognize and express conflicted feelings about his maleness. The therapist reinforced the group's explorations of male roles and expectations. In addition, limits were set early on Ronald's immature, withdrawing behaviors, and the positive value of his sensitive nature and bright mind was reinforced. These strategies enhanced his overall self-concept.

Work with Ronald's parents, particularly his father, involved a series of negotiations about what was expected of Ronald and what kinds of behaviors could be acceptable. The father's genuine positive regard for Ronald was a major factor in his eventual acceptance of Ronald's never liking or playing football. It was possible to identify alternate activities that the two could share, and Ronald's mother supported them. The therapist frequently pointed out Ronald's positive qualities and abilities in meetings with the parents. After a good relationship had been established with the parents, open discussions about changing male roles in today's society were facilitated by the therapist. On several occasions the parents were provided with reading materials as a basis for discussion. Overall, the parents' caring for Ronald and their intellectual openness permitted them to move beyond their accustomed sex-role expectations and allow Ronald to develop more comfortably in a male role that suited his needs and abilities.

Modified from Long KA: Sex-role stereotyping: implications for the mental health of school-age children, J Child Adolescent Psychia Ment Health Nursing 2:55, 1989

Nursing management. For early cross-sex behaviors of effeminacy and tomboyism, group therapy involving children with similar problems using behavior modification techniques involving self-monitoring regulation has been found most successful (Rekers, 1977b; Green, 1988). Contact with children with similar problems provides a nonrejecting social experience in which they can learn appropriate behavior from same-sexed models. Usually they are unaware of their cross-gender mannerisms to which others react negatively, and treatment goals are to expand behavioral repertoires and provide more androgynous options.

Rejection is especially strong toward young boys exhibiting what children call the *sissy boys* syndrome (Green, 1988). Girls who are tomboys do not usually experience the same derision, and little is known about the interventions and long-range implications of tomboyism.

Although limited, most clinical studies predict that approximately two thirds of children who exhibit classical prehomosexual signs later become homosexuals (Green, 1988). Their emotional distress is sufficient reason for immediate and rigorous interventions to foster less restrictive androgynous behaviors, enhancing more accepting relationships with peers.

Clinicians should avoid reassuring children that they will outgrow their problems. While clinicians need to have optimism and a developmental perspective, children should not feel that their concerns are being discounted by others (Group for the Advancement of Psychiatry, 1977).

Longitudinal and comparison case studies of markedly effeminate boys and their families showed that the early life experiences of effeminate boys differed from those of noneffeminate boys, suggesting the following areas for assessment and counseling (Green, 1967, 1979, 1988):

1. Parental indifference toward or fostering of effeminate behavior, usually first displayed as cross-dressing at the age of 4
2. Lack of psychologic separation from the mother due to excessive holding
3. Maternal overprotection and inhibition of rough-and-tumble play with other boys
4. Greater availability of female playmates and companions in the early years
5. Strong paternal rejection
6. Actual or emotional unavailability of a consistent adult male role model
7. Unusual physical beauty, influencing adults to treat them as a girl

Normal homoerotism begins during the later years of latency and often causes children great anxiety. The most common homoerotic act of both sexes is mutual masturbation, which typically occurs with peers. Because of less restrictive attitudes toward childhood sexuality and the current advocacy for more sexual freedom for children with their age-mates, an increased amount of sexual intercourse with opposite-sexed peers is also seen.

Youngsters may feel and act as if they are in love with their same-sexed friends and demonstrate intense social and psychologic bonds, including homoerotic play (Fraiberg, 1961). They assume male and female adult roles, playing out scenes from movies or television. These activities may include cross-dressing. At this age, children are aware of the stigma attached to homosexuality, and these secret interactions become a source of guilt and anxiety.

In most instances, parents react with strong disapproval and seek professional assurance once they become aware of these behaviors. Parental concerns should always be accorded serious consideration and respect, and distinctions should be made between phase-appropriate homoerotic play and activities that indicate a serious underlying problem in sexual orientation.

Clinical syndromes in physically normal children who display cross-sex behaviors are gender role-behavior disturbances that may be classified as gender identity disorder not otherwise specified. Predictive indicators of gender role-behavior disturbance in girls have not yet been established. The diagnosis is more complex because of the relatively greater social acceptance of masculine attire and preference in girls. Since the temporary phase of taking on the tomboy role is part of the healthy female emotional development, continuation of symptoms and the general emotional adjustment of girls are important considerations before viewing the following behaviors as potentially symptomatic (Rekers, 1977b):

1. Rigid insistence on wearing masculine type of clothing (for example, pants that zip in the front), with rejection of dresses, skirts, cosmetics, and jewelry
2. Masculine-appearing mannerisms, behavioral gestures, postures, and gait
3. Deviant sexual behavior or masturbation patterns associated with masculine clothing items
4. Aversion toward or avoidance of peer activities with other girls and a preoccupation with playing only with boys
5. Use of an artificially induced low voice inflection and/or predominantly masculine topics and speech content
6. Presence of the desire to be called by a boy's name or nickname

---

Gender Identity Disorders of Childhood

Females

1. Persistent and intense distress about being a girl and a stated desire to be a boy (not merely a desire for any perceived cultural advantages from being a boy) or insistence that she is a boy
2. Either a or b:
   a. Persistent marked aversion to normative feminine clothing and insistence on wearing stereotypical masculine clothing, for example, boys' underwear and other accessories
   b. Persistent repudiation of female anatomic structures, as evidenced by at least one of the following:
      (1) Assertion that she has, or will grow a penis
      (2) Rejection of urinating in a sitting position
      (3) Assertion that she does not want to grow breasts or menstruate

Males

1. Persistent and intense distress about being a boy and an intense desire to be a girl or, more rarely, insistence that he is a girl
2. Either a or b:
   a. Preoccupation with female stereotypical activities as shown by a preference for either cross-dressing or simulating female attire or by an intense desire to participate in the games and pasttimes of girls and rejection of male stereotypical toys, games, and activities
   b. Persistent repudiation of male anatomic structures as indicated by at least one of the following:
      (1) Assertion that he will grow up to become a woman (not merely in role)
      (2) Assertion that his penis or testes are disgusting or will disappear
      (3) Assertion that it would be better not to have a penis or testes

Modified from American Psychiatric Association: Diagnostic and statistical manual of mental disorders, ed 3, rev, Washington, DC, 1987, American Psychiatric Association.

The DSM-III-R criteria for gender identity disorders of childhood are shown in the box.

Children's anxiety prohibiting open communication about psychosexual issues may stem from socialization, which admonishes children for using sexual language and instills the belief that people should not discuss sexuality with strangers, adults, or nurses (Hogan, 1982). Because of their limited experiences talking about sexuality, children often lack the words to discuss and identify their sexual development.

There are many protocols for sexual assessment in health interviews and guides for sexual decision making with adults and adolescents (Group for the Advancement of Psychiatry, 1977; Tauer, 1983; Whitley and Willingham, 1978). However, most clinicians encounter these areas when health screening and evaluating young children. Communication tactics facilitating children's comfort include the following:

1. Assurance of privacy and confidentiality of the discussion
2. Deferment of the discussion of sexuality until after the examination when children are clothed and the use of comments related only to the normalcy of findings during the physical examination
3. Clarification that questions are being asked only to provide a total health assessment and emphasis on the impact of sexual and emotional concerns on other body systems
4. Demonstration of clinicians' acceptance of sexuality as a normal part of development
5. Provision of an overview of developmentally normal sexuality before elicitation of sexual history
6. Discussion of sexual myths
7. Use of a matter-of-fact approach to introduce vocabulary

The way nurses react when children seek psychosexual clarification depends on their values and attitudes toward human sexuality. Some nurses avoid socially sensitive areas such as gender identity conflicts, rationalizing that it is not their prerogative to advocate a specific lifestyle or sexual preference. The ethical rationale for intervening in psychosexual disorders is not to impose values or sexual orientations but to expand the behavior repertoire to more androgynous behaviors, reduce rigid stereotypes, increase flexibility, and diminish children's anxiety and depression (Rosen, Rekers, and Bentler, 1978).

Although the effect of therapy on adult adaptations is not known, clinical materials and intervention techniques are recommended to alleviate children's emotional distress. Psychologic testing and behavioral assessment procedures have been developed and validated that detect abnormalities in sex typing and sexual identity development. Standardized measures of masculine and feminine play have been developed, providing scores comparable to norms for boys and girls. Behavioral recordings of expressive gestures and mannerisms can be evaluated with reference to age-related norms, and because gender role behaviors are situation specific, recordings should be made in children's natural environment, including school and home (Rekers, 1982).

Intelligence tests are recommended to screen for deficits in cognitive functioning that may interfere with the identification process. The draw-a-picture story test can be analyzed for personality disturbance and compared to the norms available. Assessment of the father-child and mother-child relations can be gained by interviews and standardized tools such as the Bene-Anthony family relations test. Finally, every effort should be made to assess children's sex knowledge to determine the need for medical sex education.

Behavioral shaping and modification, play and peer groups, role modeling, and family therapy have been reported as effective interventions (Clunn, 1978; Moore, 1974). An aggressive ecologic approach strengthening participation in school and community sex-specific activities is advocated and recommends girl or boy sports, Boy Scouts and Girl Scouts, and the use of community same-sexed role models, such as the Big Brothers and Big Sisters organization.

PUBERTY

Adolescence begins when pubescence occurs, and the onset of hormonal changes psychologically confirm sexual identity. However, when early pubescence occurs in latency, children are at a high risk for sexual conflicts and psychologic distress. In some settings, such as schools, nurses are usually the only person aware of different sexual maturation patterns in peer groups. Parents do not have the opportunities to observe and compare their child's sexual maturity status with their child's classmates. Counseling early pubescent children is essential to alleviate their fears and support their vulnerable self-concept and body image distortions inherent in their obvious physical differences.

The average age of menarche in girls in the United States is 12½ years, with a normal range from 10 to 16 years. The average age of the first seminal emission for boys is 14, with the normal range of 11 to 16 years. Physical problems are usually not a concern or reason for medical referral unless puberty is more than 2 to 2½ years earlier or later than the national means (Gadpaille, 1981). The duration of pubescence is normally 4 years for boys and girls.

Both menarche and first ejaculations mark major psychologic and physical developmental milestones (Sarnoff, 1976). They are usually preceded by masturbatory fantasies, with the developmental relationship between motor activity and fantasy serving as a sexual drive discharge. Fantasy activity gradually undergoes a transformation with a dissociation between masturbation and motor activities. In some cases and usually by accident, sexual experimentation during preadolescence may uncover physical anomalies, such as vaginal agenesis, indicating surgical corrective interventions.

Early Sexual Maturation

Unfortunately, the broad age range for pubescence accentuates individual developmental differences in boys and girls at a time when identification with and acceptance by peers is critical (Berkowitz, 1985). Early genital maturation disrupts children's established peer identification and often stimulates fear.

Some early maturing boys enjoy prestige among their peers and an enhanced sexual identity. More often, boys react with fear and anxiety, aware that their genital maturation overshadows and exceeds their social and emotional growth. Early maturing girls seldom enjoy higher prestige among male or female peers, as illustrated by the case example.

Case Example

Maria experienced menarche at 10 years of age. The first in her peer group to develop breasts and menstruate, Maria was carefully questioned by her peers about her first experience and then shunned. As Maria's secondary sex characteristics rapidly developed, she felt self-conscious, different, and isolated from her female and male peers. She confided that she was aware her peers viewed her as a freak, closely observing her physical appearance each day and laughing at her. Her peers spent considerable time guessing when she was having her monthly periods, and Maria began to be absent from school and to feel sick during those days.

The parents of Maria's best friend attributed the 10-year-old's early development to sexual promiscuity and precocious heterosexual activity. They discouraged their daughter's friendship with the child with disparaging comments that their daughter's best friend had "grown up too soon." The best friend's mother disclosed that the early pubescence girl had created intense fears and bodily concerns in their daughter, and the parental interference was an effort to bolster their daughter's feelings of inadequacy.

After a year of social isolation, Maria developed friendships with several older, postpubescent girls with whom she closely identified. These older girls had the same genital maturity as Maria, partially alleviating her vulnerable body image. However, they exceeded Maria in emotional and cognitive development, and she became painfully aware of her limited social skills and judgment. Participating in their interests and social activities added to her self-doubts and social isolation, and she felt caught between two worlds.

The situation became threatening when older boys read her genital maturity and female peer associations as signs of availability for heterosexual experiences. By the age of 12, Maria became involved in activities and relationships appropriate for the social and emotional development of girls in early and midadolescence, precipitating referral to the mental health clinic.

Children who experience early pubescence are often self-conscious and embarrassed about their physical differences and usually cannot verbalize their anxieties to their peers, parents, and male health care professionals. Parental and child counseling should alleviate stress and strengthen parent-child relationships that may have weakened during the latency years. Addressing knowledge deficits and use of pictures of every stage of pubescence have been found to be effective (Conger, 1973).

Social and cultural stereotypes and expectations may have a negative effect on early pubescent children, especially if they are female. There is scientific and popular concern that children growing up in America during the 1980s are exposed to many sexual messages. The consciousness-raising edition of *Time* (1988) described the cultural pressures encouraging them to assume adult sexual behaviors, signals especially conflicting for early pubescent children. Early pubescent girls have a special attractiveness for certain males, and their allure is sometimes encouraged through their use as sexual symbols in advertising and marketing.

Adults provide important role models for early pubescent children who look to them for identification and reassurance. Unfortunately, some female teachers and nurses inadvertently reinforce peer rejection and isolation to alleviate concerns of slower maturing age mates. The transition through pubescence is eased with individual counseling and the opportunity to participate in growth groups specific for boys and girls. These groups foster peer support and same-sex relationships while focusing specifically on the different male and female physical experiences and bodily concerns. They are especially helpful for normal children negotiating this stage and are critical interventions for children who have had early childhood traumas such as sexual assaults or corrective genital surgery.

Diagnostic Criteria for Transsexualism

1. Persistent discomfort and sense of inappropriateness about assigned sex
2. Persistent preoccupation for at least 2 years with getting rid of primary and secondary sex characteristics and acquiring the sex characteristics of the other sex
3. Pubescent period
4. Specify history of sexual orientation: asexual, homosexual, heterosexual, or unspecified

Modified from American Psychiatric Association: Diagnostic and statistical manual of mental disorders, ed 3, rev, Washington, DC, 1987, American Psychiatric Association.

Transsexualism

The cross-gender identification clinical syndrome of transsexualism is a serious disorder. It indicates children's strong desire and preoccupation with changing their sex and occurs during or after puberty (see box). This diagnosis is indicated in boys if the symptoms of gender role behavior disturbance or either of the following two symptoms are manifested:

1. An expressed desire to be a girl or a woman or display of female roles in play, often including fantasies of bearing children and breast feeding infants
2. A request to have his penis removed or other sex-reassignment medical procedures performed

In girls, cross-gender identification is suggested if the DSM-III-R symptoms or the following two symptoms occur:

1. An 18 month or longer history of expressing the desire to be a boy or a man or taking predominantly male roles in play, which may include fantasies of having a penis
2. A repeated request for male hormones, breast removal, or other sex-reassignment medical procedures

Nursing management. Specialized behavioral treatment techniques have been evaluated in clinical research for the childhood problems of sexual and gender role disturbances and for excessive public masturbation. Successful treatment procedures have also been developed for preadolescent problems of transvestitism, transsexualism, homosexual orientation disturbances, exhibitionism, and heterosocial skill deficits, raising the expectation that the incidence of severe adulthood sexual deviation will decrease.

Sexual Disorders and Paraphilias

Children develop sex object preferences for exclusively opposite-sex persons, exclusively same-sex persons, or a combination of same and opposite-sex persons. The terms *heterosexual, homosexual,* and *bisexual* should not be applied until children attain adulthood and hermaphroditism and transsexualism are ruled out.

Children may indicate the beginnings of a chronic sexual deviation if they exhibit public masturbation, sexual assaultive behaviors, extreme anxiety over the process of puberty, delinquency or truancy involving sexual acting-out, and other sexual adjustment difficulties or if they have a history of sexual abuse (Gadpaille, 1981). One or more symptoms indicates a need for a thorough psychologic evaluation to determine whether psychotherapeutic intervention is necessary.

Sexual deviations are not completely developed in children so it is best to avoid labels such as *transsexual, transvestite,* and *homosexual.* Disorders of sexual desire, arousal, orgasm, and sexual pain are reserved for use in diagnosing adults because the possibility of these problems existing in children is not accepted (Adams and Fras, 1988).

Paraphilias, the second category of psychosexual disorders, include syndromes in which there is a need for unusual or bizarre acts for sexual excitement. Fetishisms, transvestitism, zoophilia, pedophilia, exhibitionism, voyeurism, sexual masochism, and sadism are disorders that often occur in conjunction with personality and other mental disorders.

Nursing management. Because many adult sexual deviations are highly resistant to therapeutic interventions, detection of symptoms and patterns during childhood to prevent the development of severe adult sexual maladjustment is most effective (Green, 1979, 1988).

It has been advocated that women professionals become active in counseling women and young females and in research in areas relating to feminine gender and sexual issues (Sherman, 1980; World Health Organization, 1975; Wright and others, 1980). McBride (1984) notes that nurses are particularly well prepared to meet the health care needs of females because they have been schooled to build their assessments on clients' perceptions of their experience and to promote self help. McBride stresses that nurses do not assume their reaction to clients are correct, appropriate, or helpful until they check their validity with clients. Her position is that nurses are the health care providers best suited to meet consumer demands for self-determination. Because nurses' professional mandate is to help clients "gain independence as rapidly as possible," nurses are best suited to facilitate self-determination.

Unfortunately, discussing gender issues and sexuality developmental issues with young male and female clients creates considerable anxiety for many nurses. Boys can seek information and clarification from same-sexed male physicians; however, the availability of female physicians for young girls is limited. When nurses abandon their role with young girls, these children are often denied the help they need.

Preparation for Gender and Sex Health Teaching

Four levels of sexual and gender health teaching and clinical interventions have been identified (Mims and Swenson, 1980). Adapted to child psychiatric nursing, these levels of nursing become increasingly complex and involve professional transformation (Benner, 1984; Light, 1981).

1. Life experience level: This minimal level of involvement is based on nurses' personal experiences. Interventions are appropriate for clients who share similar life experiences; however, different values may create problems.
2. Basic level: Nurses have self-awareness with nonjudgmental respect for other sexual beliefs, practices, and concerns. These nurses have some knowledge of

human sexual function and can intervene as a facilitator with clients' needing to discuss sexuality, for example, clinicians in prenatal clinics and teachers of childbearing classes. They can identify parents whose attitudes convey sexual and gender conflicts about the expected child. When these conflicts seem remarkable or unusual, they refer the expectant parents for counseling.

3. Intermediate level: Nurses' knowledge, self-awareness, communication skills, and use of nursing process are included. Clinicians at this level teach children and parents the stages of sexual development and screen children for further evaluation if necessary. Nurses working in schools are often responsible for gender and sex education classes and function at the intermediate level, helping children to identify concerns and assist in resolving problems.

4. Advanced level: These clinicians have specialized preparation and knowledge of sexual and gender disorders, and some meet the ANA certification requirements for Clinical Specialist in Child and Adolescent Psychiatric Nursing. Clinicians at this level may be employed in gender and sex clinics; intervene with children with gender identity problems; use behavior modification, individual play, and group psychotherapeutic interventions; counsel teachers; and conduct family therapy.

Certification by the American Association of Sex Educators, Counselors, and Therapists (AASECT) qualifies clinicians to conduct sex therapy research and develop and present formal education programs. This group defines sex counseling as helping clients to incorporate sexual knowledge into satisfying lifestyles and socially responsive behavior. Sex therapy is conducted to remove serious sexual disorders.

Many female therapists base their practice on the extensive feminist research in achievement motivation, sex-role development, sexuality, expression of power and authority, language style, nonverbal behavior, attributive styles, and life cycles, often identifying themselves as *feminist therapists*. Feminist therapy encompasses approaches from consciousness-raising groups, peer counseling of groups, and individual psychodynamic treatment with and informed by a feminist awareness.

Brodsky (1975) describes feminist health care providers as nonsexist specialists who put unique emphasis on fostering competence and independence in clients through a concentrated, egalitarian therapist-client relationship. Feminist health care providers are not defined by a specific set of techniques but by a philosophic commitment to the rethinking of traditional sex-role concepts, freeing adult and latency-aged clients from unnecessary limitations in their personal life choices, self-expressions, and self-concepts. Treatment goals foster flexibility and emphasize feminist consciousness rather than individual psychopathology as an explanatory framework.

Summary

Gender identity and sex-role distinctions begin to develop very early in life and are strongly influenced by cultural and interpersonal forces. These powerful forces can modify biologic determinants, and there is evidence that most sex differences are the result of stereotypes and child rearing.

Nurse clinicians have internalized many of the same stereotypes that affect children, modifying therapeutic thinking. Current knowledge stresses that sex-role definitions need to include a less restrictive view of female and male sexuality and should permit greater individual growth and self-actualization for both males and females.

Although nurses cannot change the cultural and social conditions and conflicts, they can contribute to a more sexually healthy society by informing and educating parents and others before predictable gender and sexual problems develop in children. Nurses' understanding of normal psychosexual development and behavior and the expected development conflicts can assist children and their parents. If sexual and gender problems have not been internalized, the need for psychotherapy will be minimal.

The younger the child, the more important it is to involve the entire family in therapy for sexual and gender problems. Young children live within the environment that usually causes, contributes, or fails to prevent the problem, and nurses and clients are limited unless the family also changes.

REFERENCES

Adams PL and Fras I: Beginning child psychiatry, New York, 1988, Brunner/Mazel, Inc.

American Psychiatric Association: Diagnostic and statistical manual of mental disorders, ed 3, rev, Washington, DC, 1987, American Psychiatric Association.

Bandura A: Social learning theory, Englewood Cliffs, NJ, 1977, Prentice-Hall, Inc.

Belenky MF and others: Women's ways of knowing: the development of self, voice and mind, New York, 1986, Basic Books, Inc, Publishers.

Bem SL: The measurement of psychological androgyny, J Consult Clin Psychol 42: 155, 1974.

Bem SL: Sex role adaptability: one consequence of psychological androgyny, J Pers Soc Psychol 31:634, 1975.

Benner P: From novice to expert, Reading, Mass, 1984, Addison-Wesley Publishing Co, Inc.

Berkowitz MS, editor: Peer conflict and psychological growth, San Francisco, 1985, Jossey-Bass, Inc, Publishers.

Block JH: Conceptions of sex role: some cross-cultural and longitudinal perspectives, Am Psychol 28:512, 1973.

Block JH: Sex differentiation. In Sherman JA and Denmark FL, editors: The psychology of women: future directions in research, New York, 1978, Psychological Dimensions, Inc.

Block JH: Gender differences and implications for educational policy. In Block JH, editor: Sex role identity and ego development, San Francisco, 1984, Jossey-Bass, Inc, Publishers.

Blumer H: Symbolic interaction: perspective and method, Englewood Cliffs, NJ, 1969, Prentice-Hall, Inc.

Brodsky A: Is there a feminist therapy? Paper presented at the Southeastern Psychological Association, Atlanta, 1975.

Casper RC and others: Disturbances in body image estimation as related to other characteristics and outcome in anorexia nervosa, Br J Psychiatry 134:60, 1978.

Clunn P: Assessment and intervention of gender identity conflict in a latency aged female, life span research. Paper presented at the fifth national conference of Advocates for Child Psychiatric Nursing, Boston, Jun 1978.

Conger JJ: Adolescence and youth, New York, 1973, Harper & Row, Publishers, Inc.

Dreyer N, Woods N, and James N: ISRO: a scale to measure sex-role orientation, Sex Roles 7:173, 1981.

Erikson E: Childhood and society, ed 2, New York, 1963, WW Norton and Co, Inc.

Erikson E: Inner and outer space: reflections on womanhood. In Lifton RJ, editor: The woman in America, Boston, 1964, Beacon Press.

Fraiberg S: Homosexual conflicts. In Lorand S and Schneer HI, editors: Adolescents: psychoanalytic approach to problems and therapy, New York, 1961, Paul B Hoeber.

Freud A: The ego and the mechanisms of defense, New York, 1946, International Universities Press, Inc.

Freud S: Analysis of a phobia in a five year old boy, London, 1955, The Hogarth Press, Ltd.

Freud S: Three essays on the theory of sexuality, London, 1959, The Hogarth Press, Ltd. (originally published in 1905).

Freud S: Some psychological consequences of the anatomical distinctions between sexes, London, 1961, The Hogarth Press, Ltd (originally published in 1925).

Gadpaille WJ: Sexual identity problems in children and adolescents. In Lief H, editor: Sexual problems in medical practice, Monroe, Wis, 1981, American Medical Association.

Gilligan C: In a different voice, Cambridge, Mass, 1982, Harvard University Press.

Gilligan C: New maps of development: new visions of maturity. In Chess S and Thomas A, editors: Annual progress in child psychiatry and development, New York, 1983, Brunner/Mazel, Inc.

Goffman E: Genderisms, Psychology Today 7:60, 1977.

Grecas V and Libby R: Sexual behavior as symbolic interaction, J Sex Res 12:33, 1976.

Green R: Sissies and tomboys: a guide to diagnosis and management. In Wahl C, editor: Sexual problems: diagnosis and treatment in medical practice, New York, 1967, Macmillan Publishing Co.

Green R: Childhood cross-gender behavior and subsequent sexual preference, Am J Psychiatry 136:106, 1979.

Green R: The sissy boy syndrome, New York, 1988, Plenum Publishing Corp.

Group for the Advancement of Psychiatry: Assessment of sexual function: a guide to interviewing, vol 3, 1977, Washington, DC, American Psychiatric Association.

Harris LJ: Sex related differences in spatial ability: a developmental psychological view. In Kopp CB, editor: Becoming female, New York, 1982, Plenum Publishing Corp.

Hogan RM: Influence of culture of sexuality, Nurs Clin North Am 17:365, 1982.

Janosik EH and Davies JL: Psychiatric mental health nursing, ed 2, Boston, 1989, Jones & Bartlett Publishers, Inc.

Kaplan M: A woman's view of the DSM-III, Am Psychol 38:786, 1983.

Kass F, Spitzer R, and Williams J: An empirical study of the issue of sex bias in the diagnostic criteria of DSM-III axis II personality disorders, Am Psychol 38:799, 1983.

Kessler SJ and McKenna W: Gender: an ethnomethodological approach, New York, 1978, John Wiley & Sons, Inc.

Klein R: Gender identity and sex-role stereotyping: clinical issues in human sexuality. In Nodelson CC and Marcotte DB, editors: Treatment interventions in human sexuality, New York, 1983, Plenum Publishing Corp.

Kohlberg L: A cognitive developmental analysis of children's sex-role concepts and attitudes. In Maccoby EE, editor: The development of sex differences, Stanford, Calif, 1966, Stanford University Press.

Kohut H and Wolf E: The disorders of the self and their treatment: an outline, Int J Psychoanal 554:413, 1978.

Light D: Becoming psychiatrists: the professional transformation of self, New York, 1981, WW Norton and Co, Inc.

Long KA: Sex-role stereotyping: implications for the mental health of school-age children, J Child Adolescent Psychia Ment Health Nurs 2:55, 1989.

Maccoby EM and Jacklin CN: The psychology of sex differences, Stanford, Calif, 1974, Stanford University Press.

Mahler M: A study of the separation-individuation process and its possible application to borderline phenomena in the psychoanalytic situations, Psychoanal Study Child 26:404, 1971.

Mason KO: Studying change in sex-role definition via attitude data, Proceedings of the American Statistical Association 8:138, 1973.

Mason KO, Czajka J, and Arber S: Changes in US women's sex role attitudes, 1964-1974, Am Sociol Rev 411:573, 1976.

McBride AB: Nursing and the women's movement, Image 14:66, 1984 (editorial).

Michael G: The development of gestures as a function of social class, educational level and sex, Psychol Record 18:515, 1968.

Mims FH and Swensen M: Sexuality: a nursing perspective, New York, 1980, McGraw-Hill, Inc.

Money J: Sin, sickness, or status? Homosexual gender identity and psychoneuroendocrinology. In Chess S, Thomas A, and Hertzig ME, editors: Annual progress in child psychiatry and child development, New York, 1988, Brunner/Mazel, Inc.

Money J and Ehrhardt AA: Man and woman, boy and girl, Baltimore, Md, 1972, Johns Hopkins University Press.

Moore WT: Promiscuity in a thirteen-year old girl, Psychoanal Study Child 29:301, 1974.

Nagera H: The developmental approach to childhood psychopathology, New York, 1981, Jason Aronson, Inc.

Phillips JL: The origins of intellect: Piaget's theory, San Francisco, 1969, WH Freeman and Co, Publishers.

Pillard RC and Wienrich JD: Evidence of familial nature of male homosexuality, Arch Gen Psychiatry 43:808, 1986.

Rekers GA: Assessment and treatment of childhood gender problems, Adv Child Clin Psychol 1:267, 1977a.

Rekers GA: Sex-typed mannerisms in normal boys and girls as a function of sex and age, Child Dev 48:275, 1977b.

Rekers GA: Play therapy with cross-gender identified children. In Schafer CE and O'Connor KJ, editors: Handbook of play therapy, New York, 1982, Wiley-Interscience.

Rieker PP and Carmen E: Teaching value clarification: the example of gender and psychotherapy, Am J Psychiatry 140:410, 1983.

Rosen AC and Teague J: Case studies in development of masculinity and femininity in male children, Psychol Rep 34:971, 1974.

Rosen AC, Rekers GA, and Bentler PM: Ethical issues in the treatment of children, J Soc Issues 32:84, 1978.

Sarnoff C: Latency, New York, 1976, Jason Aronson, Inc.

Shafer T and Gray ME: Sex and mathematics, Science 211:1, 1981.

Shepherd-Look DL: Sex differentiation and the development of sex roles. In Wolman BB, editor: Handbook of developmental psychology, Englewood Cliffs, NJ, 1982, Prentice-Hall, Inc.

Sherman JA: Problems in sex differences in space perception in aspects of intellectual functioning, Psychol Rev 74:290, 1967.

Sherman JA: Therapist attitudes and sex-role stereotyping. In Brodsky AM and Hare-Mustin RT, editors: Women and psychotherapy, New York, 1980, The Guilford Press.

Stoller RJ: Gender identity disorders in children and adults. In Kaplan H and Sadock B, editors: Comprehensive textbook of psychiatry, vol 1, ed 4, Baltimore, 1985, Williams & Wilkins.

Tauer KM: Promoting effective decision making in sexually active adolescents, Nurs Clin North Am 17:345, 1983.

Thorne B, Kramarae C, and Henley N, editors: Language, gender and society, Cambridge, Mass, 1983, Newbury House Publishers, Inc.

Through the eyes of the child: growing up in America in the 1980s, Time, p 22, Aug 8, 1988.

Tobias S: Overcoming math anxiety, Boston, 1978, Houghton Mifflin Co.

Unger RK: Toward a redefinition of sex and gender, Am Psychol 34:1085, 1979.

US Bureau of the Census: Marital status and living arrangements, Ser P20, No 389, Washington, DC, 1984, US Government Printing Office.

Whitley MP and Willingham D: Adding a sexual assessment to the health interview, J Psychiatr Nurs Ment Health Serv 8:17, 1978.

Wolman BB and Money J, editors: Handbook of human sexuality, Englewood Cliffs, NJ, 1980, Prentice-Hall, Inc.

World Health Organization: Education and treatment in human sexuality: the training of health professionals, Tech Rep No 572, Washington, DC, 1975, World Health Organization.

Wright CT and others: Psychiatric diagnosis as a function of assessors profession and sex, Psychol Women Q 5:240, 1980.

Chapter 12

Children of Dysfunctional Families

Mary Lou Scavnicky-Mylant

According to the National Center for Child Abuse and Neglect (NCCAN) (1981) the incidence of child abuse and neglect ranges from 1 to 6 million cases each year. Between 1982 and 1987 the national rate for reported cases increased 69.2% to 34 out of 1000 children becoming victims. In 1988, 2.2 million child abuse reports were filed, up 3% from 1987 (Drown These Mean Streets, 1989), and 1225 children died as a result of abuse (Child Abuse Institute of Research, 1989). The difficulty in judging the degree of child abuse and neglect from extreme to mild has led to confusion and inconsistent statistics (Campbell and Humphreys, 1984).

Establishing meaningful definitions for child abuse and neglect is complex because of different standards of parenting, especially during adolescence. Parenting behaviors that are abusive or neglectful for younger children are often considered acceptable and even necessary for adolescents. Although young children are significantly more likely to be severely injured than older children, adolescents are almost equally represented among the children who are abused and neglected (Gil, 1971; Seaberg, 1977). Children over the age of 11 are twice as likely to be maltreated than children younger than 6 years of age. More than 300,000 adolescents experience at least one form of maltreatment each year (National Center for Child Abuse and Neglect, 1981). Furthermore, 7 million children are beaten by a sibling and 10% to 20% are victims of sexual assault by a parent or parent figure (Martin, 1977). One out of every three girls today will be sexually abused, and 75% of all sexual abuse is in the form of incest (DeVine, 1980).

Current statistics emphasize the intergenerational transmission of family violence. Every 5 years the death toll of persons killed by relatives and acquaintances equals the number killed in the Vietnam War, and 80% of all men in American prisons were abused as children. In a Massachusetts study, 86% of the abusers of elderly persons were relatives (Martin, 1977).

History of Child Abuse and Neglect

Children have been mistreated by adults throughout history, and concern for the protection of children in the United States did not begin until 1874. In that year, Etta Wheeler, a nurse, and some concerned neighbors contacted the Society for the Prevention of Cruelty to Animals to remove 9-year-old Mary Ellen from her adoptive parents who routinely beat, starved, and imprisoned her. The police were unable to take action because no laws covered this abusive situation. Her case led to the development of the Society for the Prevention of Cruelty to Children in 1875 (Scharer, 1979).

Child maltreatment was rarely discussed among health professionals until 1962 when Kempe, Silverman, and Steele introduced the term *Battered Child Syndrome,* which included "any child who received nonaccidental physical injury (or injuries) as a result of acts (or omissions) on the part of his parents or guardians." The Child Abuse Prevention and Treatment Act of 1974 was passed, and it required states to enact mandatory reporting legislation before becoming eligible for grant funds. However, necessary definitions of abuse and neglect are absent from state laws because of the perceived seriousness of interfering with individual parental rights (Misener, 1986).

Definition of Abuse

Societal definitions of abuse have expanded to include not only physical abuse but also neglect, emotional abuse and neglect, verbal abuse, and sexual abuse (Hayes, 1981). Campbell and Humphreys (1984) employ a definition of child abuse to include any "harm or threatened harm to a child's health or welfare by a person responsible for the child's health or welfare which occurs through nonaccidental physical or mental injury, sexual abuse, or maltreatment." Child abuse is generally associated with acts of commission and neglect with acts of omission (Kauffman, Neill, and Thomas, 1986).

Emotional abuse has been described as an elusive crime. With a developmental approach, emotional abuse is deliberate behavior that seriously undermines the development of competence. Operationally, this means punishing an infant's operant social behavior (including attachment), punishing a child's manifestations of self-esteem, and punishing the behaviors needed for normal interaction in extrafamilial settings.

Nursing Framework

Millor (1981) presents a nursing framework for child abuse and neglect as multifactorial phenomenon involving parents, family, culture, child, and stress, with a continuum from normative and nurturing behavior to normative discipline to neglectful actions and abuse. Steele and Pollack (1968) state that abuse is more often associated with a deficit in positive parenting characteristics and neglect with parental failure due to feelings of frustration and disappointment.

Kempe and Helfer (1972) identify the parent having the potential to abuse as a commonly found characteristic within an abusive situation. The other aspects usually seen are children being viewed as different and the occurrence of a perceived crisis triggering the violent act. This model is widely used by nurses in the assessment and understanding of child abuse (Hunka, O'Toole, and O'Toole, 1985).

PARENTAL CHARACTERISTICS

Although researchers have been unable to specifically identify an abusing personality, abusive parents frequently demonstrate common characteristics (Hunka, O'Toole, and O'Toole, 1985). Neglectful parents are often apathetic and depressed, and the severity of neglect is usually proportionate to the degree of depression (Scharer, 1978).

Several attempts have been made to design and validate criteria that will assess a parent's potential for child abuse and neglect. Schneider, Pollock, and Helfer (1972) stated that abusive parents reported more severe physical punishment in their own childhood, more anxiety about dealing with their children's problems, more concern with criticism and isolation, and higher performance expectations for their children. Research findings have led to the development of a predictive questionnaire to identify potential abusers.

The high-risk family assessment tool shown in Figure 12-1 evaluates 10 common problem areas for the high-risk family: multiple crises; separation of family members; grief; guilt, blame, and anger; low self-esteem; emotional or physical exhaustion; parental role changes; discipline; sibling relationships; and finances. Developed from analysis of more than 300 families in high-risk situations, this tool may help nurses assess family strengths and problems.

Kempe and Helfer (1972) describe four categories of parental abuse potential, including ways in which parents were reared, the pattern of isolation, the interrelationship between parents, and parents' view of the child. Hunka, O'Toole, and O'Toole (1985) identified 10 dependent variables that measure the effectiveness of a self-help group for abusive parents. Variables under abuse potential included social isolation, low self-esteem, unmet dependency needs, impulsiveness, and passivity.

PARENTAL FAMILY HISTORY

Research suggests that abusive and neglectful parents frequently have experienced negative life events. Separation from birth, poor parental or substitute relationships, large families, poor school and work histories, alcoholism, physical or mental illness, low intellectual ability, criminal conviction, disturbed sexual development, marital problems, behaviorally unusual offspring, poor housing, and poverty are often seen. Not all abusive parents have been physically abused as children. However, all have been exposed to intense parental demands for support, attentiveness, submissiveness, and love at a very early age (Steele and Pollock, 1968). They often describe a lack of having been cherished as individuals with their own wants and continually having to please their parents (Schneider, Pollock, and Helfer, 1972). Thus, their self-esteem was built around meeting their parents' requirements.

Many researchers agree that parents who abuse their children have experienced developmental trauma (Campbell and Humphreys, 1984). Unmet de-

These are example questions only. They must be individualized for each family. Assess each family member individually.

Coding System

– = It is a problem.
+ = It is not a problem; instead it is a strength.
? = Unknown; it may be a problem but there is no data to show it or disprove it.

Multiple Crises

Have things been hard at home?
What have been the hard times?
Have you had "ups and downs"?
When do you think will be the next hard time?

Separation of Family Members

Who sees less of each other since the medical problem?
Who sees more of each other since the medical problem?
Are you feeling less close to someone?
Are you feeling more close to someone?
Is there someone you would like to see more (less) of?

Grief

Have you felt numb ... sad ... disbelief ... ?
Have you wanted to talk with someone about the medical problem?
Have you wanted to be left alone?

Guilt/Blame/Anger

What do you think caused the situation?
What else might have added to it happening?
Do you think you could have done something different?
Are you angry at someone else for causing it (family member, medical team, etc.)?
Do you think there is something else the medical team could have done?

Low Self-Esteem

What makes a good parent?
Who did you announce the birth to?
What things do you enjoy doing?
What things would you like to do as a parent that you have not been able to do?
What things do your family members do that make you feel important (or a good parent)?
What things do your family members do that make you feel unimportant (or a poor parent)?

Figure 12-1   Assessment tool for the high-risk family.

pendency needs for nurturant relationships drive their expectations of their children to provide the love and approval they never received. Neglectful parents also presume that their children will compensate for their neglectful or abusive background, and the role reversal is then passed onto a second generation.

Emotionally Tired/Physically Tired

Do you feel tired often?
How do you feel when you get up in the morning?
How much sleep are you getting?
Do you ever feel "about to crack"?
Do you have aches and pains?
When you are under pressure or tired, what pains do you get (headache, backache, stomach upset). Have any of these been occurring?
Do you feel like you are living day to day, one day at a time, or one hour at a time, or one minute at a time?
When you are tired, have you thought of harming yourself or your child?
What can you do in 15 minutes that refreshes you (makes you feel good)?

Parent Role Changes

Of the daily chores, who does things differently since the risk situation?
What new things do you do now that you did not do before this problem?
What things do you not do now, since this situation, that you used to do?
What things would you like your spouse or children to do that they do not do?
What things do your spouse or children do that you would prefer they not do?
Is there something small that needs to be done that a friend, neighbor, relative might be able to help with (laundry, ride, shopping, etc.)?

Discipline

How were you raised?
What would you like to do the same for your children?
What would you like to do different for your children?
How do you let your children know when they do something wrong . . . right?

Sibling Relationships

How do your children play together?
How did your children react (change) following the situation?
What do your children think caused the problem?
What do you do with each child individually that the child likes?
What do you do with the children together that they like?

Finances

Who is working?
What do you do at work?
Is someone in the family changing his/her job?
How often do you think you will have to miss work to be at the hospital or at home with your child?
How does your boss react to your being absent?
Have you discussed your insurance with the hospital billing person?
Have you discussed an arrangement for paying the bill that is comfortable for you?
Do you know who to talk to if you have questions on the costs and how you can arrange for them so that it will not put too much pressure on you?

Figure 12-1—cont'd Assessment tool for the high-risk family.

Evans' finding (1970) that abusive mothers scored significantly lower measures on the first six Eriksonian developmental stages further validates the core issue of developmental maladjustment among abusive parents, presumably resulting "from consistent early trauma which retarded resolution of the full sequence of developmental conflicts." Although the scales of the Eriksonian tool were too strongly intercorrelated, the trust versus mistrust and identity versus role confusion subscales differentiated the abusive from nonabusive mothers. Figure 12-2 helps explain the effect this developmental trauma has on initiating the next generation of violence.

Evans (1976) links Erikson's descriptions of individuals with unsuccessfully resolved conflicts of each developmental stage with character descriptions of abusive parents. These descriptions frequently mentioned isolation, mistrust, low self-esteem, role diffusion, and passivity.

Isolation and poor support systems increase the risk of poor crisis management and child abuse. Polansky and others (1979) noted that parents of similar social position were significantly less socially supported and involved if identified as being neglectful. Their lack of outside resources or their inability to use them may stem from the mistrust these parents experience (Kempe and Helfer, 1972). The degree of childhood violence they were exposed to is positively correlated with the level of difficulty they have in seeking help (Pollock and Steele, 1972). Abusive parents' behavior may also be the only way they were able to instill any control and consistency in their lives, although more often than not their efforts were unsuccessful.

Researchers have identified low self-esteem and a lack of empathy among abusive parents as basic to theories of child abuse (Disgrow, Doerr, and Caulfield, 1977). Socioeconomic stressors such as unemployment may precipitate a crisis because of their effect on parents' self-esteem. Empathy is necessary for pain cues to have an inhibitory effect on aggression (Feshbach and Feshbach, 1969).

Researchers have hypothesized that abusive parental characteristics are indicative of severe personality disorders (Spinetta and Rigler, 1972). Although most abusive parents lack impulse control, estimates identify only 5% of abusive parents as psychotic and 5% as aggressive psychopaths (Kempe, 1971). Later studies appear to support this view.

Impulsiveness is a key factor in the child abuse model, and immaturity with poor impulse control is also common (Blumberg, 1974). Komisaruk (1966) theorized that abusive parents' repressed conflicts are exacerbated by children's actions and demands. Fray (1970) views the erupting abuse as a reflexive primitive defense reaction to a sudden crisis (Bennie and Sclare, 1969). Passivity reinforces individuals' maladaptive behavior (Schiff and Schiff, 1971).

CHILD CHARACTERISTICS

The perception of a child as being special or difficult is often seen in abuse and neglect situations. It may be due to parents' negative attitude toward their child or inadequate knowledge of child development, which encourages unrealistic expectations of motor and language development, behavior, and psychologic needs (Hunka,

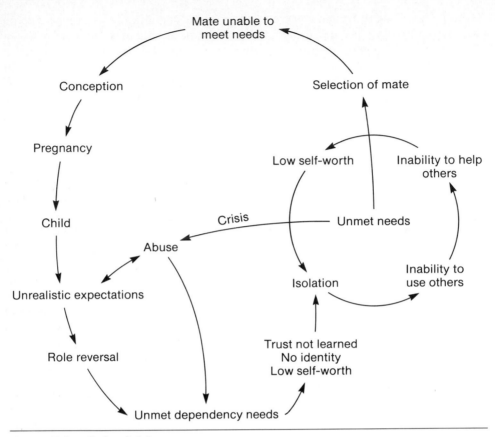

Figure 12-2 Cycle of violence.

O'Toole, and O'Toole, 1985). No one child is singled out; all are neglected until an older child can take on the parenting role (Scharer, 1978).

Negative perceptions may also be due to low birth weight (Parke and Collmer, 1975); prematurity (Elmer, 1967); illegitimacy or handicapping conditions (Kempe and Helfer, 1972); and lack of attachment (Klaus and Kennel, 1976). Abusive parents may transfer their feelings for their parents to their children, and this emotional role-reversal may cause them to view their children as deliberately not cooperating or providing them with affection (Morris and Gould, 1963). The parents display jealousy of any attention shown toward their children (Allen, 1969).

Abusive parents also rated their children as more aggressive and hyperactive (Reid, Kavanagh, and Baldwin, 1987). This exaggeration may justify the use of harsh punishment in their mind. A higher rate of emotional and behavioral problems among children of violent families has been found; however, increased parent-child aggression has also been identified among families of antisocial children (Patterson, 1982). Because positive behaviors have not been useful in getting their emotional needs met, provocative behavior and the risk of painful contact is chosen by abused children over being ignored. Neglected children often become depressed and apathetic like their parents (Scharer, 1978).

ENVIRONMENTAL FACTORS

Any stressful situation can be considered an environmental factor within the cycle of child abuse (Broome and Daniels, 1987). Neglect is not contingent on a specific crisis but may be exaggerated by the event. A family crisis can result from a seemingly trivial event such as a hair style that did not turn out right. The elements of the crisis situation are the child's behavior that has pushed the parents beyond their limit and the parent's desperate need for reassurance and nurturance. The withdrawal or alienation of a spouse often precipitates the second element (Pollock and Steele, 1972). Parents involved in an unsatisfactory marriage may displace the aggression and sadism of the relationship onto their children (Bennie and Sclare, 1969).

The quality of the relationship between the parents may be the key to the inheritance of violence (Scheider, Pollock, and Helfer, 1972). If an adult with a weak potential for abuse marries a positively-reared adult, abuse probably will not occur. If, however, two weak or moderately potentially abusive adults or one strong and one weak marry, abuse is likely. A comparison study of women who experienced incestuous relationships with their fathers during childhood found that these women often labeled their father as violent and their mother as chronically ill, disabled, or battered (Herman and Hirschman, 1981).

Poor child-rearing practices and problem-solving skills also add to the stress of abusive parents. They rely on discipline methods that are often haphazard and inconsistent (Elmer, 1967).

Many abused parents, however, do not abuse their children, and although poverty is a source of many stressors and often correlated with abuse, the majority of poor people are not abusive (Campbell and Humphreys, 1984). Their tolerance for stress and their ability to use resources protects them from abusing their children (Belsky, 1980).

Although socioeconomic problems may add to the stress of basic personality weaknesses, they are not the cause of abuse (Spinetta and Rigler, 1972). The combined effect of mental, physical, and emotional stresses underlies abuse (Simons and others, 1966).

Alcohol and Child Maltreatment

Alcoholism has been called "the family disease, for every member in such a family is affected by it—emotionally, spiritually, and, in most cases, economically, socially, and often physically" (Fox, 1962). The characteristics of violence and chemical dependency are similar. Both tend to be intergenerational problems and show personality dynamics such as low self-esteem and impulsivity. Affected families often accept the violence and alcoholism as a means of coping, which accentuates both problems (Potter-Efron and Potter-Efron, 1985). Studies have shown that almost two thirds of children referred for child abuse and neglect come from alcoholic homes

(O'Gorman, 1985). Girls are two times more likely to be sexually abused if they are raised in an alcoholic home (Black, 1985).

Parental alcoholism may be one of the most destructive risk factors for child abuse, and even a history of alcoholic drinking has been identified as a predisposing factor for severe child maltreatment (Famularo and others, 1986). The primary focus of an alcoholic family is the alcoholic. The children often feel unwanted, unloved, unimportant, and invisible (Woodside, 1988). The frequent mood swings experienced by alcoholic parents often result in their having a high tolerance for abnormal behavior and a hypervigilance and sensitivity toward predicting behavior. They are often isolated from valuable social relationships.

Their expression of feelings is either ignored or punished, which may result in the higher incidence of psychosomatic complaints (Nylander, 1960); excessive dependency (Richards, 1979); impaired self-concept and low self-esteem (Baraga, 1978); suicidal behavior (Tishler and McKenry, 1982); role reversal (Clinebell, 1968); interpersonal difficulties (Ellwood, 1980); and social isolation (Cork, 1969).

Effects of Child Abuse and Neglect

Pervasive psychiatric symptoms have been identified among abused children. Martin and Beezley (1977) studied 50 moderately battered children 4½ years after the abuse was first identified. Over half of the children had low self-esteem and symptomatic behavior, such as enuresis, aggression and avoidance, and hyperactivity, characteristics that caused peers, parents, and teachers to reject them. These children were not happy and could not enjoy themselves in play or interact in a developmentally appropriate social manner. The residual effects were not related to the type or severity of abuse but to environmental factors such as the emotional stability of their parents and family structure, permanence of their home setting (actual or perceived), and the degree of punitiveness and rejection exhibited by caretakers.

Withdrawal, opposition, hypervigilance, compulsivity, precocious behavior, and learning problems were also seen and identified as adaptations to the psychologic trauma of assault (Martin and Beezley, 1977). Withdrawn children had a low tolerance of frustration and were inattentive and uncooperative, but those with marked compulsivity often had a high tolerance of frustration and were attentive and cooperative. Precocious behavior included either caring behaviors toward adults in a pseudoempathetic way or actions that engaged adults on the adult's terms. If neglect was involved, children often showed signs of failure to thrive, developmental delay, and the depression and apathy of their parents (Scharer, 1978).

Although assumed to be stronger and more autonomous, abused adolescents demonstrated a similar pattern. Many physically abused boys with chemical dependency had been previously diagnosed as having conduct disorders, and sexually abused adolescent boys were often diagnosed as having unipolar or bipolar depression (Cavaiola and Schiff, 1988). A higher incidence of acting-out behavior, runaways, legal involvement, and sexual promiscuity was identified among the abused group, many of whom were reporting abuse for the first time. Victims are also at a higher risk for self-destructive behaviors such as chemical addiction, suicide, and accidents. A higher rate of animal cruelty and homicidal ideation were seen within incest and sexually abused groups (Kempe and Kempe, 1978).

The effects of incest may vary in intensity and may manifest immediately after the event or considerably later in life. Sexual dysfunction, promiscuity, prostitution, running away, depression, intense guilt, markedly poor self-esteem, self-destructive chemical abuse, anxiety, somatic complaints, learning difficulties, marital difficulties, and increased intergenerational risk are frequently cited problems. The wide range of behavior seen among incest victims has been attributed to chronic traumatic neurosis, continuing relational imbalances from lack of treatment, and increased intergenerational risk of incest.

Assessment

Nursing interventions with violent and dysfunctional families should be based on the nursing process and begin with an accurate assessment. Because fear may prevent them from exploring the possibility of violence with families, clinicians need to examine their feelings regarding abuse and neglect. Family strengths should be considered as the basis for nursing interventions (Campbell and Humphreys, 1984).

PRENATAL ASSESSMENT OF PARENTING

Potential problems with parenting can be predicted with some accuracy during the prenatal period and during labor and delivery (Kempe and Kempe, 1978). A prenatal assessment of parenting guide has been developed that assesses maternal attainment of the tasks of pregnancy and parent problems associated with child abuse and neglect. Nurses gather data throughout clients' pregnancy and assess parenting potential by the thirty-sixth week. Mothers who have potential parenting problems are offered additional assistance such as home visits and referrals (Josten, 1981). Women at high risk for caregiving dysfunction who were visited by nurses had fewer instances of verified child abuse and neglect during the first 2 years of their children's life.

This assessment tool should be used as a guide and not as a predictive instrument because reliability and validity measurements are not complete. However, it has an accuracy rate of 87% in distinguishing capable mothers and potentially abusive mothers (Josten, 1981).

Intervention

PRIMARY PREVENTION

Any nursing intervention that supports parent-infant attachment may prevent child maltreatment (Kuhn and Ross, 1985). Encouraging parental expression of feelings and concerns, especially any ambivalent or negative feelings; praising parents during labor; and providing opportunities for bonding are effective nursing behaviors. During the early postpartum period, nurses may also provide consistent role modeling and positive reinforcement for parenting efforts, as well as information about normal growth and development. Reassuring the parents about common variations in the newborn and guiding them during feeding, bathing, and dressing of their infant can also promote parental competence and pleasure in their new role.

Campbell and Humphreys (1984) suggest that to prevent families from becoming violent, nurses must promote nonviolence in family interactions and society. They should lobby for decreased violence in the media and gun control legislation, discourage the use of physical punishment in raising children, support the teaching of nonaggressive problem solving to preschoolers and sex education and information about violence for school-aged children, and promote healthy attitudes toward the elderly and third-party payments for nurse-administered day-care centers. Because alcoholism is a risk factor, nurses should also try to prevent this dependency in their clients (Famularo and others, 1986). Primary nursing interventions with families should assess violence, stress, poor communication, psychologic abuse, and the absence of emotional nurturance. Nurses should help families develop democratic problem-solving techniques, positive communication patterns, adequate support systems, and effective means of disciplining children. Referral to child abuse agencies and resources offering parenting education may also be indicated.

SECONDARY PREVENTION

The goals of secondary prevention involve early identification and intervention to prevent any reoccurrence of abuse or neglect. If violence involves children, a report to child protective services is mandatory. Crisis intervention includes helping family members express their feelings about the situation and clarifying misinformation. Clinicians need to develop or activate support networks, emphasize healthy coping mechanisms and family strengths, and make referrals. They should expect but not encourage denial and support initial insight. Families are often open to learning new methods of coping and eliminating violence in their homes during the 4 to 6 weeks after the crisis event (Campbell and Humphreys, 1984). Nurses can manage parents' defensive behavior by separating caregivers from the abuse and by being nonjudgmental and empathetic (Scharer, 1978; Smith, 1981).

Table 12-1 delineates the nursing subroles in secondary interventions (Scharer, 1979). The primary task of the initial phase of treatment is to build a trusting relationship, and children should not be included in the nurse-parent sessions until trust and rapport are established. Parents may become extremely dependent during this initial phase, indicating that trust is developing (Hayes, 1981). However, it may also activate nurses' desire to rescue the family, negating the family's attempt to grow and develop.

If a multidisciplinary approach is necessary, the number of individuals on the treatment team should be limited because of the parents' difficulty relating to and trusting people (Hayes, 1981). As the trust develops between the family and nurse, other subroles become more significant. The initial application of the teacher role must be judicious and use role modeling to give advice, and the nurse psychotherapist role is employed only after a trusting relationship has evolved (Scharer, 1979). Completion of the socializing role is essential before termination of the interventions.

A research study found that nursing-led, behaviorally oriented intervention teams are successful (Carter, Reed, and Reh, 1975). Researchers found that mothers in a

Table 12–1   Nursing Roles in the Treatment of Abusive and Neglectful Families

Role	Description	Goal
Mother-surrogate	Includes focusing on needs of parents; providing support while setting limits; teaching appropriate methods to meet personal needs	To develop relationship with family; reparent abusive caregiver; protect child from further abuse; improve self-image and competency of parents
Manager	Involves coordinating activities and providing positive physical environment (Scharer, 1979); making necessary referrals; helping family identify and prioritize needs; developing system to meet parental needs (Hayes, 1981)	To build competence and self-worth in parents
Technical	Includes using medical interventions	To improve the health of client
Teacher	Includes using role modeling, play; disclosing feelings while addressing parental specific needs; emphasizing positive parenting behaviors (Hayes, 1981)	To help parents identify and apply methods of coping; teach importance of play; educate parents about normal developmental growth and milestones
Nurse psychotherapist	Includes using behavioral therapy model (Campbell and Humphreys, 1984); allotting responsibility for violent behavior to family members; establishing realistic consequences of actions; reinforcing nonviolent behaviors; teaching methods of coping with stress and conflict; analyzing communication and power distribution in family members; employing group therapy	To extinguish violent behavior
Socializing agent	Includes socializing with parents; assisting them with forming friendships; teaching socializing skills	To eradicate parents' isolation and loncliness

long-term (5 to 6 months) intervention group demonstrated significant improvement on all variables of concern except safety. None of their children were hospitalized, but 90% of the control group children were rehospitalized within a 6 month period because of parental abuse or negligence. Interventive techniques included building a relationship with the mothers and children, role-modeling appropriate child care, providing support, using behavioral-educational approaches concerning discipline, and collaborating with mothers.

TERTIARY PREVENTION

Tertiary prevention is necessary when the abusive and neglectful family cannot function safely. The goals of nursing interventions are help the family achieve healthy functioning and process the grief for the lost family member or total family unit. Tertiary prevention also involves working with children so that the emotional effects of violence are identified and treated and alternate coping mechanisms are presented (Campbell and Humphreys, 1984). Maltreated children need assistance in expressing feelings, improving self-esteem, becoming more spontaneous, and learning to have fun (Martin and Beezley, 1977). This level and focus of intervention is extremely important to interrupt the cycle of violence.

Smith (1981) identifies objectives for working with hospitalized children as providing a trusting environment incorporating a consistent caregiver, warmth and affection accompanied by reasonable limits, socialization with peers and adults, organized play and school environments, recovery from illness or injury, maintenance of the parent-child relationship, and opportunities to express their feelings.

The most important intervention for children is to secure a positive and loving home so that they receive developmentally appropriate, positive stimulation as quickly as possible (Campbell and Humphreys, 1984). Rescue fantasies are the biggest problem for nurses working with abused or neglected children (Scharer, 1978). Clinicians often give children extraordinary attention, fail to set appropriate limits, and reject them when they do not respond as expected. Children may respond with exaggerated, provocative behavior or be nondiscriminate in giving affection. Nurses should not encourage either form of behavior but should teach the appropriate methods of receiving attention and providing warmth and affection.

Abused or neglected children may be developmentally delayed and may regress further because of the separation and trauma related to intervention. Regression may interfere with socialization and promote later aggression. It is normal and should be accepted but not promoted. Clinicians must set appropriate limits.

Children often feel responsible for the abuse or neglect. Nurses need to point out the inconsistencies of children's previous home life and not arouse expectations that parents can never meet.

Many negative thought patterns of abused and neglected children can be expressed through drawing, which is a natural mode of expression and especially helpful in identifying and sharing feelings. Children from dysfunctional homes often cannot express themselves verbally because of their developmental level and fear of retribution for discussing sensitive issues. Because drawings are not subject to children's defense mechanisms, a request to draw is likely to reduce tension.

Scavnicky-Mylant (1986) identified denial, poor self-image, powerlessness, and feelings of responsibility in the drawings of children of alcoholics. One child drew

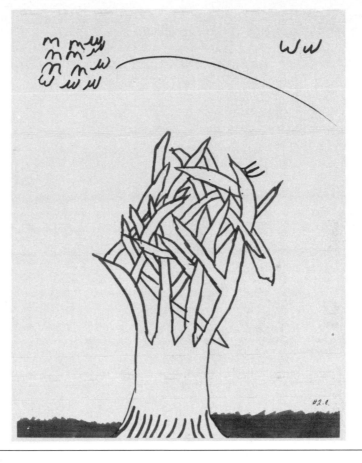

Figure 12-3

"a dog dreaming that he was a person" after describing his alcoholic father beating and starving him in the past. Another child explained that his picture was just for the interviewer and that it was a tree "you won't believe" (Figure 12-3). The branches of the tree were bare, spiked, and twisted, conveying hurt, abuse, and lifelessness. This child drew the tree after describing a fight that his friend had started and he had finished, a common discussion topic during his sessions. He also frequently talked about his father's physical aggression toward him and his brothers.

Another child described a fight he had been in and later drew an owl and a tree. This boy stated, "There's a hole in the tree and he's a night owl" (Figure 12-4). Hammer (1958) identifies this depiction as a desire for a withdrawn, warm, and protected environment. The client had been in the custody of his father while separated from his mother and described her as inattentive. The traditional leaved tree, reflective of hopeful feelings and protection, is absent in these tree drawings.

Asking children to draw a picture of their family's life and their views on violence may help them avoid denying the existence of an alcoholic problem. Drawings are

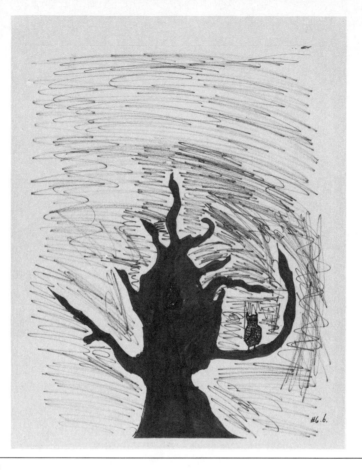

Figure 12-4

also useful with sexually abused children. In both situations a major family secret is being disclosed by children who may have been threatened not to tell. Drawing decreases the associated anxiety by providing them with a motor activity and develops the relationship between therapists and clients. Verbal techniques, such as the use of a third-person situation, also encourage sharing of painful situations (Triplett and Arneson, 1983).

Discussing the realities of a violent family situation and appropriate developmental tasks with children may lead to more successful outcomes and positive self-esteem. The assumption of responsibility for unrealistic expectations and resulting failures are avoided, and mastery of developmental tasks is facilitated. Felker (1974) suggests emphasizing positive and minimizing negative aspects, acting as a role model, respecting children's feelings, and assisting with learning experiences to increase children's self-esteem.

Coping behaviors may involve children's disengaging from family, developing positive and supportive relationships with peers and other adults, taking responsibility for their actions, and viewing reality on a continuum. Information about ways

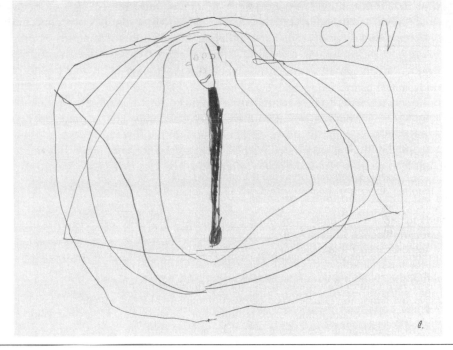

Figure 12-5

in which violence affects families and art therapy can improve their feeling of control. For example, a 5-year-old boy who drew a "tree man getting smashed" by surrounding circles was offered a pair of scissors to cut the tree man out (Figure 12-5). The child readily accepted and seemed somewhat relieved (Scavnicky-Mylant, 1986). They begin to realize that they do have choices despite their parents' or another person's behavior and feelings. Support groups, such as Alateen and Alatot for children of alcoholics, can also provide alternate coping strategies and a sense of worthiness and trust and alleviate feelings of isolation and embarrassment. Children's usual coping style, however, must never be deprived, especially if the home situation does not allow flexibility; instead, they are given additional choices (Black, 1983).

Legal Issues

Clinicians are obligated to know enough about child abuse and neglect to recognize it (Rhodes, 1987). All states presently have legislation allowing them to remove children and become their guardian (Munro, 1984). Criteria for reporting abuse and neglect has been set at the federal level through the Child Abuse Prevention and Treatment Act of 1974, which states must follow to qualify for federal funds. Although reporting statutes vary, a report is generally required in cases of physical abuse, emotional abuse, some forms of neglect, and sexual abuse. Nurses need to obtain a copy of the state law affecting their community (Munro, 1984).

In all 50 states, nurses are considered mandatory reporters—required by law to report child abuse. Although state laws vary, anyone who examines or treats children is usually classified as obligated. These individuals are liable to monetary or criminal sanctions if they knowingly or willfully fail to report child abuse. A permissive reporter is anyone in the community who believes that a child has been abused (Rhodes, 1987).

Nurses do not have to be certain that a child is being maltreated; "well-founded suspicion is sufficient cause" (Munro, 1984). Statutes that create mandatory reporting laws give immunity from civil and criminal liability if a report was made in good faith. Health care providers are also protected when privileged information is divulged in reporting child abuse (Munro, 1984; Rhodes, 1987).

REFERENCES

Allen H: The battered child syndrome: social and psychiatric aspects, Minn Med 52:539, 1969.

Baraga DJ: Self-conception in children of alcoholics, Dissertation Abstracts International 39:368B, 1978.

Belsky J: Child maltreatment: an ecological integration, Am Psychol 35:320, 1980.

Bennie E and Sclare A: The battered child syndrome, Am J Psychiatry 128:975, 1969.

Black C: Children of alcoholics. Paper presented at the advanced winter workshop of the Psychotherapeutic Associates, Colorado Springs, Colo, 1983.

Black C: Adult children of alcoholics. Paper presented at the advanced winter workshop of the Psychotherapeutic Associates, Colorado Springs, Colo, 1985.

Blumberg M: Psychopathology of the abusing parent, Am J Psychother 28:21, 1974.

Broome M and Daniels D: Child abuse: a multidimensional phenomenon, Holistic Nurs Pract 1:13, 1987.

Campbell J and Humphreys J: Nursing care of victims of family violence, Reston, Va, 1984, Reston Publishing Co, Inc.

Carter B, Reed R, and Reh C: Mental health nursing intervention with child abusing and neglecting mothers, J Psychiatr Nurs 13:11, 1975.

Cavaiola A and Schiff M: Behavioral sequelae of physical and/or sexual abuse in adolescents, Child Abuse Negl 12:181, 1988.

Child Abuse Institute of Research: Child abuse update, Cincinnati, 1989, The Child Abuse Institute of Research.

Clinebell HJ: Understanding and counseling the alcoholic, New York, 1968, Abingdon Press.

Cork M: The forgotten child, Ontario, Can, 1969, General Publishing.

DeVine AR: The sexually abused child in the emergency room. In Jenstrom L and MacFarlane K, editors: Sexual abuse of children: selected readings, DHHS Pub No 78-30161, Washington, DC, 1980, US Government Printing Office.

Disgrow M, Doerr H, and Caulfield C: Measuring the components of parents' potential for child abuse and neglect, Int J Child Abuse Negl 1:279, 1977.

Drown these mean streets: violence by and against America's children, USHR Fact Sheet, May 1989.

Ellwood JC: Effects of alcoholism as a family illness on child behavior and development, Milit Med 145:188, 1980.

Elmer E: Fragile families, troubled children: the aftermath of infant trauma, Pittsburgh, 1967, University of Pittsburgh Press.

Evans A: An Eriksonian measure of personality development in child-abusing mothers, Psychol Rep 44:963, 1970.

Evans A: Personality characteristics of child-abusing mothers, doctoral dissertation, East Lansing, Mich, 1976, Michigan State University.

Famularo R and others: Alcoholism and severe child maltreatment, Am J Orthopsychiatry 56:481, 1986.

Felker DW: Building positive self-concepts, Minneapolis, 1974, Burgess International Group, Inc.

Feshbach N and Feshbach S: The relationship between empathy and aggression in two age groups, Dev Psychol 1:102, 1969.

Fox R: Children in the alcoholic family. In Bier W, editor: Problems in addiction: alcohol and drug addiction, New York, 1962, Fordham University Press.

Fray P: Crimes and offenses by primitive reactions, Psychol Abstracts 45:8540, 1970.

Hammer EF: The clinical application of projective drawings, Springfield, Ill, 1958, Charles C Thomas, Publishers.

Hayes P: The long-term treatment of victims of child abuse, Nurs Clin North Am 16:139, 1981.

Herman J and Hirschman L: Families at risk for father-daughter incest, Am J Psychiatry 138:967, 1981.

Hunka C, O'Toole A, and O'Toole R: Self-help therapy in parents anonymous, J Psychosoc Nurs 23:24, 1985.

Josten L: Prenatal assessment guide for illuminating possible problems with parenting, MCN 6:113, 1981.

Kauffman C, Neill M, and Thomas J: The abusive parent. In Johnson S, editor: Nursing assessment and strategies for the family at risk: high-risk parenting, ed 2, Philadelphia, 1986, JB Lippincott Co.

Kempe C: Pediatric implications of the battered baby syndrome, Arch Dis Child 46:28, 1971.

Kempe C and Helfer R, editors: Helping the battered child and his family, Philadelphia, 1972, JB Lippincott Co.

Kempe R and Kempe C: Child abuse, Cambridge, Mass, 1978, Harvard University Press.

Kempe C, Silverman F, and Steele B: The battered child syndrome, JAMA 181:17, 1962.

Klaus M and Kennel J: Mother-infant bonding, St Louis, 1976, The CV Mosby Co.

Komisaruk R: Clinical evolution of child abuse: scarred families, a preliminary report, Juvenile Court Judges Journal 17:66, 1966.

Kuhn J and Ross M: Primary prevention of child abuse, MCN 10:198, 1985.

Martin D: Battered wives, New York, 1977, Pocket Books.

Martin H and Beezley P: Behavioral observations of abused children, Dev Med Child Neurol 19:373, 1977.

Millor G: A theoretical framework for nursing research in child abuse and neglect, Nurs Res 30:78, 1981.

Misener T: Toward a nursing definition of child maltreatment using seriousness vignettes, Advances in Nursing Science 8:1, 1986.

Morris M and Gould T: Role reversal: a necessary concept in dealing with the battered child syndrome, Am J Orthopsychiatry 33:298, 1963.

Munro J: The nurse and the legal system: dealing with abused children. In Campbell J and Humphreys J, editors: Nursing care of victims of family violence, Reston, Va, 1984, Reston Publishing Co, Inc.

National Center for Child Abuse and Neglect: Study findings: national study of incidence and severity of child abuse and neglect, DHHS Pub No 81-30325, Washington, DC, 1981, US Government Printing Office.

Nylander I: Children of alcoholics: a role-theoretical perspective, J Soc Psychol 115:237, 1960.

O'Gorman P: An historical look at children of alcoholics, Focus on the Family 8:5, 1985.

Parke R and Collmer C: Child abuse an interdisciplinary analysis. In Hetherington EM, editor: Review of child development research, Chicago, 1975, University of Chicago Press.

Patterson GR: Coercive family process, Eugene, Ore, 1982, Castalia.

Polansky N and others: Isolation of the neglectful family, Am J Orthopsychiatry 49:149, 1979.

Pollock C and Steele B: A therapeutic approach to the parents. In Kempe C and Helfer R, editors: Helping the battered child and his family, Philadelphia, 1972, JB Lippincott Co.

Potter-Efron R and Potter-Efron P: Family violence as a treatment issue with chemically dependent adolescents, Alcoholism Treatment Q 2:1, 1985.

Reid J, Kavanagh K, and Baldwin D: Abusive parents' perceptions of child problem behaviors: an example of parental bias, J Abnorm Child Psychol 15:457, 1987.

Rhodes AM: The nurse's legal obligations for reporting child abuse, MCN 12:313, 1987.

Richards TM: Working with children of an alcoholic mother, Alcohol Health Res World 3:22, 1979.

Scavnicky-Mylant M: The use of drawings in the assessment and treatment of children of alcoholics, J Pediatr Nurs 1:178, 1986.

Scharer K: Rescue fantasies: professional impediments in working with abused families, Am J Nurs 78:1483, 1978.

Scharer K: Nursing intervention with abusive and neglectful families within the community, MCN 8:85, 1979.

Schiff AW and Schiff JL: Passivity, Transactional analysis J 1:71, 1971.

Schneider C, Pollock C, and Helfer R: Interviewing the parents. In Kempe C and Helfer R, editors: Helping the battered child and his family, Philadelphia, 1972, JB Lippincott Co.

Simons B and others: Child abuse: epidemiologic study of medically reported cases, N Y State J Med 66:2783, 1966.

Smith J: Care of the hospitalized abused child and family: a framework for nursing intervention, Nurs Clin North Am 16:127, 1981.

Spinetta J and Rigler D: The child-abusing parent: a psychological review, Psychol Bull 77:296, 1972.

Steele B and Pollock C: A psychiatric study of parents who abuse infants and small children. In Helfer R and Kempe CH, editors: The battered child, Chicago, 1968, University of Chicago Press.

Tishler C and McKenry P: Parental negative self and adolescent suicide attempts, J Am Acad Child Psychiatry 21:404, 1982.

Triplett J and Arneson S: Working with children of alcoholics, Pediatr Nurs 9:317, 1983.

Woodside M: Children of alcoholics: helping a vulnerable group, Public Health Rep 103:643, 1988.

Chapter 13

Emotional Consequences of Chronic Physical Illness

Catherine Ayoub

Leaders among health care professionals argue that chronically ill children merit national attention (Pless and Perrin, 1985). Children with chronic illnesses are the recipients of a sizable public investment, and consume a large portion of the total dollars spent on child health. They also require special service and educational systems to meet their physical and emotional needs. Because an increasing number of children with chronic illnesses are living to adulthood, they need longer care and the assessment of the quality of life becomes more complex.

Consequently, health care professionals and educators designing and implementing physical, psychologic, and educational interventions must consider the processes affecting the emotional adjustment of children with a chronic illness across their life span. Knowledgeable assessment and treatment plans, comprehensive educational programs, and sensitive mental health programs must be developed to support their special needs and maximize their potential of becoming a productive adult.

Nurses can contribute substantially because they understand children's medical and psychosocial needs and frequently have the most contact with children and their family. Although nurses are in these critical roles, there is relatively little documentation of their impact (Hymovich, 1985).

Child psychiatric nurses can contribute to the assessment and treatment of children with physical illnesses only if they become involved in primary health care settings. They must also have a solid physiologic base in the disease processes involved, a working knowledge of adaptive and maladaptive coping strategies, and the ability to interrelate children's emotional and physical needs. As part of the multidisciplinary team, child psychiatric nurses are helpful in roles as therapists, consultants, and liaisons for other nurses and professionals with primary responsibility for the care of ill children.

Definitions and Concepts

Handicapping conditions of childhood are divided into the classifications of chronic illness, loss of physical or sensory ability, and terminal illness. Chronic illness is any illness with a protracted course. It may be progressive and fatal or associated with a normal life span, and the degree of physical or mental impairment varies. Common chronic childhood diseases include juvenile diabetes melitus, cystic fibrosis, and asthma.

The permanent loss of a physical or sensory ability as a result of congenital or acquired disorders is the second category of handicapping conditions. Blindness, spina bifida, and cleft lip and palate are examples. The last category is the terminal stage of an illness, which may involve an acute or chronic disease process. Although increases in the incidence of some diseases have been seen, this trend is not expected to continue. However, because many children are living longer, health care and mental health providers need to focus on children's long-term normative adjustment.

Emotional Impact

Chronic illnesses of childhood affect from 10% to 15% of the population under 18 years of age. Of these children, 10% have disabilities severe enough to interfere with the completion of tasks appropriate for their age (Pless and Roghmann, 1971). Pless and Pinkerton (1976) estimate that 17% to 20% of children with chronic physical illness demonstrate emotional distress or maladjustment, from transient adjustment reactions to severe depression and psychosis.

The diagnosis of psychologic factors affecting physical condition on Axis I of the DSM-III-R is specific to children with illness (American Psychiatric Association, 1987). The diagnostic criteria shown in the box refer to aspects that contribute to the initiation or exacerbation of a physical condition, and the category applies to children who develop anxiety or panic linked to specific medical procedures or eating or elimination problems because of physical changes or medical treatment.

The physical condition listed on Axis III may be a symptom or a diagnosis and is associated with chronic pain or painful procedures seen with tension headache, migraine headache, rheumatoid arthritis, leukemia, and other metastatic diseases. Conditions requiring long-term medication administration and multiple invasive procedures, such as cystic fibrosis, diabetes, and asthma; those involving loss of physiologic function (particularly of the bowel and bladder) including spina bifida

---

DSM-III-R Diagnostic Criteria for Psychologic Factors Affecting Physical Illness

1. Psychologically meaningful environmental stimuli are temporarily related to the initiation or exacerbation of a specific physical condition or disorder (recorded on Axis III).
2. The physical condition involves either demonstrable organic pathology (for example, rheumatoid arthritis) or a known pathologic process (for example, migraine headache).
3. The condition does not meet the criteria for a somatoform disorder.

Modified from American Psychiatric Association: Diagnostic and statistical manual of mental disorders, ed 3, rev, Washington, DC, 1987, American Psychiatric Association.

and cerebral palsy; and disorders affecting the upper digestive tract including nausea, vomiting, and failure to thrive are other commonly listed physical conditions.

This diagnostic category is also used to describe disorders that were referred to as *psychosomatic* or *psychophysiologic* in the past. The new organization reflects the current thinking that no specific psychiatric syndromes accompany disease entities.

Although most researchers agree that chronically ill children are at an increased risk for difficulties with emotional adjustment the type, cause, and extent of maladjustment and its specificity to individual diseases is still an issue of debate (Pless and Roghmann, 1971; Simmonds, 1971; Wallander and others, 1989). Some researchers suggest that no definitive pattern of behavior is associated with chronic illness but that the stress experienced by chronically ill children is similar, regardless of the specific ailment (Wallander and others, 1989). Others believe that there are marked differences in ways in which competence is assessed depending on the illness, influencing professionals' appraisal of maladjustment (Perrin, Ramsey, and Sandler, 1987). Because of this lack of agreement, psychiatric nurse clinicians must be aware of the specific nature of the illness and the other individual, family, and community variables that can affect emotional adjustment.

The promotion of emotional health in chronically ill children focuses on a developmental approach to intervention planning and treatment, normalization, and increased family participation and control. A developmental approach implies that developmental competence rather than chronologic age or specific illness characteristics will be used to orient teaching and communication. Piaget's theoretic framework of cognitive development (1929) serves as the basis for progressive cognitive understanding of the concepts of illness, its causality, and the meaning of death.

The concept of normalization contends that children lead as normal a life as possible within the constraints of their illness and places emphasis on their interacting with normal peers, attending school regularly, and participating in recreational activities appropriate for their age. This view distinguishes between the disease and the illness behaviors that its symptoms may exacerbate. One objective in the approach is to minimize illness behaviors—actions that emphasize being ill rather than well. Two children with the same type of chronic illness can display strikingly different behavior, increasing or reducing dysfunction. Also included in the concept of normalization is the emphasis on participation and the control of interventions by children and their family. Motivation research shows that when people participate in and control a situation, they are more likely to develop a personal investment, which adds to self-competence and knowledge.

Using these concepts as guiding principles, targeted preventive programs have been developed to help children adjust to the hospital environment and cope with difficult symptoms and procedures. Active hospital orientation programs for children, support groups for parents, and outreach services to ensure that children can negotiate both school and recreational activities minimize the risk of emotional difficulties developing.

Children's Concepts of Illness and Death

Chronic illness poses a significant challenge to normal developmental processes at all ages; however, the impact of diagnosis, treatment, and impending death differ based on children's cognitive understanding. Toddlers and preschoolers function at a preoperational stage of cognitive development and are mainly aware of present experiences. They differentiate poorly between themselves and the external world, and their thinking is focused on externally perceived events. Because they often concentrate on a single aspect of an experience, they are unable to understand global processes and see the world from their own limited perspective. Consequently, they do not have an understanding of the concepts of illness and death but respond to the physical pain of procedures and the physical separation from parents. Immobilization, regression to a less independent state, separation from primary caregivers, intrusive procedures, and alterations in their routine cause them the most anxiety.

Robertson (1958) describes three phases displayed by young children in hospitals in which parental visitation was minimal. They respond first with protest — crying, kicking, and yelling for the absent parent, and this behavior may be prolonged. After being left repeatedly, they become passive, withdrawn, depressed, and disinterested, entering the stage of despair. If the separations continue, toddlers may become detached and resigned, a condition that can result in long-term behavioral disturbance. Hospitalization lasting over a week and repeated hospitalizations were associated with an increased risk of behavioral disturbance (Douglas, 1975). This progressive withdrawal is sometimes interpreted by parents and health care providers as improved adjustment. Children are praised for being good and not crying when left or exposed to a painful procedure. Invasive procedures and the lack of an environment in which they can use play to deal with feelings are also damaging. Again, withdrawal coupled with anxiety and intermittent outbursts may signal difficulty in adjustment.

Preschoolers often perceive death as departure and cannot grasp the permanence of it, regarding it as a reversible process. Preschoolers often see their condition as a punishment, and painful treatments and prolonged separations strengthen these beliefs. Parents reinforce or affirm these feelings through denial or direct statements, adding to children's stress. If children hear that they are going to die, they may assume it will happen immediately. Similarly, when the adults around them are saddened by the prospect of future loss, young children interpret the reason for the grief as immediate and may reflect the adult sadness with little understanding of the potential outcome.

School-aged children have mastered concrete operations and usually define illness as a set of multiple, concrete symptoms. They begin to understand causal relationships and often interpret illness as resulting from some action or attribute of their own, producing feelings of guilt and sadness. They often misconstrue feelings and take responsibility for actions over which they have no control. Some children feel responsible for their parents' emotions as well.

Because mastery is a primary goal of school-aged children, the loss of control that accompanies some illnesses is a serious threat to ego integrity. Children may be verbally uncooperative and suffer from significant anxiety and panic attacks, especially when confronted with an invasive or painful procedure. Children who perceive themselves as different or are absent from school and outside activities for an extended time may have difficulty reintegrating with peers. Depression, school phobia, anxiety disorders, and disruptive behavior disorders are not uncommon in this age group.

School-aged children have an expanded concept of death; however, they may personify it as the "bogey man" or the "ghost." They fear the reason for their illness; its effect on their competence, ability, and function; and the process of dying. Children at this age are often passive and do not ask questions about their conditions, but they seem to want and need more concrete descriptions about their illness, hospital procedures, and the process of dying.

Many children of 9 or 10 years of age have developed the adult conception of death as being universal, irreversible, and inevitable. However, the ramifications of dying may not be understood. One of the most frightening revelations of death to these children is that their parents cannot prevent their death from occurring, which may cause anger toward parents for their helplessness.

At approximately 12 years of age, children function at the formal operational stage. They can differentiate between self and the external world and can understand illness as an internal psychologic structure and system in which dysfunction is manifested by external symptoms. They usually define illness in abstract terms and can comprehend that there are many interrelated causes of illness.

At some level, children acknowledge their own illness and impending death. They often use symbolic language and work through their feelings in play, dreams, or art. The importance of symbolic communication should not be underestimated, and they should be offered the opportunity to express their feelings in their own time and in their own way. A family's ability to communicate and allow expression in accordance with age and personality will influence the way in which feelings are shown. Children who cannot express their feelings often display depression or acting out behaviors.

Crisis, Loss, and Grief

The reactions of crisis, loss, and grief should be recognized as expected and adaptive in children with chronic illness and their family. Coping behavior is used in a crisis to adapt to this life event in a way that will promote continuous, positive growth and interaction (Mattsson, 1972). This approach empowers the family and the provider by placing increased value on the process through which each person must progress.

All families experience the feelings of loss and grief. The loss of having a normal child is universally traumatic, and the grief process begins with the identification of the physical problem and continues throughout the family's socialization. The diagnosis and prognosis will have a primary effect on the child and the parenting process. The more visible the problem and energy the treatment requires, the more active the grief process will appear. Mourning the loss of normalcy and health of an infant or child includes feelings of failure, inadequacy as a procreator and protector, and helplessness at the situation. Anger at self and others is common. Ambivalence and resentment at the loss of time spent in care of the handicapped child, the financial drain due to the cost of care, and the social isolation that results also occurs.

Researchers believe that people progress through predictable sets of emotional responses to traumatic life events (Bowlby, 1961; Gunther, 1969). The best known pattern of normal human grief includes denial, anger, bargaining, depression, and reorganization or acceptance (Kubler-Ross, 1969). Grief responses are anticipatory or reactive behavioral indicators of distress that can foster normalization and growth with appropriate understanding and support. Because human response is both variable and complex, grieving behaviors should be considered as reactions rather than rigid stages through which individuals should or will pass.

For chronically ill children and their families, grief may occcur repeatedly as a disease progresses and children suffer increased loss of physical function. When they reach new levels of developmental awareness, they may also further recognize the physical limitations that accompany their illness.

Because coping is modulated by each person's special role and perspective within the family unit, the way in which family members express their grief and progress through the grief process can be very different. Some family members work through their grief in ways that lead to sharing and mutual support. The coping styles and progression through the process of grieving of others can lead to conflict and even dissolution of a family. Sensitive and responsible intervention throughout the process helps families through a tremendously painful and difficult time and builds positive relationships in the family unit.

The diagnosis of a chronic or terminal illness usually initially results in shock and denial, which can last from days to months. Parents may continue their daily routines, respond with little emotion, or physically avoid the issue. Parents report that they did not hear professionals' statements following the news of the diagnosis because of shock; therefore, basic information needs to be repeated before it can be assimilated by the family.

Common responses at the time of diagnosis include physician shopping, attributing symptoms of the actual illness to a minor ailment, acting happy despite the diagnosis, refusing to believe the laboratory tests, refusing to tell anyone about the illness, and asking few or no questions about the diagnosis or prognosis. These responses are normal reactions to loss and become a concern only if they are prolonged and interfere with the course of treatment.

Children will respond based on their developmental level, the given information, their level of support, previous experiences, and their family's belief system. Siblings will also react to the same factors but often suffer additional difficulties because they lose their parents to the task of caring for their sick family member. Siblings are the family members most frequently omitted from the information exchange process. Taylor (1980) reports that only 1 sibling out of 25 had received information directly from a health care professional. Including siblings (based on the situation and their cognitive ability) at the time of diagnosis is effective in reducing their isolation.

The characteristic of denial in children has been discussed as a positive factor in their ability to cope with a diagnosis (O'Malley and others, 1979). Some denial is an adaptive mechanism to help individuals maintain hope in the face of overwhelming odds. However, some reality adjustment is necessary for children to participate positively in treatment. Balancing reality and hope is difficult for chronically ill or terminal children, especially if they are not comfortable asking questions about their illness and its ramifications and the process of dying.

At the time of diagnosis, the goal is to promote honesty and awareness of family member's feelings. Nurses and other health care professionals often feel obligated to convey information as quickly as possible so that treatment can begin, yet one of the most significant roles of nurses at this time is to be an active listener. Staff members need to know what the family has understood and the ways factual information is being integrated with the family's belief system, past experiences, and coping mechanisms. Children's understanding can be assessed through listening and the symbolic languages of play and art. Children sense that there is sadness and anxiety and, depending on their age, realize that they are the focus of those feelings. By allowing them to express their feelings in a comfortable way, nurses communicate the appropriateness of their fears. Neither children nor their family should be pushed into insight, rather they should be accepted and supported.

The anger that often follows the shock may be directed inwardly at the child or family or outwardly at professionals or others. If this anger lessens family communication and creates isolation, it can drive families apart and impede treatment. If it is directed and understood through expression, it can integrate families and communities.

Children and adults often ask, "Why me?" and become resentful toward professionals who are seen as strong and healthy yet ineffective in eradicating the disease. Because nurses usually conduct the painful procedures included in treatment, children identify them with such procedures and react with anger. Involving nurses in pain management will alter children's perspective.

The painful feelings that gradually follow shock and denial may either accompany or succeed anger. Most parents feel that they have failed when their child is not perfect and that they have been cheated. For chronically ill children the adjustment that usually follows shock presents as chronic sorrow and leads to only partial acceptance, especially in families in which the illness is prolonged and medical interventions are either intermittently intense or constant (Young, 1977). Parents also suffer more difficulties when they cannot explain their child's condition.

Guilt is frequently a strong component of this emotional process. If hereditary factors are present, guilt is intensified, and if the handicap is the result of an action of the parent, guilt may be overwhelming. It may occur as parents or children become angry or bargain for more time and plays a role in the depression that commonly occurs during the grieving process.

Clinicians need to understand the different forms of depression in chronically ill children and their families. Children with conditions such as cerebral palsy or facial deformities often receive the message that they are different and deformed at an early age. Similarly, children with leukemia or other cancers react to the visible changes such as hair loss and loss of a limb or other bodily functions, which frequently lead to a reactive depression—a response to present events. A second type of depression is the result of the anticipatory grief at a future loss of a bodily function, family members, and ultimately life. To direct therapeutic interventions appropriately, nurses need to differentiate between reactions to a specific present deprivation and behaviors responding to a future loss.

For many families the next step is characterized by the reintegration of family roles with the illness or disability and the development of realistic expectations. For children with a chronic illness, this process is active and continuous as the disease progresses. Acceptance or reorganization is gradual, and the mastery of tasks involved in the care of handicapped children can create changes that improve self-image (Voysey, 1972). For children, overcoming a handicap and becoming a functional, contributing member of society can strengthen character and build confidence.

Anticipatory acceptance occurs when children and their family accept the possibility and probability of death and make plans for the event. At this stage, families focus on their child's comfort, decide whether the child should go home to die, and discuss their fears and requests.

For example, a 10-year-old girl in the terminal stages of cystic fibrosis selected the dress she wanted to be buried in and planned her funeral. For mother and child this was a loving, shared experience that offered some control over the helplessness they felt at the child's impending death. A 12-year-old child made a video tape for other children with leukemia to help them through the painful procedures. Parents often manage their grief by giving to others in similar circumstances. Many disease-specific support groups were founded by parents who had experienced the loss of a child from the disorder.

Children who seem to cope effectively may still develop problems such as depressive reactions, panic reactions during procedures, acting out behavior, and family communication inhibitions (Koocher and Sallen, 1978). Some children and families cope well during the active treatment periods but become anxious, angry, or depressed once active treatment ends (Koocher and O'Malley, 1981).

When children die, the anticipatory grief process transforms into acute and chronic grief. Even when death is viewed as an end to suffering, the responses are similar to the reactions to sudden, unexpected death.

The usual pattern of the mourning process includes shock and disbelief; the expression of grief characterized by loneliness, sadness, guilt, and a focus on the deceased; disorganization and despair producing feelings of emptiness, depression, and isolation; and reorganization and recovery from loss (Lindemann, 1944). The process is gradual and the duration of stages varies. Reorganization occurs once individuals find meaning in living again, progress through a day or days without overwhelming thoughts of their dead child or sibling, and remember the deceased with less pain. Forgetting the pain of the loss often takes years, and anniversaries of the death and other special times can intensify distress even after years of reorganization.

Children who have lost a sibling may demonstrate the grief reactions of tearfulness, social and emotional withdrawal, loss of interest in favorite pastimes or toys, decreased attention span, development of tics, loss of appetite, persistent insomnia or nightmares, decreased effectiveness in school, unfocused activity levels, and expressions of guilt over past activities, especially in relationship to the deceased (Koocher, 1973). Children's potential for magical thinking and their increased dependency increases the risk of prolonged negative psychologic consequences. Interventions should be aimed at helping children disclose their feelings about the loss, including their guilt, feelings of responsibility, sadness, and fears. Clinicians also need to assist children in differentiating between their fate and the early death of their sibling.

Impact on Families

Families with children suffering from chronic illnesses experience considerable stress and adverse effects (Burton, 1975; Ireys, 1981). Their psychologic resources are important to the emotional well being of their children (Hauser and others, 1985; Wallander and others, 1989). Regardless of children's medical status or illness, family functioning is a powerful predictor of adjustment (Perrin, Ayoub, and Willett, 1989; Rutter, 1981). Individual parental support systems, self-concept, coping styles, and attitudes toward health also contribute to children's adjustment (Rutter, 1981; O'Grady and Metz, 1987). The marital relationship has been cited by some researchers as the best predictor of parental coping behaviors (Friedrich, 1979). If spouses can discuss their feelings and negotiate role changes supportively, less guilt, anger, blame, and isolation results. In contrast, families who are unable to talk about their child's physical problem and its implications have internally isolated themselves from each other's support, and feelings are expressed through nonverbal communication. Marital relationships that are stressed before the crisis are more likely to result in dissolution during or after the experience.

Single parent families are particularly vulnerable to the increased stress because one person must handle the work and responsibility for the ill child alone. Extended family, friends, and formal support networks can be vital to their continued function.

Because of increased survival rates, families must deal with rigorous medical regimens that are time consuming and often painful and that only reduce the rate of physical deterioration. Focusing on meeting present needs and anticipating long-term adjustment are also concerns. Ordinary events are more difficult and have a greater than normal impact. For example, moving to a new house or going to a new school may be severely disruptive.

Families with chronically ill children often reorient their lives around the care of the ill child and consequently reduce their communication and social interaction with others. As a chronic illness continues (particularly if it is progressive or involves a visible handicap), communication occurs only with individuals immediately involved with the child's care. In cases of serious illness and death, isolation naturally increases. The presence of a helpful social network assists with successful coping, and health care providers often become a powerful component of this resource (Stein and Jessop, 1984).

Mothers of chronically ill children differed from mothers with healthy children in their health locus of control beliefs. They demonstrated greater beliefs in powerful others and less in the perception that events were contingent on their own behavior (Perrin and Shapiro, 1985). Their perceived degree of control over behavioral outcomes may influence the family belief system and affect children's emotional adjustment. Therefore, assessment of children and their family must include information about the illness and the psychologic aspects affecting the family.

Obtaining the needed care for physically handicapped children is also difficult and frequently requires parents to serve as child advocates. Children of families that lack the necessary knowledge and organization may not receive optimal care. Families may need to travel to attend clinics or receive other care, further disrupting family life, and the illness may also interfere with parents' work responsibilities and limit their activities.

The other issue involved in special services is the cost. The financial burden of having a handicapped child is tremendous. Insurance policies are inadequate, and eligibility for public funds necessitates that a family exhaust its resources almost completely before help can be provided.

Clinical Nursing Implications

Clinicians need to identify children's cognitive stage of development before discussing illness or death with them. Nurses can evaluate concepts of body function and illness causality by having children draw body outlines. Drawings aided the staff in understanding the quiet silence of a 9-year-old boy who thought that the mass in his lower bowel was a "mask" and the fears of a 7-year-old boy with congenital heart disease who thought that his heart was being hit by a drumstick every time it "beat."

Toddlers and preschoolers at the preoperational stage need to hear about immediate expectations and consequences. For these children, preparation for a later procedure may increase their anxiety. In contrast, school-aged children can be prepared for procedures ahead of time, which may alleviate their anxiety if they are taught specific skills such as relaxation or distraction for dealing with the event.

Clinicians need to also consider children's prior experiences with death, which can have a direct impact on their adjustment. If they have encountered a small death — the death of an animal or a person not close to them — they may have some preconceptions that need to be understood (Whaley and Wong, 1987). For example, a 6-year-old boy was told that his grandfather just "got old and went to sleep in the hospital." When he was later diagnosed with leukemia, he was terrified to fall asleep in his hospital bed for fear he would die. Children's ethnic, social, and religious background and their family's perception of the illness and potential death are other critical factors in clinical care.

Honesty should be the central concept in discussing children's illness and prognosis. Children who are chronically ill have a special need to trust adults, particularly those that are central in their lives. This trust must be carefully built, regularly reinforced, and constantly nurtured. Failure to talk to children about their illness often leads to fears and anxiety about implied or misinterpreted meanings of the illness and hospitalization.

Clinicians should encourage children to ask questions and provide support and information to parents so that they will be prepared to talk with their ill child. Failure to include parents in discussions restricts them and their child from offering mutual support.

Cruel truth dispels all hope, increases anxiety, and destroys the will to survive. It is often used as the excuse for not telling children about their disease. *Gentle truth* allows hope without negating the facts of the illness or prognosis. It can be told in terms of the illness, its effect on their body function, and the reason for treatment, often leading to questions about the benefits and limitation of interventions. It also desensitizes families to emotionally loaded words such as *cancer, tumor,* and *incurable* (Whaley and Wong, 1987). Families and clients who are given concrete information about an illness and ensuing procedures participate more effectively in the process of care.

Maximizing the control and involvement for children and their family by providing information, offering support, and interfacing with the health care system includes them in decision making and ameliorates their ability to cope with disease (Langer and Rodin, 1976).

Loss of control is frequently expressed with acting-out behaviors. Children may refuse to take medication or participate in medical regimens. Difficult and painful procedures are less traumatic if children are given options about where they sit or lie or who will be with them during a test. Children are often comforted when they can bring a familiar toy or book or perform a procedure on a doll or stuffed animal before or during the intervention. Adults may act out by challenging medical regimens and criticizing their child's care. Unfortunately, staff members often ignore or avoid oppositional parents instead of acknowledging their feelings of helplessness and implementing steps to reduce the parental perception of loss of control. To accomplish this, clinicians can assist parents in planning their child's day in the hospital or include them in painful procedures as a source of support for the child.

Nurses are responsible for coordinating the efforts of the multidisciplinary team. Regular meetings focusing on both children and families as well as on staff roles, interventions, and their interface are effective measures. Staff members must define and operationalize their role in the care of each family, often requiring negotiation and compromise among health professionals, which can be facilitated by mental health nurses. Mental health nurse clinicians also serve as the facilitator for the provision of on-going services and as the developer of systems of communication sensitive to the emotional needs of children, families, and providers.

NURSING GUIDELINES

Preparation for hospitalization before and at the time of admission is effective in reducing children's anxiety. Many hospitals offer routine preadmission tours involving the surgical suite, equipment, and the process of anesthesia for children scheduled for surgery. For chronically ill children, specific information regarding scheduled procedures is essential, and play equipment that illustrates tests is commonly used. Ideally, the nurse that is providing primary care to the client prepares the child. Mental health nurse consultants are often involved, especially when children are frightened or uncomfortable.

Clinicians should recommend visitation of parents and siblings and parental participation in the daily routine. Parental involvement provides continuity and security for their child and gives parents an increased sense of involvement and understanding of the process and procedures. Sibling visitation can dispel fears of the unknown for siblings and foster normalization for clients.

To promote normalization, many hospitals provide child life programs involving therapeutic play and intervention for hospitalized children. These programs are usually staffed by professionals with backgrounds in child development and experience with ill children. Children's continued participation in school-related activities also facilitates normalization and their transition into school. If teachers are available to a hospital unit, nurses must coordinate these services with children's hospital care. If not, nursing staff is often responsible for encouraging the completion of school work.

Health education is a vital part of maximizing children's hospital experience and should include parents whenever possible. Nurses are often the central provider of information about the medical regimen, and their skill in conveying the necessary data and their knowledge of a family's relationships, beliefs, and resources are vital for the continuation of the therapeutic process at home.

Maladaptive Responses to Chronic Childhood Illness

The responses of overprotection, extended denial, rejection, and morbid grief are often seen in chronically ill children and their families. They result from the interaction between personalities and responses to stress, the family system's issues and beliefs, past experiences, the perception of the illness for children and families, available resources, and past and present involvement with the health care system. Maladaptive patterns occur when the parent-child-caregiver interaction system does not progress toward change and positive growth for the family. A pathologic balance is seen in which homeostasis is achieved by perpetuation of positive feedback loops that do not lead to behavioral change (Hoffman, 1981).

Responses that are initially seen as expected coping mechanisms within the grief process may become prolonged or exaggerated and are then considered maladaptive. In other cases, initial responses are identified as clearly inappropriate and signal serious distress. Families that cannot differentiate between feelings and actions experience difficulty with the grief process. Families that are unable to acknowledge the impact of an illness over time are also more likely to demonstrate maladaptive responses.

Overprotection is a common initial response to diagnosis and is not considered as maladaptive if the behavior does not continue. It is illustrated by parents catering to children's every wish, failing to set limits, and controlling the environment so that children cannot achieve new skills. Their benevolent overreaction perpetuates a cycle of guilt and fearfulness in parents and leads to dependency, demands, and immaturity from children (Boone and Hartman, 1972). This behavior creates resentment, hostility, and frustration in the parents and results in increased insecurity in ill children. If the pattern is prolonged, children intensify their illness behavior to gain attention, causing the process to repeat itself. A positive balance between normalization and realistic adjustment to the illness is therefore impeded. Overprotected children learn little independence but can sense parental anxiety and helplessness through the gifts and superficial gaiety, which heightens their fear.

Parental behaviors that signal overprotection include the following:
1. Sacrificing themselves and other family members for the child
2. Continually assisting the child, even when the child is capable
3. Providing inconsistent discipline, especially applying different rules for the ill child and siblings
4. Calling attention to every detail and overpraising the child
5. Restricting play to protect the child from every possible discomfort
6. Monopolizing the child's time by sleeping with the child, permitting few friends, and keeping the child home from school or other outside activities

Child behaviors include the following:
1. Constantly demanding attention
2. Refusing to perform daily functions
3. Fearing new experiences
4. Demonstrating anger and hostility toward parents and others
5. Increasing illness behaviors including overreaction to pain, medical procedures, and activities that require physical effort
6. Viewing self as inadequate and unable to cope without the immediate presence of a parent

Overprotection is often associated with unresolved parental guilt or fear. Ambivalent feelings regarding desire for a child during pregnancy, perceived responsibility for the disorder, or memories of a previous death of a loved one may exacerbate guilt. Conditions that may have occurred because of a parental act or illness such as alcohol intake during pregnancy, a chronic condition resulting from an accident in which a parent was responsible, and genetic disorders often result in the maladaptive response of overprotection. It may also occur when parental aspirations for their children are denied.

Bitterness and anger can build as daily care becomes more burdensome. Parents may envy parents of normal children and reinforce their feelings of worthlessness by seeing their child's problem as punishment for their sins. Other parental reactions may include depression to the extent of being unable to participate in family interaction and defensiveness in which parents are acutely aware of implied criticism and respond by denying the need for help.

Denial, a central element in the initial reaction to a loss or traumatic event, may become maladaptive. Some partial denial is a healthy coping mechanism and is accompanied by hope that motivates the acceptance of treatment. However, global denial in which parents completely refuse to accept that their child is ill interferes with treatment. Parents demand that their child compensate for the illness with impossible requests.

For example, seeking a second opinion is common and should be encouraged if it will aid the grief process and strengthen treatment decisions. If it continues and becomes the primary focus of the parents, it is seen as dysfunctional. Other behaviors that may signal include insisting that children not be informed of their illness or prognosis; subversion of their medical regimen by not obtaining or giving medication or following dietary requirements and by missing medical appointments; and promoting activities that have been specifically prohibited. These responses are classified as *avoidance behaviors* (see box).

Parents absorbed by their own anger or withdrawal to the degree of not accepting the prognosis may need more intense help. These parents are often uncomfortable with discussing death on any level and may use religion to relinquish their own responsibility or feelings. Isolation of the family from the community heightens these reactions. The use of avoidance leads to misconceptions about the meaning and significance of the event, often producing unnecessary guilt and anger.

Children may not receive needed care because of parental denial and may feel deserted and rejected. They must not only manage their illness without adult support but also balance the conflict between their family's response and others who

---

Assessment of Coping Behaviors

Approach behaviors

Asks for information regarding diagnosis and child's present condition
Seeks help and support from others
Anticipates future problems; actively seeks guidance and answers
Endows the illness or disability with meaning
Shares burden of disorder with others
Plans realistically for the future
Acknowledges and accepts child's awareness of diagnosis and prognosis
Expresses feelings, such as sorrow, depression, and anger, and realizes reason for the emotional reaction
Realistically perceives the child's condition; adjusts to changes
Recognizes own growth through passage of time, such as earlier denial and nonacceptance of diagnosis
Verbalizes possible loss of child

Avoidance behaviors

Fails to recognize the seriousness of the child's condition despite physical evidence
Refuses to agree to treatment
Intellectualizes about the illness, but in areas unrelated to the child's condition
Is angry and hostile to members of the staff, regardless of their attitude or behavior
Avoids staff, family members, or child
Entertains unrealistic future plans for child, with little emphasis on the present
Is unable to adjust to or accept a change in progression of disease
Continually looks for new cures with no perspective toward possible benefit
Refuses to acknowledge child's understanding of disease and prognosis
Uses magical thinking and fantasy, may seek "occult" help
Places complete faith in religion to point of relinquishing own responsibility
Withdraws from outside world; refuses help
Punishes self because of guilt and blame
Makes no change in life-style to meet needs of other family members
Resorts to excessive use of alcohol or drugs to avoid problems
Verbalizes suicidal intents
Is unable to discuss possible loss of the child or previous experiences with death

From Whaley L and Wong D: Nursing care of infants and children, ed 3, St Louis, 1987, The CV Mosby Co.

---

acknowledge the illness. They are frequently used by charlatans and fakes who prey on parental needs. Many parents waste needed emotional and financial resources searching for false cures.

Children may be overtly or covertly rejected by their parents for their handicap. They are seen as a handicap first and an individual second, and their pain intensifies because of their lessened self-worth. Depression, and acting-out behavior may be seen in children's response to the rejecting parent. The dependency they have on their caretaker adds to the rejection.

Coping through distance is often found with parents of premature infants. This coping style reduces the acquaintance process in the hospital and forces parents to rely on the experts to care for their infant. Parents express more fear, anxiety, and denial before they accept their infants and demonstrate emotional withdrawal from the child, with or without attention to the child's physical needs; constant nagging or scolding, often with the implication that the child is imposing on the family; and freezing out, the phase in which children are relinquished by their parents because of their handicaps.

Because of the limitations of their handicap, children may unintentionally exacerbate the situation. Premature infants are unpredictable, sleepy, immature, hypotonic, and fragile. They sleep more than normal newborns, and their patterns of sleep may be unpredictable. When awake, they engage less often. They are harder to feed due to a weak suck, small stomach, and poor gag reflex. They may vomit because of a weak cardiac sphincter and lax abdominal muscles. Premature infants' inability to respond normally interferes with positive attachment and results in the need for increased care. Mothers may view their child as defective or imperfect and feel a sense of failure (Cramer, 1982).

The possibility of death or a permanent or progressive handicap also increases the risk of rejection and withdrawal. Although the prognosis for many children is positive, many parents experience prolonged stress. As with denial, the values placed on abilities such as intellect or athletic prowess will determine the type and extent of rejection.

Delayed grief and distorted grief reactions are also indicative of maladaptive grief work. The former is illustrated by lack of the expected psychosomatic responses immediately after death, grief for an unresolved earlier loss, a strong reaction that begins on the anniversary of the death, and acute grief that is postponed because of the individual's need to support others (Lindemann, 1944). Some of the distorted reactions include the following:

1. Overactivity without a sense of loss
2. Acquisition of symptoms of the illness
3. Social isolation and a radical change in relationships with family and friends
4. Unjustified intense hostility toward specific people
5. Repression of hostility, including altered affect and conduct, often resembling psychotic symptoms
6. Prolonged lack of decision and initiative
7. Presence of behavior detrimental to social and economic existence
8. Agitated depression with or without signs of suicide

Families that have focused their lives around the care of ill children and those that have been overprotective or have largely denied the illness will experience continued difficulty with the grief process. Because they cannot effectively progress through the process, many families dissolve after the death of a child. Siblings often need help in coping with the death. They may show prolonged difficulties expressed through psychologic disorders, especially depression, fearfulness, and acting-out behavior. Nursing guidelines for maladaptive responses are shown in the box.

Nursing Implications for Maladaptive Responses

1. Clinicians should offer supportive, sensitive intervention as quickly as possible.
2. Nurses need to explore parents' belief systems, individual experiences, and present stressors before implementing interventions. Provision of a central person to provide support and reduction of changes in caregivers are also essential actions.
3. Nurse clinicians or therapists can be helpful in working with staff members to reduce their anger and frustration toward both parents and child and promote coordination of professionals. They must also be available when families are in crisis, interact with them during hospitalization, and manage outpatient and home-based care if necessary.
4. Nursing staff should be available to model alternative behavior for parents. Parents should be given as much control as possible but should not be forced into making noncritical decisions.
5. Clinicians should recommend outside support groups involving parents of children with similar problems.
6. Nurses need to provide early, consistent interaction to improve reality testing and assist parents in the grief process.
7. Clinicians should make an on-going system of support available to parents and children so that it can respond in times of family crisis.
8. Nurses need to consider intervention by child protection authorities if maladaptive reactions are seriously impeding children's physical and emotional health.

Pain

Children may experience pain as a result of the illness, such as the acute pain of sickle cell crisis or the joint pain associated with rheumatoid arthritis. Pain may result from observable trauma or injury such as burns or fractures. It may also occur from the assessment and treatment of the disease. For example, children with leukemia are subjected to periodic bone marrow aspirations and IV chemotherapy, children with diabetes mellitus take a daily dose of insulin by injection, and children with facial disfigurement or other orthopedic deformities require multiple reconstructive surgical procedures.

Pain assessment requires an interdisciplinary, multidimensional approach. When assessing children's pain, clinicians must consider children's cognitive developmental level, physiologic responsiveness, previous experiences, individual coping styles, parent-child interaction, and supports offered.

Pain assessment tools have been developed to aid in the interpretation of pain in children by quantifying the intensity of pain. The validity and reliability of such measures is not well documented; however, these assessment tools are clinically useful if used with care and in conjunction with the history and other observations.

PAIN MANAGEMENT AND NURSING INTERVENTIONS

The first step in developing a pain management program is to obtain a comprehensive assessment. Most important is listening to children, parents, and medical personnel.

Nonpharmacologic Pain Management in Children

General strategies

Prepare children in advance of potentially painful procedures but avoid "planting" idea of pain. For example, instead of saying "This is going to (or may) hurt," say "Sometimes this feels like pushing, sticking, or pinching and sometimes it doesn't bother people. You tell me what it feels like to you." This allows for variation in sensory perception, avoids suggesting pain, and gives children control in describing reactions.

Avoid evaluative statements or descriptions, such as "This is a terrible procedure" or "It really will hurt a lot."

Stay with children during a painful procedure; parents are often a neglected source of support for them and can be involved in distraction efforts.

Use the power of positive suggestion by saying "I am giving you a medicine that *will* take the hurt away."

Reinforce the effect of the analgesic by telling children they will begin to feel better in a certain amount of time (according to drug use); use a clock or timer to measure onset of relief; reinforce the cause and effect of pain analgesic so that children become conditioned to *expecting* relief.

Avoid saying "I am going to give you a shot for pain," since this is another pain in addition to the existing pain; if children refuse an injection, explain that the little hurt from the needle will take away the bigger hurt for a long time.

Give children control whenever possible (for example, choosing which leg for an injection, taking bandages off, holding the tape or other equipment).

Educate children about the pain, especially when explanation may decrease anxiety (for example, that the pain children are experiencing is expected after surgery and does not indicate that something is wrong; reassure children that they are not responsible for the pain).

For long-term pain control give children a doll that becomes "their patient" and allow them to do everything to the doll that is being done; pain control can be emphasized through the doll by stating, "Dolly feels better after her medicine."

Continued.

Nurses need to believe children when they say they are experiencing pain because they are capable of describing their discomfort. The erroneous belief that they lack the verbal ability to describe pain or remember past painful experiences has been discounted (Ross and Ross, 1984).

Regardless of the intervention strategy, the second step involves rehearsal. Clinicians convey information regarding a procedure or an upcoming hospitalization, including where they will be and the events that will occur. The timing of such rehearsal is developmentally based: Younger children require rehearsal just previous to the activity, and older children need time to work through some of their concerns.

Nonpharmacologic approaches to pain-perception regulation have been used effectively. These include distraction, relaxation, guided imagery, thought stopping, cutaneous stimulation, and behavioral contracting (see box).

Nonpharmacologic Pain Management in Children — cont'd

Specific strategies

Distraction. Involve parents and children in identifying strong distractors.

Involve children in play; use radio, tape recorder, record player; have them sing or use rhythmic breathing.

Have them concentrate on yelling or saying "ouch" by focusing on "yelling loud or soft as you feel it hurt; that way I know what's happening."

Relaxation. With infants or young children:

Hold in comfortable, well-supported position, such as vertically against chest and shoulder.

Rock in wide, rhythmic arc in rocking chair or sway back and forth, rather than bouncing.

Repeat one or two words softly, such as "Mommy's here."

With slightly older children:

Ask to take deep breath and "go limp as a rag doll" while exhaling slowly, then ask children to yawn (demonstrate if needed).

Help children assume comfortable position (for example, pillow under neck and knees).

Begin progressive relaxation: starting with the toes, systematically instruct children to let each body part "go limp" or "feel heavy;" if they have difficulty with relaxing, instruct them to tense or tighten each body part then relax it.

Guided imagery. Have children identify some highly pleasurable experience.

Have them describe the details of the event, write down the script, or record it.

Encourage them to concentrate only on the pleasurable event during the painful time and/or enhance the image by recalling specific details, such as reading the script or playing the record.

Combine with relaxation.

Thought-stopping. Identify positive facts about painful event, such as "It does not last long."

Identify reassuring information, such as, "If I think about something else, it does not hurt as much."

Condense positive and reassuring facts into a set of brief statements and have children memorize them.

Have children repeat the memorized statements whenever they think about or experience the painful event.

Cutaneous stimulation. Includes simple rhythmic rubbing; use of pressure: electric vibrator, massage with hand lotion, powder, or menthol cream; application of heat or cold, such as ice cube on site before giving injection or application of ice to site opposite the painful area (for example, if right knee hurts, place ice on left knee).

Is most effective if rhythmic or constant and moderate in intensity.

Behavioral contracting. May be used informally with children as young as 4 or 5; use stars or tokens as rewards. For example, if children are uncooperative and procrastinate during a procedure, give them a limited amount of time (measured by a visible timer) to complete the procedure and if they are unable to comply, proceed as needed; if procedure is accomplished within the set time, reinforce cooperation with reward. With older children a written contract may be used.

REFERENCES

American Psychiatric Association: Diagnostic and statistical manual of mental disorders, ed 3, rev, Washington, DC, 1987, American Psychiatric Association.

Boone D and Hartman B: The benevolent over-reaction, Clin Pediatr 11:268, 1972.

Bowlby J: Processes of mourning, Int J Psychoanal 42:317, 1961.

Burton L: The family life of sick children: a study of family coping with chronic childhood disease, London, 1975, Routledge & Kegan Paul, Inc.

Cramer B: Interview with parents of premature infants. In Klaus MH and Kennell JH: Parent-infant bonding, St Louis, 1982, The CV Mosby Co.

Douglas J: Early hospital admission and later disturbances of behavior and learning, Dev Med Child Neurol 17:456, 1975.

Friedrich W: Predictors of the coping behavior of mothers of handicapped children, J Consult Clin Psychol 47:1140, 1979.

Gunther MS: Emotional aspects. In Ruge D, editor: Spinal cord injuries, Springfield, Ill, 1969, Charles C Thomas, Publisher.

Hauser S and others: The contribution of family environment to perceived competence and illness adjustment in diabetic and acutely ill adolescents, Family Relations 34:99, 1985.

Hoffman L: Foundations of family therapy, New York, 1981, Basic Books, Inc, Publishers.

Hymovich D: Nursing services. In Hobbs N and Perrin J, editors: Issues in the care of children with a chronic illness, San Francisco, 1985, Jossey-Bass, Inc, Publishers.

Ireys H: Health care for chronically disabled children and their families. In Department of Health and Human Services: Better health for our children: a national strategy, DHHS Pub No 70-55071, Washington, DC, 1981, US Government Printing Office.

Koocher G: Childhood, death, and cognitive development, Dev Psychol 9:369, 1973.

Koocher G and O'Malley J: The Damocles syndrome: psychological consequences of surviving childhood cancer, New York, 1981, McGraw-Hill, Inc.

Koocher G and Sallan S: Psychological issues in pediatric oncology. In Magrab P, editor: Psychological management of pediatric problems, College Park, Md, 1978, University Park Press.

Kubler-Ross E: On death and dying, New York, 1969, Macmillan Publishing Co.

Langer E and Rodin J: The effects of choice and enhanced personal responsibility for the aged: a field experiment in an institutional setting, J Pers Soc Psychol 32:951, 1976.

Lindemann E: Symptomatology and management of acute grief, Am J Psychiatry 101:141, 1944.

Mattsson A: The chronically ill child: a challenge to family adaptation, Med College Va Q 8:171, 1972.

O'Grady D and Metz R: Resilience in children at high risk for psychological disorder, J Pediatr Psychol 12:3, 1987.

O'Malley J and others: Psychiatric sequelae of surviving childhood cancer, Am J Orthopsychiatry 49:608, 1979.

Perrin E and Shapiro E: Who's in charge? Health locus of control beliefs of healthy children, children with a chronic physical illness, and their mothers, J Pediatr 16:76, 1985.

Perrin E, Ayoub C, and Willett J: Adjustment of children with a chronic illness: parent's, child's, and teacher's perspective on family influences. Paper presented at the meeting of the Society for Research in Child Development, Kansas City, Mo, Apr 1989.

Perrin E, Ramsey B, and Sandler H: Competent kids: children and adolescents with a chronic illness, Child Care Health Dev 13:13, 1987.

Piaget J: The child's conception of the world, New York, 1929, Harcourt Brace.

Pless I and Perrin J: Issues common to a variety of illnesses. In Hobbs N and Perrin J, editors: Issues in the care of children with chronic illness, San Francisco, 1985, Jossey-Bass, Inc, Publishers.

Pless I and Pinkerton P: Chronic childhood disorders—promoting patterns of adjustment, London, 1976, Henry Kimpton.

Pless I and Roghmann K: Chronic illness and its consequences: some observations based on three epidemiological surveys, J Pediatr 79:351, 1971.

Robertson J: Young children in hospital, New York, 1958, Basic Books, Inc, Publishers.

Ross D and Ross S: The importance of type of question, psychological climate and subject set in interviewing children about pain, Pain 19:71, 1984.

Rutter M: Stress, coping and development: some issues and some questions, J Child Psychol Psychiatry 22:323, 1981.

Simmonds J: Psychiatric status of diabetic youth matched with a control group, Diabetes 26:921, 1971.

Stein R and Jessop D: Relationship between health status and psychological adjustment among children with chronic conditions, Pediatrics 73:169, 1984.

Taylor SC: The effects of chronic childhood illness upon well siblings, MCN 9:109, 1980.

Voysey M: Impression management by parents with disabled children, J Health Soc Behav 13:80, 1972.

Wallander J and others: Children with chronic disorders: maternal reports of their psychological adjustment, J Pediatr Psychol 13:197, 1988.

Whaley LF and Wong DL: Nursing care of infants and children, ed 3, St Louis, 1987, The CV Mosby Co.

Young R: Chronic sorrow: parent's response to the birth of a child with a defect, MCN 2:38, 1977.

Chapter 14

Anxiety and Depression in Preschool and School-Aged Children

Deborah Kay Brantly
Donna J. Takacs

Definitions and Concepts

Attempts to clarify the relationship between anxiety and depression have been made. Spitz and Wolf (1946) identified *anaclytic depression* as a syndrome that was etiologically associated with separation. Bowlby (1960) identified a similar syndrome in children, which is currently known as separation anxiety. Current thought holds that anxiety and depression are distinct syndromes, with overlapping characteristics are linked (Ganellen, 1988). In one study, 50% of adolescent school refusers were found to fulfill criteria for both anxiety and depression (Bernstein and Garfinkel, 1986).

Both anxiety and depression may be operationalized as discrete symptoms, syndromes, and disease states. The symptomatology involves subjective feelings and physiologic manifestations. When these symptoms become associated with others, a syndrome emerges. Once the underlying cause of the syndrome becomes evident, a disease state is identified.

As a symptom, anxiety is a subjective feeling of apprehension or nervousness that may be considered normal. According to Carpenito (1987), it is a "state in which the individual experiences feelings of uneasiness (apprehension) and activation of the autonomic nervous system in response to a vague, nonspecific threat." As a syndrome, it presents signs associated with the subjective feeling of anxiousness, and as a primary, independent disease, its severity is inappropriate, it occurs under inappropriate circumstances, or it is qualitively atypical (Cameron, 1985). Anxiety disorders appear when affected people attempt to resist their symptoms, leading to phobias or compulsions and include separation anxiety disorder (SAD), avoidant disorder, and overanxious disorder (OAD) in children (American Psychiatric Association, 1987; Campbell, 1981).

As a symptom, depression presents as a sad affect and subjective feelings of sadness. In children, depressive symptoms are thought to be transient and to occur normally as part of the developmental process in which children strive to gain mastery. However, depression may present itself as a primary affect for some individuals (Bemporad and Wilson, 1978). As a syndrome, depression manifests itself with clusters of behaviors such as loss of interest or pleasure in daily routines and activities; feelings of hopelessness, guilt, and worthlessness; sleep disturbances; fatigue; and changes in appetite and weight. In addition, suicidal ideation can be associated with depressive symptomatology. As a disease, the syndrome is acknowledged as a formal disease process with an etiologic basis that can be seen in physiologic functioning and that is confirmed by laboratory testing, response to treatment, course of the illness, and familial pattern of the illness (Nelms, 1986). In one study, 100 children who were admitted to a hospital for orthopedic procedures were evaluated to determine the rate and symptomatology of depression. Researchers found that 23% were diagnosed as depressed. Of those, 100% exhibited depressed mood, 87% exhibited loss of interest or pleasure, 80% exhibited feelings of guilt, and 22% exhibited suicidal ideation.

The prevalence of anxiety is difficult to ascertain because it is frequently considered a normal phenomena, and may not be reported or treated. In a recent cross-sectional study, psychopathology was evaluated in children of 8, 12, and 17 years of age using the child assessment schedule (CAS). Approximately 33% of the children met the criteria for a DSM-III disorder; however, the level of severity did not necessarily warrant treatment. In approximately 20% of cases, the DSM-III disorder diagnosed was anxiety (Kashani and others, 1989). In preadolescents, one of the most frequently occurring diagnoses is SAD, with OAD being the least prevalent. In adolescents, the reverse is true (Kashani and Orvaschel, 1988). The frequency of the occurrence of anxiety was not dependent on age; however, the incidence of separation anxiety decreases with age, and specific fears and social concerns appear to increase with age. Males and females show similar trends except that females demonstrate greater anxiety related to their personal competencies (Kashani and others, 1989).

It is estimated that over 400,000 children suffer from depression each year in the United States. The studies available show discrepant results—from 1% to 60% of clinical populations thought to suffer from it, with typical results falling between 10% and 20%. Discrepencies may exist because of differences in frequency of depression in the sampled ages (for example, younger children exhibited lower rates than older children), inconsistency in measures used, and differences in criteria for depression (Mash and Terdal, 1988). Gender-related variations initially manifest in adolescence, with more females exhibiting depression than males.

Diagnosis

ASSESSMENT

Assessment of anxiety and depression occurs subjectively and formally and involves observation of behavior. Nursing diagnoses of depression and anxiety are frequently

---

Nursing Diagnoses Related to Depression

Ineffective individual coping
Disturbance in self-concept
   and self-esteem
Alteration in thought processes
Potential for self-harm

Self-care deficit
Alteration in nutrition
Alteration in activity and rest
Alteration in elimination
Alteration in sexuality

---

made, but there is a need for greater specificity of the disorders (Whitley, 1989). Other nursing diagnoses are used to address the symptomatology present with depressive disorders or to identify reactions with depressive features. Nursing diagnoses that may result from a depressed state are listed in the box, and Table 14-1 presents potential characteristics of anxiety and depression that may be found after a comprehensive nursing assessment.

Parents' evaluation of depression showed a lower rate of DSM-III disorders than clinical assessment using children's interviews, and nurses need to be aware of discrepancies in the perception of anxiety. Clinicians should also realize that information regarding the measurement of children under the age of 6 is not found in current literature and that the most comprehensive picture of clients is gained by using various methods to gather data.

Anxiety Scales

Several measures for testing anxiety in children have been developed. Generally, the methods devised for children have been adapted from adult scales. A commonly used anxiety scale is the children's manifest anxiety scale (CMAS). The CMAS was developed for children's self-report of experiences of general or chronic anxiety in different situations. The scale consists of 53 items, including 42 anxiety items and 11 items that formulate a lie scale. A revised edition of the CMAS was produced in 1978 and was renamed *What I Think and Feel*. It includes 28 anxiety items and 9 lie items, is reliable, and can be used for grades 1 through 12. Reading level is geared for third graders, and questions are read to younger children. Although identifying the type of anxiety is difficult, it may measure trait anxiety and tendencies toward chronic anxiety reaction. (Goldman, Stein, and Guerry, 1983; Hoehn-Saric and others, 1987).

The state-trait anxiety inventory for children (STAIC) is a self-report inventory designed for elementary school-aged children. Two scales, one measuring trait and one measuring state, are administered individually or in groups and are each composed of 20 statements. The state scale describes the present status of psychic anxiety, and the trait scale describes the general tendency to respond to stressful events with anxiety (Hoehn-Saric and others, 1987). Further research is indicated to extend the norms to a broader age range and to different ethnic groups (Goldman, Stein, and Guerry, 1983).

Structured or semistructured interviews have also been developed that yield more comprehensive and reliable data than free-form interviews, including the Interview for Children and Adolescents (DICA), the Kiddie-SADS, the Mental Health

Table 14-1   Characteristics in Children with Anxiety and Depression

Characteristic	Depression	Anxiety
Behavior	Predominately sad facial expression with absence or diminished range of affective response Solitary play, work, or tendency to be alone; disinterest in play Lowered grades in school; lack of interest in doing homework or achieving in school Diminished motor activity; tiredness Change in appetite resulting in weight loss or gain Alterations in sleeping pattern Tearfulness or crying	Lack of initiative Increase in motor activity resulting in irritability and nervousness Inability to relax Inability to concentrate Inability to remember Rumination Tendency to blame others
Internal states	Utterance of statements reflecting lowered self-esteem, sense of hopelessness or guilt Suicidal ideations	Utterance of statements reflecting self-depreciation, helplessness, worry Apprehension Fear of unspecific consequences Inordinate concern with health or illness
Physiology	Constipation Nonspecific complaints of not feeling well Lowered urinary excretion of 30 methoxy-4-hydroxyphenyl-glycol (MHPG) Abnormal dexylmethazone supporession test (DST) Hypersecretion of growth hormone during sleep Blunting of growth hormone to insulin-induced hypoglycemia (ITT), suggestive of endogenous depression	Elevated heartrate, palpitations Increased blood pressure Diarrhea

Assessment Form, the Child Assessment Schedule (CAS), and the Interview Schedule for Children (ISC). In general, the interview format is not used for children under the age of 6 years.

Some researchers measure anxiety in children by gathering information using several methods. The Children's Anxiety Evaluation Form (CAEF) involves examining the history of the present illness, its symptoms, and its signs. Interviewers initially review client documentation for the presence of anxiety symptoms. They use a checklist of items as a guideline and rate the severity of the symptoms on a five-point scale, based on the findings from a semistructured interview.

Depression Scales

Several depression scales have been devised for children. The Children's Depression Inventory (CDI) is a widely used, self-rating scale yielding a global assessment of children's depression. It is employed primarily to evaluate young school-aged children, and its test-retest reliability is 0.87. It can be modified to be used by adults to rate children's depression.

Research on the CDI has found a high rate of internal consistency, the ability to distinguish clinic from nonclinic groups of children, and positive correlation with related constructs, such as self-esteem, negative cognitive attributions, and hopelessness. However, the CDI does not necessarily predict depression or differentiate depression from other psychopathology (Mash and Terdal, 1988).

Other self-report measures commonly used include the Schedule for Affective Disorders and Schizophrenia for School-Aged Children (K-SADS or Kiddie-SADS), the Children's Depression Scale (CDS), the Children's Depression Rating Scale (CDRS), the Peer Nomination Inventory for Depression (PNID), and the Childhood Depression Assessment Tool-Revised (CDAT-R). These scales quantify the symptoms present, measure specific depressive symptoms, and assess concepts associated with childhood depression.

Theoretic Considerations

THEORIES OF ANXIETY

Researchers have proposed several hypotheses to explain the etiology of anxiety. It is thought to result from the appraisal of a threatening situation that continues until coping efforts are mobilized to deal with the event (Lamontagne, Mason, and Hepworth, 1985). Learning theorists believe that anxiety is a conditional part of fear and serves as a secondary drive (Klein, 1980). An unconditioned stimulus such as pain causes an unconditioned response such as fear, which then serves as the primary drive and leads to escape behavior. When experienced repeatedly, a stimulus that precedes an unconditioned response becomes conditioned and produces anxiety, which then serves as a secondary drive and incites avoidance behavior. Successful avoidance behavior reduces anxiety and reinforces the avoidance response. The learning theory explains some anxieties; however, most phobias do not start with a traumatic incident. In addition, the range of phobic objectives is limited, and behaviors may also be learned through the observation of others (Schwartz and Johnson, 1985).

The psychoanalytic theory of Freud posited that rising instinctual impulses, if ungratified, would produce traumatic excitation, similar to the unconditioned stimulus in learning theory. Infants learn to recognize that certain situations, for example, the absence of the mother, regularly precede the lack of gratification. Therefore, the absence of the mother becomes a conditioned stimulus producing anxiety.

Klein (1980) believes that learning and psychoanalytic theories are deficient because neither addresses the distinction between panic attack and chronic anticipatory anxiety. He postulated an ethologic theory in which a relationship between agoraphobia and separation anxiety exists, with the latter being the root of the problem. In reviewing histories of agoraphobic clients, he found approximately 50% of them had experienced separation anxiety in childhood. Protest, a normal response to separation in children, appears similar to the anxiety attack, which is also characterized by pleading, clinging, and demanding.

Although the ethologic theory is presently the most common, it and other theories do not explain all characteristics of anxiety. Further research and investigation is necessary.

THEORIES OF DEPRESSION

Definitions of depression in children are still being developed because it was not viewed as a distinct disorder until the 1960s. Theories of depression either address depressive symptomatology and the existence of the disorder in children or focus on etiologic models.

Symptomalogic Theories

Before the 1960s, psychoanalytic theory asserted that the disorders of depression necessitated a well-developed superego and that children could not experience them because their superego was still developing. Current psychoanalytic views acknowledge depressive disorders in children and view them as evolving from psychosexual development, childhood and early experiences, and cognitive or perceptual skills (Mash and Terdal, 1988).

The theory of masked depression emerged and was dominant in the 1960s. It posited that the symptoms inherent in adult depression (such as dysphoric mood and lack of interest) may not be observable in children. Depression may instead manifest itself in depressive equivalents such as running away, delinquency, irritability, hyperactivity, and temper tantrums. Because of the difficulty in designing research studies that could link depressive equivalents to depression, this theory lost momentum but did influence the identification of depression as a distinct disorder.

Lefkowitz (1980) proposed that depressive symptoms in children are part of the normal process of childhood development and that if they are not seen over a period of time, they should not be viewed as pathologic. Although some studies have supported this theory, opponents note that the depressive symptomatology is being pinpointed, not depression as a syndrome or disorder.

The most commonly accepted view is described by the DSM-III-R. This position accepts the existence of childhood depression and proposes that depression has essential features common to all age levels and that associated features differ according to developmental level. Similar manifestations in children and adults include low self-esteem, an external locus of control, a general unhappiness, and an abnormal DMST. However, disturbances in the REM cycle of sleep are found in adults with depression but not in children.

Etiologic Theories

The genetic predisposition theory states that depression is a result of a dominant gene. NIH studies show that adopted children and their biologic parents demonstrate more depression than adoptive parents. Identical twin studies reveal that when one twin has depression, the other twin is 70% more likely to develop depression, compared with 15% for other siblings, parents, and children of affected individuals and 7% for aunts, uncles, and grandparents. According to this theory, a family history of depression predisposes children for the disorder.

The biochemical theory states that biochemical factors are associated with depression. The biogenic amine hypothesis postulates that serotonin and norepinephrine are responsible for regulating mood and controlling drives such as hunger, sex, and thirst. Increased amounts of these amines at the receptor sites cause elevation of mood, and decreased amounts cause depression of mood. Levels of cortisol are also altered in depressed individuals. These levels usually increase in the early morning, remain constant during the day, and decrease in the evening. In depressed people, cortisol levels peak earlier and remain high throughout the day and evening.

According to this theory, biochemical factors would be confirmatory, rather than predictive, of the disease. Differential diagnoses of types of depression are thought to be more effectively substantiated. An effort is being made to discriminate between state factors, biochemical results found during the acute phase of the illness, and trait factors, biochemical findings in a nonacute phase.

The object-loss theory posits depressed individuals have sustained a major loss in life, which causes depression and a lowered self-esteem. Losses commonly occurring in childhood include loss of parents through death or divorce, loss of bodily control from a chronic disease process, loss of friends resulting from moves, and loss of status in the family through the addition of family members.

Associated Disorders

Other syndromes often coexist with depression and may confuse practitioners identifying diagnostic criteria. In a study by Alessi and Magen (1988), 52% of the children with depressive disorders had three or more additional psychiatric diagnoses. The Axis I diagnoses of adjustment disorder, attention deficit disorder, and anxiety disorder and the Axis II diagnoses of specific developmental disorders and personality disorders occurred at a rate of 25% or more. Researchers proposed the following explanations for the additional psychiatric disturbances (Alessi and Magen, 1988):

1. They are preexisting disorders leading to the development of depressive disorders.
2. They are a shared diathesis or genetic predisposition with an expression dependent on environmental mediating variables.
3. They occur by chance.

SEPARATION ANXIETY DISORDER

DSM-III-R criteria for the recognition of SAD includes the presence of excessive anxiety for at least 2 weeks. When children are separated from parents or significant others, they may experience anxiety to the extent of panic. The onset of the disorder may occur during the preschool period or in adolescence but must be found before the age of 18 to be classified as SAD. Presenting behaviors include uneasiness when in unfamiliar surroundings, refusal to visit friends' homes or attend school, and clinging activity. Physical complaints such as headaches, stomaches, nausea, and vomiting are common when separation is anticipated, and the cardiovascular symptoms of dizziness and faintness are rare in children but may occur in adolescents (American Psychiatric Association, 1987). SAD may be associated with fears of animals, monsters, potentially harmful situations, death, and dying. Fears of younger children are generally more vague and become more specific and focused with age. Fear of the dark is common in younger children, and accompanying nightmares may occur.

Depressed mood is an associated feature of SAD, which may become more persistent and justify an additional diagnosis of dysthymia or major depression. Periods of exacerbation and remission are common, and evidence of SAD may be seen in later situations, such as an avoidance of leaving home.

In most cases, SAD develops after a life stress such as a loss of a pet or relative or a change in environment. The families of children with SAD are often close-knit and caring, and a familial pattern may be found. The disorder is not uncommon and seems to appear equally among boys and girls, with a greater frequency in children of mothers with panic disorder. An illustration of the manifestation of SAD is shown in the case example.

Case Example

Susan, an 8-year-old girl, experienced difficulty remaining at school. She complained of high-level anxiety with no identifiable reason, nausea, and the inability to breathe. Susan was sent home several days in a row because of her complaints. The results of a physical exam were negative for any physiologic explanation, but Susan resisted returning to school. She preferred to accompany her mother at all times and became upset when separation was imminent. It was learned during counseling that Susan's father, with whom she was close, had died suddenly several months before. Susan had appeared to cope with her father's death until recently when she became alarmed with the knowledge that her mother faced a minor routine surgical procedure.

STEREOTYPIC/HABIT DISORDERS

According to the DSM-III-R, the essential feature of this disorder is that specific behaviors are intentional and repetitive and serve no constructive, socially acceptable purpose. Children with the disorder may rock their body, bang their head, hit or bite parts of their body, such as their thumb, pull their hair, pick their skin, grind their teeth, perform body manipulations, hold their breath, and use noncommunicative, repetitive vocalizations.

The diagnosis is applied when the behavior causes physical injury to children or markedly interferes with normal activities. The diagnosis is not made when a pervasive developmental disorder or a tic disorder is present. In its more severe forms, it is frequently associated with mental retardation (American Psychiatric Association, 1987).

The pathologic disorder is usually first seen in childhood, may intensify in adolescence, and may lead to interference with self-care and social rejection. In most cases, the disorders are triggered by underlying conditions.

Thumb Sucking

The estimated frequency of thumb sucking is from 15% to 60% in infants, and it is not considered a problem unless it persists in school-aged children. It often occurs at bedtime or during other periods of separation and when children are lonely, sad, or depressed. Thumb sucking may be related to loss or separation and be a symbolic attempt to overcome pain and anxiety by stimulating the sensation of being full and satisfied. It also may represent withdrawal from a situation that is too frightening or overwhelming to face (Noshpitz, 1979).

Nail Biting

Parents rarely seek medical help for nail biting unless it is accompanied by other habits or problem behaviors. The usual onset is approximately at the age of 3, and incidence peaks at the age of 6 and again at the age of 13 to 15. Nail biting is found in 40% to 45% of children and has been associated with motor restlessness, restless sleep, tics, and other body manipulations. It usually occurs during periods of fear or stress (Noshpitz, 1979).

Rhythmic Body Movements

Rocking and head banging are common activities among infants and toddlers and may occur together or separately. Normal rhythmic body movements usually decrease at approximately age 2, and when seen in older children, they may signal a more serious problem such as organic brain syndrome, mental retardation, and autism.

The lack of emotional factors in the environment may cause the movements, and the single habit of body rocking does not appear to lead to later personality disturbances (Noshpitz, 1979).

Trichotillomania

Hair pulling is common but is not usually a psychiatric issue unless other symptoms are present. In many cases, children experience a significant object loss before the onset of the behavior, and approximately 65% of clients reported moderate to severe depression preceding it. Family histories often indicate pathologic conditions. Mothers of children with trichotillomania have been described as ambivalent and competitive. The mothers reported experiencing unmet dependency needs and held their parents in poor regard (Noshpitz, 1979). Mother-daughter relationships were generally characterized by hostile dependency and mutual fears of separation.

OVERANXIOUS DISORDER

According to the DSM-III-R, OAD appears during childhood, and the predominant feature is unrealistic anxiety lasting 6 months or longer. Children with the disorder are self-conscious and worry about future events such as the possibility of injury, examinations, and inclusion in peer group activities. Anxiety may also occur when meeting deadlines or thinking about past behaviors. Children may ask repeatedly about expectations and require more reassurance. In some cases, physical signs of anxiety such as headaches and stomachaches are present.

The diagnosis is not applied if the anxiety occurs only during the course of a psychotic or mood disorder. It is normally seen in connection with SAD in children under 13 years of age, and children older than 13 are more likely to display overanxious disorder alone (American Psychiatric Association, 1987).

Social and simple phobias may be present concurrently, as well as refusal to attend school. Excessive motor restlessness such as nail biting or hair pulling is also observed. Children may be reluctant to engage in age-appropriate activities in which demands are made for performance (American Psychiatric Association, 1987).

OAD may develop gradually or suddenly, and the age of onset is unknown. It may persist into adult life as an anxiety disorder. Impairment is severe if children cannot meet demands at home or school. Because physical signs of anxiety have no physiologic basis, unnecessary physical evaluations may be performed (American Psychiatric Association, 1987).

The incidence of OAD is higher in the oldest child of small families, upper socioeconomic class families, and families where there is concern about achievement even when children are functioning at an adequate or superior level. Anxiety disorders appear to be more common among mothers of children with OAD than among mothers of children with other mental disorders (American Psychiatric Association, 1987).

Dysthymia and Major Depression

Major depression can occur as a single episode or as a recurrent event. It is not, however, related to a chronic state of depression. The DSM-III-R identifies major depression as a disorder in which at least five of the identified depressive symptoms have occurred in a 2 week period and represents a change in functioning. The identified symptoms include the following:
1. Depressed mood
2. Markedly diminished interest or pleasure in activities
3. Significant weight loss or gain (more than 5% of body weight in a month) or increased or decreased appetite
4. Insomnia or hypersomnia
5. Psychomotor agitation or retardation
6. Fatigue or loss of energy
7. Feelings of worthlessness or excessive or inappropriate guilt
8. Diminished ability to think or concentrate
9. Recurrent thoughts of death

At least one of the first two symptoms needs to be displayed to make the diagnosis.

Dysthymia was once labeled *depressive neurosis* and is considered chronic. The DSM-III-R describes the symptoms of dysthymia as the following:
1. Poor appetite or overeating
2. Insomnia or hypersomnia
3. Low energy level

4. Low self-esteem
5. Poor concentration or difficulty making decisions
6. Feelings of hopelessness

The diagnosis of dysthymia is made after individuals demonstrate symptoms for 2 years and are not symptom-free for more than 2 months during the 2 year period. The diagnosis is not made when symptoms exist in conjunction with a specific organic cause, major depressive episode, or chronic psychotic condition (American Psychiatric Association, 1987).

SUICIDAL BEHAVIOR

Suicidal behavior is often associated with a diagnosis of depression. Some experts argue, however, that suicidal behavior is independent of depression in children and more often a result of family conflicts. Some researchers believe that children view suicide as their only escape and that it is an acting-out behavior representing a cry for help or a true desire to die (Finn, 1986). Children's suicidal attempts are usually impulsive or accidental events, but they are the second-leading cause of death in children aged 1 to 14 (U.S. Department of Health and Human Services, 1983). The case example illustrates some behaviors associated with suicidal potential.

Case Example

Jana is an 11-year-old girl who had been referred to the nurse therapist for outpatient therapy. Jana's mother described her grades as dropping in the last 9 weeks from A's and B's to C's, D's, and an F. Jana's mother described her as becoming more of a loner — not socializing as much with her friends or her older brother. Jana's parents were separated 10 months previously, and their divorce had been final for 2 months. Jana has not seen her father for 3 months, and her mother frequently found her in her room crying and asking about her father. Jana's mother was especially concerned when Jana became upset and stated, "It would have been better if I hadn't been born." She had lost 5 lbs in the previous 2 months and frequently picked at her food. The nurse therapist initially assessed Jana for suicide and depression. The assessment revealed a high potential for suicide, demonstrated by Jana's plan to take her mother's sleeping pills and a depressive rating on the CDI. She was referred to an inpatient unit for evaluation of depression and stabilization of suicidal ideation. The outpatient nurse therapist maintained a therapy relationship with Jana and her mother during the course of treatment.

RISK FACTORS

Risk factors have been identified for children with depression and suicidal ideations and include the following (Achenbach, 1980; Finn, 1986; Nelms, 1986):

1. Academic pressures
2. Stressful social relationships
3. Social isolation
4. Parental absence or loss
5. Low socioeconomic status

6. Dysfunctional family relationships
7. Family disruptions
8. Inadequate childrearing practices
9. Parental or family history of depression, suicide, or other psychopathology
10. Parental alcoholism and substance abuse
11. Hospitalization and chronic illness

In one study of 80 chronically ill children, 30 were classified as depressed (Nelms, 1986). Depressed children have also been found to manifest a low self-esteem, general unhappiness, and an external locus of control on self-report measures, but they did not significantly evidence behavioral manifestations of depression during play and task completion observations. They also demonstrate less sociable and soothable ratings on a temperament rating scale. Kovacs and others (1981) suggest that mild depression places children at risk for major depression.

Prevention of Anxiety and Depression in Children

PRIMARY PREVENTION

Primary prevention of disease is the most effective method to decrease the incidence or severity of disorders. Clinicians may offer classes on parenting skills, normal growth and development, depression, anxiety, and suicidal behavior in children in schools and clinics and may act as speakers for organizations involving parents. School nurses can identify student populations at risk.

Once a problem has been identified, clinicians can facilitate individuals' coping. For example, when a child commits suicide, nurse therapists support the children in the deceased child's class by assisting in their addressing the feelings gendered by suicide. Support groups can be organized, and nurses may refer parents or clients when necessary.

Access to information and guidance is an important primary prevention intervention. Organizations maintaining suicide prevention hot lines provide timely support measures, as do psychiatric emergency rooms in hospitals. Emergency room nurses should be able to assess physiologic and psychosocial problems.

For prevention during infancy, staff members in therapeutic nurseries can identify children that need help early in life and support parents in their management of problem areas. For preschoolers, programs such as Head Start and television shows such as *Sesame Street* and *Mister Rogers* that discuss feelings and relationships are effective sources of prevention.

Strengthening children's awareness of their inner states and increasing their self-esteem is termed *affective education* and is a source of primary prevention of anxiety, depression, and suicidal behavior in school-aged children (Finn, 1986). Because many childhood suicides are related to family problems, programs in local mental health centers that focus on strengthening the family unit, improving parenting skills, increasing communication among parents and children, and promoting consistent discipline and limit setting increase self-esteem and decrease children's distress. Education through groups such as Al-Anon support children with a family history of substance abuse.

A study by Nelms (1986) reveals that parental recognition of depression in children with a chronic illness was justified as illness-related and not as depression-related. Primary prevention should include education of chronically ill children and their parents addressing the common manifestations of the disorder so that the depressive symptomatology is recognized and assistance is sought early in the disease. Parents need to understand the importance of children discussing their common depressive feelings, and clinicians should promote positive rehabilitation measures, that is, encourage families to emphasize children's strengths and normalization. Assisting parents in their awareness of normal behaviors during infancy and childhood provides an essential perspective and prevents parental anxiety.

SECONDARY PREVENTION

Physiologic Interventions

Pharmacologic intervention for anxiety and depressive disorders is common and involves the use of antidepressants such as imiprimine. Medication-teaching considerations are of paramount importance for children and families, and nurses must monitor common and dangerous side effects of the antidepressants. Pharmacologic measures are also discussed in Chapter 16.

Safety is another area affecting physiologic functioning. For example, chronic head-bangers should have a complete physical, neurologic, and psychologic evaluation. In severe cases a helmet may be used to protect children's head. For suicidal children, several nursing interventions relating to safety have been identified as appropriate:

1. Have children write a no-suicide contract in their own handwriting.
2. Provide a room near the nurses' station for close observation.
3. Place children on suicidal precautions based on suicidal potential and continue to assess their potential for suicide by asking about their feelings and suicidal plans.
4. Provide frequent, documented, one-on-one contact and check their status every 15 minutes.
5. Remove any items that might be considered dangerous and search their belongings for harmful objects.
6. Use seclusion to provide an adequate level of safety, if necessary.
7. Observe for checking of medications or use liquid forms whenever possible.
8. Ask children to commit to verbalization when feeling suicidal.
9. Stay with children who are experiencing a suicidal crisis.

Another aspect of physiologic intervention is diet. Excessive amounts of stimulants such as tea or cola may produce physiologic changes demonstrated as anxiety (Emery, 1981). Adequate nutrition and correct body weight may also affect depressed children.

Psychosocial Interventions

In crisis intervention the goal is not to resolve all underlying problems but to provide stabilization. Therapy interventions with older, school-aged children should include careful evaluation to determine issues related to the symptomatology and counseling and/or psychotherapy to address causes and relieve symptoms. Play therapy is frequently used for younger children because it is less threatening than one-on-one talk therapy. When using individual therapy with older children, clinicians should provide an avenue of self-expression or distraction, such as playing cards and board games, sorting papers, and drawing. This activity defocuses children's attention on the subject and the adult that may feel threatening. Family therapy is another important modality of treatment in children.

Focusing on symptoms may only increase anxiety and depression. Parents can use distraction to lessen tension and provide an outlet of expression. Clinicians can assist clients in correcting thinking errors and understanding that anxiety is normal, often unavoidable, and helpful in certain circumstances. Thinking errors in depression are common, especially in suicidal thinking. Individuals develop a tunnel vision in which they have difficulty endorsing any options other than suicide. In addition, discussing misperceptions about fears can decrease them (Emery, 1981).

Visual imaging is another effective intervention. It provides mastery of or experience in common developmental tasks through fantasy. For example, children who cannot walk can image themselves dancing or running. Anxious children can imagine upcoming events and, by being aware of or communicating the fantasies to others, can overcome possibly stressful situations with coping images. Visual imaging can be accompanied by relaxation training.

Milieu Services and Treatments

The implementation of a behavior modification program is frequently successful with children because they are reward oriented. All should provide immediate feedback for the younger children. The use of star charts providing positive reinforcement is a system that may be successful in diminishing symptoms (Noshpitz, 1979).

Occupational therapy provides a forum for mastery of tasks that are developmentally appropriate, enhancing self-esteem and conquering fears. Participating in recreational outings allows children to experience community activities with peers, especially important for anxious children who may use positive visualization before the event. For depressed children, movements involved in recreational activities decrease depression. Rhythmic motor activities such as dangling and swinging should be encouraged for children demonstrating head-banging behaviors.

TERTIARY PREVENTION

Adjustment into the community (rehabilitation) is the primary aim of tertiary prevention. Partial hospitalization programs facilitate reentry into the community for hospitalized children. A community-based approach maximizes children's positive outcomes at home, and outpatient therapy services perpetuate the supportive relationship. Nurses may recommend support groups and use clergy to assist parents in organizing neighborhood interventions. The involvement of school nurses and counselors to identify potential crisis behavior is also essential.

REFERENCES

Achenbach T: DSM-III in light of empirical research of the classification of child psychopathology, J Am Acad Child Psychiatr 19:395, 1980.

Alessi N and Magen J: Comorbidity of other psychiatric disturbances in depressed, psychiatrically hospitalized children, Am J Psychiatry 145:1582, 1988.

American Psychiatric Association: Diagnostic and statistical manual of mental disorders, ed 3, rev, Washington, DC, 1987, American Psychiatric Association.

Bemporad J and Wilson A: A developmental approach to depression in childhood and adolescence, J Am Acad Psychoanal 6:325, 1978.

Bernstein GA and Garfinkel MD: School phobia: the overlap of affective and anxiety disorders, J Am Acad Child Psychiatry 25:235, 1986.

Bowlby J: Grief and mourning in infancy and early childhood, Psychoanal Study Child 15:9, 1960.

Cameron OG: The differential diagnosis of anxiety, Psychiatr Clin North Am 8:3, 1985.

Campbell R: Psychiatric dictionary, ed 5, New York, 1981, Oxford University Press, Inc.

Carpenito L: Nursing diagnosis: application to clinical practice, ed 2, Philadelphia, 1987, JB Lippincott Co.

Emery G: A new beginning: how you can change your life through cognitive therapy, New York, 1981, Simon & Schuster, Inc.

Finn P: Self-destructive behavior in school-aged children: a hidden problem? Pediatr Nurs 12:198, 1986.

Ganellen R: Specificity of attributions and overgeneralization in depression and anxiety, J Abnorm Psychol 97:83, 1988.

Goldman J, Stein C, and Guerry S: Psychological methods of child assessment, New York, 1983, Brunner/Mazel, Inc.

Hoehn-Saric E and others: Measurement of anxiety in children and adolescents using semistructured interviews, J Am Acad Child Psychiatry 26:541, 1987.

Kashani J and Orvaschel H: Anxiety disorders in mid-adolescence: a community sample, Am J Psychiatry 145:960, 1988.

Kashani J and others: Psychopathology in a community sample of children and adolescents: a developmental perspective, J Am Acad Child Adolesc Psychiatry 28:701, 1989.

Klein DF: Anxiety reconceptualized, Compr Psychiatry 21:411, 1980.

Kovacs M and others: Depressive disorders in childhood: II. a longitudinal study of risk for a subsequent major depression, Arch Gen Psychiatry 41:643, 1981.

Lamontagne LL, Mason KR, and Hepworth JT: Effects of relaxation on anxiety in children: implications for coping with stress, Nurs Res 34:289, 1985.

Lefkowitz M: Childhood depression: a reply to Costello, Psychol Bull 87:191, 1980.

Mash E and Terdal L: Behavioral assessment of childhood disorders, ed 2, New York, 1988, The Guilford Press.

Nelms B: Assessing childhood depression: do parents and children agree? Pediatr Nurs 12:23, 1986.

Noshpitz J, editor: Basic handbook of child psychiatry, vol 2, New York, 1979, Basic Books, Inc, Publishers.

Schwartz S and Johnson JH: Psychopathology of childhood, New York, 1985, Pergamon Press, Inc.

Spitz R and Wolf K: Anaclytic depression, Psychoanal Study Child 314:85, 1946.

Taylor E: Childhood hyperactivity, Br J Psychiatry 149:562, 1986.

US Department of Health and Human Services: Monthly vital statistics report, Washington, DC, 1983, US Government Printing Office.

Whitley G: Anxiety: defining the diagnosis, J Psychosoc Nurs 27:7, 1989.

Part IV

Psychotherapeutic Interventions

Chapter 15

Crisis Intervention: Children with AIDS

Donna C. Aguilera

The Chinese characters that represent the word *crisis* mean both danger and opportunity. Crisis may occur when people encounter a problem they cannot solve, causing a rise in inner tension, signs of anxiety and inability to function, and extended periods of emotional upset (Caplan, 1961). Crisis is a danger because it threatens to overwhelm individuals or families and may result in suicide or a psychotic break. It is also an opportunity because individuals are more receptive to therapeutic influence during times of crisis.

The usual coping mechanisms of people in crisis are ineffective, and they feel incapable of taking action on their own. Prompt and skillful intervention may not only prevent the development of a serious, long-term disability but also allow the emergence of coping patterns that facilitate functioning at a higher level of equilibrium. Crisis intervention is an inexpensive, short-term therapy that focuses on solving the immediate problem. Increasing awareness of sociocultural factors precipitating crisis situations has led to the rapid evolution of crisis intervention methodology.

Brief Psychotherapy

Brief psychotherapy as a treatment form developed because of the increased demand for mental health services and the lack of personnel trained to meet this need. Initially, it was largely conducted by psychiatric residents as part of their training, and psychiatric social workers and psychologists later became involved.

Brief psychotherapy is rooted in psychoanalytic theory but differs from psychoanalysis in terms of goals and other factors. It is limited to removing or alleviating specific symptoms. Intervention may lead to some reconstruction of personality, although this is not considered the primary goal. As in more traditional forms of psychotherapy, an orderly series of concepts directed toward beneficial change must guide therapy. The degree of abatement of the symptoms presented and the return to or maintenance of individuals' ability to function adequately are major goals, and people may choose to become involved in a longer form of therapy. Another goal is assistance in preventing the development of deeper neurotic or psychotic symptoms.

Modified methods of free association, interpretation, and the analysis of transference are used in brief psychotherapy. According to Bellak and Small (1965), free association is not a basic tool in short-term therapy but may arise in response to a stimulus from therapists. Interpretation is modified by the time limit and the immediacy of the problem. Although it may occur in brief psychotherapy, it is commonly used with medical or environmental intervention.

Researchers also believe that positive transference should be encouraged (Bellak and Small, 1965). Clients must view therapists as likeable, reliable, and understanding people who will help them. This type of relationship is necessary to accomplish treatment goals in a short time. Clinicians address negative transference feelings but do not analyze them in terms of defenses.

Therapists assume a more active role in brief psychotherapy than in the traditional methods. They avoid trends not directly related to the presenting problem and accentuate positive aspects. Clinicians confine difficulties by using clients' environmental positions to facilitate self-evaluation of situations and encourage productive behavior.

Diagnostic evaluation is extremely important in short-term therapy. Its aims are to understand symptoms and clients dynamically and to formulate hypotheses that can be validated by historical data. The result of the diagnosis enables therapists to select factors most susceptible to change and the appropriate method of intervention. The evaluation should address the degree of discrepancy or accord between clients' fantasies and reality and their ability to tolerate past and future frustrations. The adequacy of past and present relationships is also pertinent. Clinicians need to analyze clients' present situation and expectations and realize that meaningful emotional necessities motivate their request for help.

Once therapists choose an intervention, they carefully interpret behaviors and use direct confrontation sparingly. They strengthen clients' ego and increase self-esteem by promoting feelings of equality in the relationship and calling attention to the prevalence of problems in others. This technique not only relieves clients' anxiety but also facilitates communication, Therapists may also use catharsis, drive repression and restraint, reality testing, intellectualization, reassurance and support, counseling and guidance, and conjoint counseling (Bellak and Small, 1965). The general philosophic orientation necessary for therapists to be fully effective has been identified:

1. Clinicians must not view the therapy as a second-best approach but as the treatment of choice with persons in crisis.
2. An accurate assessment of the presenting problem and not a thorough diagnostic evaluation is essential to an effective intervention.
3. Both therapists and clients should be aware that treatment is time limited and should persistently direct their energies toward resolution of the presenting problem.
4. Clinicians should avoid dealing with material not directly related to the crisis.
5. Therapists must be willing to take an active and sometimes directive role in the intervention.

6. Maximum flexibility of approach is often appropriate.
7. Clinicians should direct all their energy toward returning clients their precrisis level of functioning.

The ending of treatment is an important phase in brief therapy. Clients must possess a positive transference and the feeling that they may return if necessary. Reinforcement of the skills learned in therapy by the clinician and demonstration of this reinforcement by clients will promote their self-esteem and ability to recognize possible future problems.

Drug therapy may be used as an adjunct in selected cases. Clinicians consider environmental manipulation when it is necessary to remove or modify an element causing disruption in the life pattern. It involves a close scrutiny of family and friends, job and job training, education, and plans for travel (Bellak and Small, 1965).

Brief psychotherapy is indicated in cases of acutely disruptive emotional pain or severely destructive circumstances and in situations endangering the life of a client or others. Life circumstances can also have an impact. If clients cannot participate in the long-term therapeutic situation, which suggests a stable residence and job, brief therapy is advocated to alleviate disruptive symptoms.

Clients must feel relief as quickly as possible, even during the first therapeutic session. The span of treatment usually involves more than 6 but less than 20 visits. Clients can attain treatment goals in this short time if they are seen quickly and intensively after requesting help. Therapists need to understand that the circumstances associated with disrupted functioning are more easily accessible if recent and that only active conflicts are amenable to therapeutic intervention. Similarly, therapy resolves disequilibriated states more easily before they have crystallized, acquired secondary gain features, or developed into highly maladaptive behavior patterns.

Crisis Intervention

The minimum therapeutic goal of crisis intervention is psychologic resolution of the immediate crisis and restoration of individuals' previous level of functioning. A maximum goal is improvement in functioning above the precrisis level.

Crisis is characteristically self-limiting and lasts from 4 to 6 weeks (Caplan, 1964). This transitional period both increases the danger of psychologic vulnerability and provides an opportunity for personality growth. Outcomes may largely depend on the ready availability of appropriate help during this time, with interventions lasting an average of 4 weeks (Jacobson, 1980).

Therefore, therapeutic climates mandate the concentrated attention of both therapists and clients, and the goal-oriented commitment develops in sharp contrast to the more modest pace of traditional treatment modes.

METHODOLOGY

Jacobson (1980) states that crisis intervention may be divided into two major categories, designated as *generic* and *individual*. Table 15-1 lists the major differences between the two approaches.

Table 15-1   Differences between Brief Psychotherapy and Crisis Intervention

	Brief psychotherapy	Crisis intervention
Goals of therapy	Removal of specific symptoms	Resolution of immediate crisis
Focus of treatment	Genetic past as it relates to present situation; repression of unconscious; restrainment of drives	Genetic present only; restoration to precrisis level of functioning
Usual activity of therapists	Suppressive techniques; participant observer; indirect manner	Suppressive techniques; active participant; direct manner
Indications	Acutely disruptive emotional pain and severely disruptive circumstances	Sudden loss of ability to cope with life situation
Average length of treatment	1-20 sessions	1-6 sessions

Generic Approach

A leading proposition of the generic approach is that certain recognized patterns of behavior occur in most crises. For example, studies of bereavement identified necessary grief work after the death of a relative (Lindemann, 1944). Researchers studying the effect on the mother of the birth of a premature baby designated four phases or tasks that she must work through to ensure healthy adaptation to the experience (Caplan, 1964; Kaplan and Mason, 1960). Janis (1958) suggested several hypotheses concerning the psychologic stress of impending surgery and the patterns of emotional response that follow a diagnosis of chronic illness, and Rapoport (1963) defined three subphases of marriage, during which unusual stress could precipitate crises.

The generic approach focuses on the characteristic course of a particular kind of crisis rather than on the psychodynamics of each individual in crisis. The goal of treatment plans and specific intervention measures is to resolve the crisis, and both are designed to be effective for all people affected by the type of crisis.

Tyhurst (1957) suggested that knowledge of patterned behaviors in transitional states occurring during intense or sudden changes in life situations may provide an empirical basis for the management of these states and the prevention of subsequent mental illness. He cites as examples the studies of individual responses to community disaster, migration, and retirement of pensioners.

Generic approaches include encouragement of adaptive behavior, general support, environmental manipulation, and anticipatory guidance (Jacobson, Strickler, and Morley, 1968). They emphasize (1) specific situational and maturational events occurring to significant population groups, (2) crisis-oriented intervention related to these specific events, and (3) intervention conducted by nonmental health professionals. This approach can be learned and implemented by nonpsychiatric physicians, nurses, and social workers because it does not require complete knowledge of the intrapsychic and interpersonal processes of individuals in crisis.

Individual Approach

The individual approach differs from the generic in its emphasis on assessment of the interpersonal and intrapsychic processes of persons in crisis by professionals. It is used in selected cases, usually for those not responding to the generic approach. Clinicians plan interventions to meet the unique needs of an individual in crisis and to resolve the particular situation and circumstances that precipitated the crisis.

Unlike extended psychotherapy, the individual approach rarely addresses clients' developmental past. Information from this source is only relevant when it results in a better understanding of a present crisis situation. Assessment emphasizes the immediate causes for disturbed equilibrium and the processes necessary for regaining a precrisis or higher level of functioning. The approach's inclusion of family members or other important persons in the process differs from most individual psychotherapy techniques (Jacobson, Strickler, and Morley, 1968).

STEPS IN CRISIS INTERVENTION

There are certain specific steps involved in the technique of crisis intervention (Morley, Messick, and Aguilera, 1967). Although the phases cannot be categorized, typical interventions frequently follow a defined sequence:

1. Assessment: Therapists use active focusing techniques to obtain an accurate assessment of the precipitating event and the resulting crisis that led to the seeking of professional help. They may have to judge the risk of suicidal of homicidal behaviors occurring. If clinicians identify a high risk, they refer the client to a psychiatrist for consideration of hospitalization. The initial hour of assessment may focus solely on the circumstances of the immediate crisis situation.
2. Planning of therapeutic intervention: After completing an accurate assessment, clinicians plan the intervention and determine the length of time since the onset of the crisis which is usually 1 to 2 weeks. Therapists identify ways in which the crisis has disrupted clients' life and the effects of this disruption on others. They also evaluate clients' strengths, coping skills that have been used successfully in the past but are not being employed presently, and sources of supports.
3. Intervention: Techniques for intervention depend on the preexisting skills, creativity, and flexibility of therapists and include the following (Morley, Messick, and Aguilera, 1967):
   a. Clinicians help clients to gain an intellectual understanding of their crisis by using a direct approach that describes the relationship between a crisis and the life event.
   b. Therapists assist clients in revealing present inaccessible feelings to reduce tension by providing the means for self-recognition or promoting an emotional catharsis.
   c. Clinicians explore alternative coping mechanisms.

   d. Therapists attempt to reopen clients' social world by introducing new people to replace the loss and supporting role of a significant person.

 4. Resolution of the crisis and anticipatory planning: Therapists reinforce and summarize adaptive coping mechanisms, assist in the formulation of realistic plans for the future, and discuss the ways in which the therapeutic experience can help in future crises.

Paradigm of Intervention

According to Caplan (1964), a crisis has four developmental phases:

 1. Clients demonstrate an initial rise in tension as they attempt habitual problem-solving techniques.

 2. Clients' coping is unsuccessful as the stimulus continues and they experience more discomfort.

 3. A further increase in tension acts as a powerful internal stimulus and mobilizes internal and external resources, resulting in the clients' use of emergency problem solving. They may redefine the problem or classify certain aspects of their goal as unattainable.

 4. If the problem continues and clients can neither solve nor avoid it, their tension increases and they experience a major disorganization.

Whenever a stressful event occurs, certain recognized balancing factors can cause a return to equilibrium; these are perception of the event, available situational supports, and coping mechanisms (Figure 15-1). A stressful event is seldom defined so clearly that its source can be determined immediately. Internalized changes occur concurrently with externally provoked stress, and some events may therefore cause a strong emotional response in one person and not affect another.

Acquired Immune Deficiency Syndrome

No infectious condition of recent times has had the psychosocial impact of human immunodeficiency virus (HIV) disease. A near AIDS hysteria has developed throughout the country as the informative as well as the sensational media have bombarded the public with reports about AIDS. AIDS clients must cope not only with their own adjustment to a terminal diagnosis but also to discrimination caused by society's fear (Johnson, 1988).

AIDS IN CHILDREN

Social, Psychologic, and Ethical Aspects

The AIDS virus has affected the child and adolescent population, although in relatively low numbers to date. Infection for children and teenagers occurs from maternal transmission in utero or in the perinatal period, blood transfusions and use of blood products, sexual activity, and shared needles during IV-drug use.

 The increasing incidence of AIDS, ARC, and the AIDS antibody in children evokes difficult ethical issues. Conflicting concerns include the need for research to provide an adequate treatment and cure, the provision of humane and sensitive

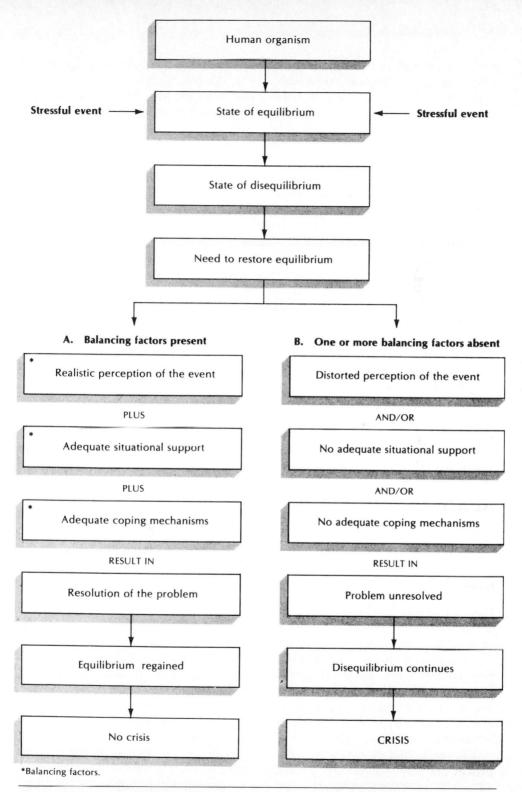

*Balancing factors.

Figure 15-1   Paradigm: The effect of balancing factors in a stressful event. (From Aguilera D: Crisis intervention: theory and methodology, ed 6, St Louis, 1990, The CV Mosby Co.)

treatment as well as protection for the individual child, and the need to protect other people and prevent the spread of the disease.

Adults' emotional reactions to AIDS result from the association of the disease with sexuality, homosexuality, illicit drug use, promiscuity, and prostitution, eliciting strong societal condemnation, prejudice, and discrimination. These feelings can affect not only the general public but also caregivers, service providers, public officials, and scientists. *AIDS hysteria* results from adults' fear of the unknown and the actual consequences of AIDS, which can activate their psychologic need to segregate the sources of contamination.

The emotional reactions of adults are important for several reasons: (1) The social and psychologic implications for children who have AIDS or ARC, or are seropositive will largely depend on the reactions and responses of the adults in their life; (2) policies, regulations, and procedures that profoundly affect the lives of children are promulgated by adults subject to these psychologic influences; and (3) fear and prejudice are difficult to counter with reason (AIDS Project Los Angeles, 1990). When children develop AIDS, parents and especially mothers may be overwhelmed by a sense of guilt for having been the source of infection. For school-aged children the inability to attend school, participate in activities with other children, and be accepted and included in a group may lead to serious psychologic and social adjustment difficulties.

Medical experts generally recommend that children with AIDS attend school. Although classmates aware of their condition may tease and discriminate against them, children excluded from school or other activities may be encouraged to keep the reason for their isolation secret. This action can have detrimental results in developing a positive sense of self and being accepted and integrated. Health professionals need to counsel parents on ways to discuss AIDS and its effects with their child.

Many issues that apply to school-aged children also affect teenagers, such as the problem of being excluded, handicapped, and socially isolated. They are becoming more aware of and frightened by AIDS. In addition, many of the social and psychologic factors that affect adults also influence teenagers. If teenagers are seropositive and their family is informed, educated guesses about their sexual life or drug use may result in additional psychologic trauma for teens and families. They may experience painful discrimination from peers because teenagers frequently struggle with their sexual identity and prejudice against homosexuality can be profound in this age group. If they have AIDS or ARC or are seropositive, they may be seen as tainted or associated with homosexuality by others.

Homeless and runaway youth are especially vulnerable to exposure to AIDS and need education and supportive counseling regarding sexual practices and drug use. However they may be extremely difficult to reach because of their lifestyle. Explaining the meaning of a positive AIDS antibody test to teenagers is a complicated undertaking and may be more than they can tolerate. The possibility of behavior disturbances, flight into promiscuity, and suicidal activity is great.

Efforts to educate the public are critically important because of the complex psychologic and social effects. The implications of AIDS may differ among children with AIDS, children with ARC, and those who are seropositive, but the major concerns are similar for each group. The case example illustrates a family's and child's reaction to the disease.

Case Example

Melie, a 9-year-old girl, and her parents were referred to the crisis center by Melie's pediatrician. Melie had been repeatedly sexually molested and had contracted AIDS. The pediatrician had contacted the Child Protection Agency.

The therapist initially spoke with the parents and discovered that Melie had been sexually molested by her uncle, who had lived with the family for a year. The parents were unaware of the abuse until Melie's pediatrician informed them that Melie had chlamydia and was HIV positive. The parents then spoke with Melie and learned of the abuse. The father blamed himself for her disease because the molestor was his brother.

The therapist then met with Melie alone and briefly explained the pediatrician's findings. The therapist reassured her that her parents did not blame her for the abuse and told her she would receive medications. Because both parents admitted that they knew little about AIDS, the therapist gave them brochures with information and contacted a family support group through an AIDS intervention center. A summation of the paradigm of this case is shown in Figure 15-2.

Modified from Aquilera D: Crisis intervention: theory and methodology, ed 6, St Louis, 1990, The CV Mosby Co.

Confidentiality

An important issue for children with AIDS, ARC, or confirmed exposure is the question of confidentiality. Different jurisdictions are enacting regulations for reporting results, dissemination of information, and quarantine options. A public opinion poll conducted by the *Los Angeles Times* found that 48% of the participants favored mandatory identification cards for adults with positive results to the AIDS antibody test, 51% supported quarantine, and 15% endorsed tattooing people with AIDS. Interestingly, 55% stated that they would send their child to a classroom even if a classmate had AIDS (AIDS Project Los Angeles, 1990).

Vaccines and Foster Homes

Infected infants and young children with a compromised immune system should probably not be immunized with the live virus used in mumps, measles, and some polio immunizations but need to be protected from exposure to infection. Therefore, primary caretakers, physicians caring for them, and foster parents should be aware of test results.

An additional concern is the possible reticence of foster parents to care for these children and the effect on the foster-care system, which is presently significantly lacking in adequate foster homes. If children develop AIDS while in foster care, the likelihood of them being returned to the system is great, creating another trauma for childhood victims.

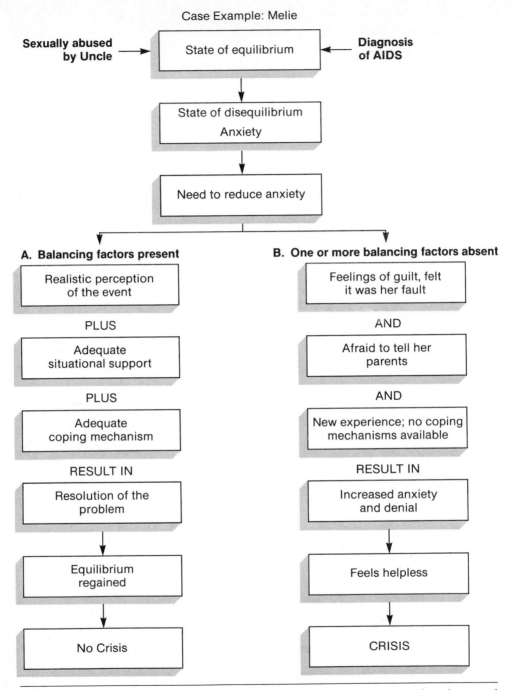

Figure 15-2   Summation of the paradigm.(From Aquilera D: Crisis intervention: theory and methodology, ed 6, St Louis, 1990, The CV Mosby Co.)

Recommendations

Legislators need to be aware of the social and psychologic implications of AIDS when developing public policies, and discussions of school adminissions must consider possible psychologic effects on children. Health professionals should test infants of mothers at risk for AIDS to prevent dangerous immunizations, and society must provide skilled and trained counselors to help both children and families to understand and adjust. Caregivers, parents, and children need education and support to lessen the psychologic and social effects of AIDS.

REFERENCES

Aquilera D: Crisis intervention: theory and methodology, ed 6, St Louis, 1990, The CV Mosby Co.

AIDS Project Los Angeles: Personal communication, Jan 1990.

Bellak L and Small L: Emergency psychotherapy and brief psychotherapy. New York, 1965, Grune & Stratton, Inc.

Caplan G: An approach to community mental health, New York, 1961, Grune & Stratton, Inc.

Caplan G: Principles of preventive psychiatry, New York, 1964, Basic Books, Inc, Publishers.

Jacobson G: Crisis theory, New Dir Ment Health Serv 6:1, 1980.

Jacobson G, Strickler M, and Morley WE: Generic and individual approaches to crisis intervention, Am J Public Health 58:339, 1968.

Janis L: Psychological stress, New York, 1958, John Wiley & Sons, Inc.

Johnson J: AIDS-related psychosocial issues for the patient and physician, JAOA, 88:23, 1988.

Kaplan DM and Mason EA: Maternal reactions to premature birth viewed as an acute emotional disorder, Am J Orthopsychiatry 30:539, 1960.

Lindemann E: Symptomatology and management of acute grief, Am J Psychiatry 101:101, 1944.

Morley WE, Messick JM, and Aguilera DC: Crisis: paradigms of intervention, J Psychiatr Nurs 5:537, 1967.

Rapoport R: Normal crises, family structure, and mental health, Fam Process 2:68, 1963.

Tyhurst JA: Role of transition states — including disasters — in mental illness, Washington, DC, 1957, US Government Printing Office.

Chapter 16

Psychopharmacology

Norman Keltner

By definition, psychotropic drugs act on the central nervous system and pass the blood-brain barrier to affect the brain. When individuals have distressful thoughts, feelings, and behaviors, psychotropic drugs are often prescribed. Some concerns about prescribing and administering psychotropic drugs to children include the potential for altered pharmacokinetics (absorption, distribution, metabolism, and excretion) and the potential for developmental risk. As a result, weight-based extrapolations of child dosages from adult dosages are potentially dangerous. As children grow, their reactions and responses to drugs begin to approximate those of adults.

The first specific drug used for a childhood psychopathologic disorder was reported by Bradley in 1937, who found that amphetamine benefited behavior-disordered children. In the following years a series of pharmacologic approaches to childhood disturbances evolved (Wiener and Jaffe, 1985). In the 1950s methylphenidate (Ritalin) was found effective in the treatment of hyperkinesia, which is now referred to as ADHD.

In 1952, Delay and Deniker reported that the aliphatic phenothiazine chlorpromazine (thorazine) was first used in public mental hospitals (Weiner and Jaffe, 1985). It quickly found advocates among people who were caring for disordered children. By 1953 Heuyer and others described the value of chlorpromazine in treating psychomotor excitement (Weiner and Jaffe, 1985). During the 1960s, many new drugs were introduced for pediatric psychopharmacologic use. These new drugs included two more subclasses of phenothiazines—the piperidines (for example, thioridazine [Mellaril]) and the piperazines (for example, triofluperazine [Stelazine]); two nonphenothiazine antipsychotics—the thioxanthenes (such as thiothixene [Navanel]) and a butyrophenone (haloperidol [Haldol]); and antidepressants. In the 1970s antidepressants were used to treat separation anxiety (school phobia), enuresis, and attention deficit disorders. With FDA approval in the late 1960s, lithium gained acceptance as a therapeutic agent for children. In the 1970s it was used to treat bipolar affective disorder (not recommended for children under 12), autism, aggression, and undersocialized conduct disorders (Campbell and Pali, 1985). The 1980s, however, have assessed the ethical issues that relate to childhood psychopharmacology, and in the 1990s effects and effectiveness of these drugs continues to be a priority in pediatric psychopharmacologic research.

In 1986, Gadow reported that 15% to 30% of all emotionally disturbed school children received psychotropic drugs, that 1% to 2% of all elementary school children received psychotropic drugs for attention deficit disorder, and that 5% of moderately, and 13% of mildly mentally retarded children received these drugs.

This chapter provides a useful guide for nurses in pediatric psychopharmacology. The material is organized by disorders, not by chemical agent.

ADHD

ADHD is the most common of all pediatric behavioral disorders. The drugs most commonly used for treatment are central nervous system (CNS) stimulants. ADHD is characterized by deficiencies in social behavior, cognition, and attention. Specific problems include abnormal motor movements, restlessness, emotional problems, social skills deficits, impulsiveness, and learning disability. These deficits cause problems for the child in school, and they may afflict 20% of all school-aged children (LaGreca and Quay, 1984).

ADHD, in contrast to most childhood behavior disorders, has been well studied. For 10 to 20 years clinicians have debated the use of stimulants in children. Currently, CNS stimulants are important tools in the treatment of ADHD.

CNS STIMULANTS

The most commonly used drugs in the treatment of ADHD are the amphetamines (usually dextroamphetamine [Dexedrine]) and methylphenidate (Ritalin). Methylphenidate is used more often. When used in conjunction with counseling, cerebral stimulants improve approximately 70% to 80% of ADHD patients. Improvement means the ability to control behavior, to pay attention, and to learn.

In normal adults these drugs cause stimulation and euphoria. Hyperactive children, however, paradoxically become less hyperactive. Some attribute the effect of amphetamines on hyperactivity to low drug levels' preferential stimulation of inhibitory efferent neurons in the cerebral cortex, (logically causing a decrease in motor activity). Others believe that low levels stimulate the afferent neurons of the reticular activating system. Because of increased input *constancy,* the brain is enabled to concentrate longer on a particular task, and is not as easily distracted by other stimuli. CNS stimulants work by increasing the synaptic levels of dopamine, norepinephrine, and serotonin; the adrenergic component, especially norepinephrine, probably has the greatest effect. Many drugs used in the treatment of childhood behavior disorders simply make children more manageable; CNS stimulants directly affect the problem behavior.

Dextroamphetamine and methylphenidate are well absorbed from the GI tract and distributed throughout the body. They begin to have an effect within an hour or less. Dextroamphetamine is excreted unchanged in the urine, and methylphenidate is completely metabolized in the liver.

Side effects include nervousness, tachycardia, insomnia, anorexia, stomachache, symptoms of depression (sadness, crying), weight loss, and temporary growth retardation (height and weight). Insomnia and anorexia are best handled by timing the dosage. For example, anorexia is minimized by giving the drug with meals, and insomnia by giving it at least 6 hours before bedtime. Methylphenidate has less sympathomimetic effect than amphetamines. Despite concerns about their dangers, these drugs are among the safest psychotropics in use.

A number of significant drug interactions occur with stimulants. By acidifying the urine with ascorbic acid or fruit juices, amphetamine's excretion will be enhanced. On the other hand, sodium bicarbonate, which alkalinizes the urine, will promote reabsorption, and amphetamine action will be prolonged due to decreased elimination. Children taking amphetamines (but not methylphenidate) should not be given agents that alkalinize the urine, such as sodium bicarbonate, or other adsorbed over-the-counter products for upset stomach. This would prolong the elimination, and thus intensify the effect of amphetamine. CNS stimulants increase the serum levels of antidepressants interfere with the effects of antihypertensives, increasing blood pressure. When they are given with antipsychotic drugs or CNS depressants, the effects of the CNS stimulants are reduced. In fact, antipsychotic drugs can be used to treat CNS stimulant overdoses. MAO inhibitors and sympatho-mimetics (including OTC preparations) cause hypertension when given with CNS stimulants.

Dextroamphetamine (Dexedrine). Dextroamphetamine is not recommended for children under 3 years of age. The dosage for children from 3 to 5 years old is 2.5 mg daily as a tablet or elixir taken with, or immediately after, meals. The dosage may be raised in 2.5 mg/day increments at weekly intervals as needed. Children who are 6 years old and older may be given 5 mg once or twice a day, with an increase of 5 mg/day at weekly intervals as needed. Spansules (a slow-releasing preparation) may be given once daily in the morning to prevent insomnia. Children should not be given a supply of more than 40 mg of dextroamphetamine daily, because of its potential for abuse, especially by those who have access to the child's supply. Amphetamines are Schedule II drug.

Methylphenidate (Ritalin). Methylphenidate is not recommended for children under the age of 6. In children over 6 years of age, 5 mg before breakfast and lunch is recommended. If necessary, the daily dose may be increased by 5 to 10 mg increments at weekly intervals. The optimal daily dose is 0.3 mg/kg. This may not correct all behavioral problems, but it will increase learning ability. Children should not receive more than 1 mg/kg/day or a total of more than 60 mg/day regardless of weight. A single daily dose of the sustained-release form (Ritalin-SR) can be used instead of divided doses of the regular product. Abuse potential exists with methylphenidate. It is a Schedule II drug.

Pemoline (Cylert). Pemoline differs chemically from the amphetamines and methylphenidate. It is used exclusively for ADHD. It is well absorbed, has a 12-hour duration of action, and is excreted 50% unchanged in the urine.

Pemoline also causes less cerebral stimulation than the other two CNS stimulants. Its side effects are similar to those of the amphetamines and methylphenidate. The dosage for children over 6 years of age is 37.5 mg daily in the morning. Pemoline has a long half-life and can be given once per day. The daily dose may be increased by 18.75 mg at weekly intervals up to a maximum of 112.5 mg/day. The usual maintenance dose is 56.25 to 75 mg/day. Pemoline has low abuse potential and is a Schedule IV drug.

Other drugs used in the treatment of ADHD. Tricyclic antidepressants (TCAs) have been used for ADHD but have more side effects and shorter-lived results than the CNS stimulants. The phenothiazine tranquilizers and haloperidol have been tried but are less effective than the stimulants. Lithium, diphendydramine (Benadryl), phenobarbital, and the benzodiazepines have been used with less than satisfactory results. CNS stimulants remain the drugs of choice for ADHD. However, for ADHD sufferers who do not respond to stimulants, these drugs are alternatives.

NURSING IMPLICATIONS

Interactions. The nurse must take a thorough history to be aware of other drugs being taken by the client. A history reduces the possibility of drug interactions. For example, since stomachache is a side effect of amphetamines, a parent might unwittingly give a child sodium bicarbonate alkalinizing the urine and intensifying the effect of amphetamine. OTC drugs for colds and hay fever also contain sympatho-mimetic agents and should be avoided.

Toxic effects. Amphetamine overdose can be fatal. The typical overdose picture is a hyperalert, talkative child that may have tremors, exaggerated startle reflex, paranoia, hallucinations, confusion, and tachyarrhythmias. If a child on amphet-amines presents with some of these symptoms, clinicians should notify the physician and arrange for hospitalization. Urinary acidification speeds up elimination, activated charcoal slows absorption, and gastric lavage can rid the body of un-absorbed drug. The nurse should monitor vital signs and reduce environmental stimuli.

Side effects. Anorexia can be reduced by giving these drugs immediately after meals. Insomnia is reduced by giving the last dose at least 6 hours before bedtime. Nurses should assess the child for side effects. Sometimes ADHD can worsen paradoxically with methylphenidate. If this occurs, the drug should be withheld.

Parent teaching. Parents are ultimately responsible for compliance to dosage schedules. They play an important role in psychopharmacology and need to know general information about their child's medication, their side effects, and their abuse potential.

Parents may have to tolerate some hyperactivity in their child and should not increase dosages on their own to further reduce unwanted behavior. Even optimal dosages of these stimulants will not always induce immediate acceptable social behavior. Pemoline's therapeutic effect is not evident for 3 to 4 weeks, and parents should be informed of this to prevent their assuming that lack of immediate improve-ment means treatment has failed. Parents should weigh the child weekly because of the potential for appetite suppression and temporary growth retardation. Long-term growth problems apparently do not occur. As with all psychotropics, an occasional drug-free holiday will help determine if drug administration should be continued.

Psychotic Disorders

Schizophrenia can occur in 5- to 8-year-old children. Symptoms may include hallucinations, delusions, thought disorder, anxiety, and inappropriate affect. Speech idiosyncracies such as mutism, echolalia, and an inability to understand the spoken word may also be present, along with morbid thoughts and a lack of friends and concrete thinking. It is a rare disorder, more common in boys. There are obvious developmental delays. Some people believe that a highly functioning mind is present; however, evidence seems to indicate the opposite.

Autism is a pervasive developmental disorder, diagnostically differentiated from schizophrenia by its earlier onset (possibly birth) and lack of hallucinations, delusions, and schizophrenic thought processes. By comparison, the schizophrenic child has experienced a normal life, while the autistic child has not. The autistic child is unemotional, anxious, and unresponsive to normal speech. The autistic child has a number of disturbing stereotypic behaviors, such as rocking, biting, hand flicking, and head banging. Both diagnostic groups of children exhibit very little spontaneous behavior and are social isolates.

ANTIPSYCHOTIC DRUGS

The goals of psychotropic intervention are primitive when compared to the goals of drug intervention in ADHD. The goal for the schizophrenic child is to decrease thought disorganization to restore a normal level of functioning. The goal for the autistic child is to decrease anxiety or stereotyped behaviors. These drugs are used in both groups of clients to manage aggressive, assaultive, or self-destructive behavior. However, psychotropic drugs are never used as the sole treatment measure. Drugs are merely one aspect of a treatment plan that includes therapeutic communication, milieu management, parental involvement, and education.

Phenothiazines are often the first drugs used to treat childhood psychoses (Weiner, 1977). The aliphatic chlorpromazine (Thorazine), is the prototype antipsychotic, although little evidence exists that one antipsychotic is more effective than another.

The phenothiazines are usually taken orally and are absorbed rapidly in the GI tract. A tranquilizing effect occurs in about an hour. Chlorpromazine accumulates in fatty tissues and is slowly released. It is 95% to 98% protein bound and is extensively metabolized in the liver. Its renal excretion is negligible: only 1% is excreted unchanged.

Two effects account for the beneficial results of antipsychotic therapy—a *neuroleptic* effect and an *antipsychotic* effect. The neuroleptic effect is characterized by sedation, emotional quieting, and psychomotor slowing. The antipsychotic effect is characterized by normalization of thought, mood, and behavior. The neuroleptic effect may be more significant for the autistic child, and the antipsychotic effect for the schizophrenic child. Their effectiveness is probably linked to their ability to block dopamine receptors. Excessive levels of the neurotransmitter dopamine could be related to schizophrenia. As dopamine is blocked by phenothiazines, schizophrenic symptoms are reduced. The well-known antiemetic properties of the phenothiazines are related to this antidopaminergic effect.

Two categories of peripheral autonomic side effects are related to these drugs: *anticholinergic* side effects and *antiadrenergic* side effects. These drugs also produce central side effects in the extrapyramidal system (EPS), which are essentially *antidopaminergic* side effects. Low potency antipsychotic drugs, such as Thorazine and Mellaril, tend to produce more autonomic side effects. High potency drugs, such as Haldol and Prolixin, tend to produce more central side effects or extrapyramidal symptoms (EPS).

Anticholinergic side effects include dry mouth, blurred vision, tachycardia (usually reflexive), constipation, and urinary hesitancy. Antiadrenergic side effects include hypotension, reflex tachycardia, and cardiac stimulation.

EPS side effects include problems such as rigidity; tremors; bradykinesia; akathisia, a subjective imperative to movement; and dystonias, a rigidity of muscles controlling posture or gait. The occurrence of oculogyric crisis is a particularly frightening dystonic reaction. This is the result of neck and eye muscle spasm in which clients are frozen in position, eyes straight up and rolled back and neck tensed. This is not only terrifying to the clients, it is a medical emergency; due to the position and rigidity of the neck, obstruction of the airway is a nursing concern.

EPSs are caused by the imbalance of the acetycholine/dopamine ratio by the dopamine-blocking effects of antipsychotic drugs. A balance of the two neurotransmitters is necessary for muscle tone. Another EPS, dyskinesia, is an incomplete muscle action. Dyskinesias are a major concern in children. Facial muscles become motionless and the eyes stare ahead without blinking or emotion. Although children are clear-headed, they appear dazed. Although rare in children and usually seen in long-term antipsychotic treatment, tardive dyskinesia is a serious uncoordinated rhythmic movement of the mouth and face that disappears during sleep. Tardive dyskinesia is usually permanent. Although other EPSs mentioned are caused by disruptions in the aceytylcholine/dopamine balance, dyskinesias seem to be caused by a drug-induced sensitivity to dopamine, which is irreversible in many people. Since dyskinesias are caused by a sensitivity to dopamine, it not unusual for them to be hidden while the client is on antipsychotics, only to emerge once the drug is withdrawn. Some researchers have concluded that these withdrawal emergent symptoms appear to be tardive dyskinesia but are actually reversible (Engelhardt and Polizos, 1978).

Neuroleptic malignant syndrome (NMS) is a relatively new but serious adverse effect of antipsychotic drugs (Keltner and McIntyre, 1985). Its incidence in children is not yet clear. NMS is characterized by severe muscle rigidity and high fever. If a child receives antipsychotic drugs and has either of these symptoms, the drug should be held and the physician notified.

Finally, sedation and weight gain are side effects of many antipsychotic drugs. Sedation is caused by the drugs' ability to depress the CNS. Unfortunately, drowsiness can interfere with other important therapies.

Drug interactions of these antipsychotics are numerous. Alcohol and other CNS depressants increase sedation and CNS depression. Amphetamines tend to decrease antipsychotic effects. Anticholinergic drugs, including many OTC varieties, increase the risk of anticholinergic side effects. If antipsychotics are given with lithium, a decrease in antipsychotic serum levels occur, the antiemetic effect can mask nausea and vomiting (early signs of lithium toxicity), and there is a possible neurotoxic reaction. When combined with benztropine (Cogentin) (an anticholinergic drug used to treat and prevent EPS), an increase in anticholinergic side effects and a decrease in antipsychotic effect have been reported.

Phenothiazines. There are three subclasses of phenothiazines: the aliphatics, the piperidines, and the piperazines. Chlorpromazine (Thorazine), an aliphatic phenothiazine, is not recommended for children under 6 months of age. If a child is agitated, overexcited, or overactive, an aliphatic may be preferable because they are more sedating than other antipsychotics. Chlorpromazine is usually prescribed at 0.25 mg/lb every 6 to 8 hours and is gradually increased to an oral dose of 50 to 100 mg a day for severely ill and hospitalized children. Rectal suppositories are also available. For acutely disturbed children who require immediate treatment, an IM dose of 0.25 mg/lb every 6 to 8 hours is appropriate. A 2- to 5-year-old child should not receive more than 40 mg per day, and a 5- to 12 year-old child should not receive more than 75 mg per day.

Thioridazine (Mellaril), a piperidine phenothiazine, is used by many clinicians. It is not recommended for children under 2 years of age. The dosage for treating psychosis in 2- to 12-year-old children is 0.5 to 3.0 mg/kg/day. This usually translates into 10 mg BID or TID for mild symptoms and 25 mg BID or TID for severe symptoms. No child should receive more than 3 mg/kg per day.

Trifluoperazine (Stelazine), a piperazine phenothiazine, is not recommended for children under 6 years of age. In 6- to 12-year-old children who are hospitalized or closely supervised, clinicians should start therapy with 1 mg once or twice per day and increase it slowly until the symptoms are resolved or until side effects occur. For rapid control of symptoms, 1 mg (0.5 ml) IM once or twice a day can be given. Dosage should not exceed 15 mg per day.

Some drugs are used in childhood psychiatric disorders that are not approved for pediatric use in the *Physician's Desk Reference* (PDR) (PDR, 1990). Use of these drugs (fluphenazine, thiothixene, molindone, and loxapine) should be done with care and parental approval. A signed informed consent form is advised.

Fluphenazine (Prolixin), a commonly used piperazine in adults, is not recommended for children under 12 years old. Nonetheless, clinicians, prescribe the drug and find it effective for children over 6 years of age. Werry (1978) recommends a starting dose of 0.025 to 0.05 mg/kg up to 0.3 mg/kg per day (3 to 6 mg/day). Joshi, Capozzoli, and Coyle (1988) found low maintenance dosages of 0.04 mg/kg per day to effect significant results.

Thioxanthenes. The two thioxanthenes are structually related to phenothiazines and are generally less sedating and cause fewer EPS. Thiothixene (Navane) is used more often in adults and is not recommended for use in children under 12 years of age. Werry (1978) recommends an average dose of 0.15 to 0.3 mg/kg per day. Chlorprothixene (Taractan) is not recommended for children under 6 years of age. For children 6 to 12 years old, 10 to 25 mg TID or QID is recommended.

Butyrophenones. Haloperidol (Haldol), a high potency antipsychotic, is structurally unrelated to the phenothiazines. It can be given to children between the ages of 3 and 12 years (weight 15 to 40 kg). Its antipsychotic use in children causes a significant amount of EPS when compared with chlorpromazine. However, it is the least sedating antipsychotic. A dose of 0.05 to 0.15 mg/kg per day is recommended for children. Joshi, Capozzoli, and Coyle (1988) found that low maintenance doses of neuroleptics have a significant effect. They recommend 0.04 mg/kg/day. Doses typically should not exceed 6 mg per day.

Other antipsychotic drugs. The dihydroindolone, molindone (Moban), is not recommended for children under 12 years of age, the dibenzoxapine, loxapine (Loxitane), is not recommended for use in children under 16 years of age, and the diphenylbutylpiperidines, pimozide (Orap), is not recommended for children under 12 years of age and is used primarily for the treatment of tics.

NURSING IMPLICATIONS

Nurses need to understand the variation in the bioavailability of antipsychotic drugs. Another brand should not be used if clients' supply is depleted because the new brand's bioavailability may be different. For example, it may not dissolve or be absorbed at the same rate, which can result in high or low serum levels. Compliance is a problem with adult clients and is a potential problem with children. It is important for clients to swallow the medication. If noncompliance is suspected, a liquid form may be advisable. IM injections should be given *deep* IM because of their potential irritation. Nurses should always aspirate to avoid IV administration, and contact dermatitis is not uncommon.

Side effects. EPS should be reported to the physician for possible prescription of antiparkinson-anticholinergic drugs such as benztropine (Cogentin) or trihexyphenidyl (Artane). The anticholinergic drugs are effective for most EPSs but are not effective for tardive dyskinesia. The abnormal involuntary movement scale (AIMS) is an easily used tool for assessment.

Sedation, weight gain, and autonomic side effects can be treated with dose modification. Sedation is prominent in psychotic children and, although welcomed at times in the hyperactive child, interferes with other psychotherapeutic interventions. A shift to a less sedating drug such as trifluoperazine (Stelazine) might be required. In children, the autonomic side effects are not as prominent as they are in adults (Campbell, 1985). Drowsiness and weight gain are more common. Dose modification and the consequent side effect reduction must be weighed against an increase in disturbed behavior.

Generally anticholinergic side effects and antiadrenergic side effects can be resolved by dose modification. Antidopaminergic side effects can be resolved both by dose modification and by antiparkinson-anticholinergic drugs.

Interactions. Children taking antipsychotic drugs should not be given other medications containing alcohol, including OTC sleeping aids and cough syrups. Clinicians should assess for drowsiness if such preparations are taken. Nurses should also guard against ingestion of OTC anticholinergics such as cold or hay fever medications and assess for blurred vision and constipation if necessary. Because anticholinergic drugs prescribed to reduce EPS can potentiate anticholinergic side effects and mask the development of tardive dyskinesia, they must assess for increased anticholinergic effects. Nurses should question any order combining antipsychotic drugs and lithium.

Toxicity. Deaths solely from antipsychotic drug overdose have been rarely reported in any age group. Overdose usually results in CNS depression, hypotension, and EPS. Treatment is symptomatic and supportive. Gastric lavage may help rid the body of unabsorbed drug. Vomiting is not induced because of the potential for dystonias of the head and neck, which may compromise the ability to vomit and cause aspiration. Antiparkinson-anticholinergic drugs may be given to treat EPS.

Parent teaching. When children are living at home, parents must be committed to compliance to the drug regimen. Psychotropic drugs are only part of a comprehensive treatment program. Parents must also be given a realistic understanding of the drug's expected and side effects to recognize when they should contact the physician. Parents should be taught to assess for muscle rigidity, inability to remain still, vague subjective complaints such as a need to move, and any abnormal involuntary movements. Parents should also be taught to monitor bowel and bladder function and to encourage appropriate fluid intake.

Parents must clear OTC medications with physicians or nurses. Nurses should ensure that parents know antipsychotic drugs are not addicting. Antipsychotic drugs should not be used for nonapproved indications, the lowest effective dose for maintenance therapy should be employed because of the relationship between dose and EPS, and children should be placed on physician approved drug-free holidays occasionally (Keltner, 1989a).

Depression and Mania

Until 10 years ago, many clinicians debated whether depression actually occurred in children. Rutter and others (1976) carefully studied the 10- to 11-year-old children on the Isle of Wight (a total of 2199 children) and found only 3 that could be described as depressed. Today there is consensus that childhood depression is a mental health problem. However, much less is known about the clinical picture of childhood depression than the features of adult depression. Childhood depression can be dichotomized into primary and secondary depression. *Primary* or *endogenous* depression is defined as a mood disorder in which depression is the presenting problem, and the cause cannot be traced to external events. *Secondary* or *reactive* depression is a reaction to a real life event, situation, or illness and can evolve into a primary depression (Weiner, 1977). The reaction often takes the form of grief or *anhedonia,* the inability to experience joy, which is a major symptom of the depressed child. Even when surrounded by a series of unpleasant and depressing events, most children will display happiness at times.

The existence of mania in children is not as easy to recognize, and its incidence is not clear. Once adolesence is reached, manic symptoms more closely resemble the adult illness. Puig-Antich (1985) identified the following symptoms in children with mania: (1) elation, (2) unrealistic optimism, (3) more activity than usual without fatigue, (4) grandiosity, (5) decreased need for sleep, (6) racing thoughts, (7) flight of ideas, (8) distractibility, and (9) motor hyperactivity.

Although the psychopharmacologic treatment of depression is known, drug treatment for mania is not as well established. Lithium, an antimania drug and the drug of choice for adult mania, has been used in childhood mania with mixed results. It is *not recommended* for use in children under 12 years of age.

ANTIDEPRESSANT DRUGS

There are two major antidepressant drug classes: the tricyclic antidepressants (TCAs) and the monoamine oxidase inhibitors (MAOIs). These two classes of drugs have different mechanisms for accomplishing the same neurophysiologic result of an increase in catecholamine availability (norepinephrine, dopamine, serotonin) at the receptor site (Keltner, 1989b). MAOIs have potentially life-threatening side effects and are not recommended for children under 16 years of age. TCAs were developed in the late 1950s and gained acceptance for treatment of childhood depression in the 1960s.

TCAs are well absorbed from the GI tract. The prototype TCA is imipramine (Tofranil). It is 90% to 95% bound to plasma protein, and is metabolized in the liver into many other compounds, some of which have their own antidepressant properties. For example, desipramine (Norpramin, Pertrofrane), is a metabolite of imipramine and is excreted in the urine. Physical problems that cause incomplete metabolism (hepatic problems) or interfere with excretion (renal problems) can prolong the half-life of imipramine.

By increasing catecholamine availability at the receptor site, TCAs cause central and peripheral effects. The most obvious central response is the *antidepressant effect*. Less obvious is the sedative quality of some TCAs. Peripheral side effects are caused by the increased availability of the neurotransmittors in the periphery. Increased levels of norephinephrine cause a sympathomimetic response such as tachycardia and elevated blood pressure. TCAs are cardiotoxic and overdose can be fatal. Orthostatic hypotension is a common side effect.

An anticholinergic response also occurs with TCAs, and a comparison of the sedative and anticholinergic effects of TCAs are shown in Table 16-1. All anticholinergic side effects associated with antipsychotic drugs occur with TCAs, that is, dry mouth, blurred vision, constipation, and urinary hesitancy. The last side effect is used in the treatment of enuresis. Hematologic disorders caused by TCAs are uncommon.

TCAs interact with many other drugs, and drugs with anticholinergic properties such as atropine, antihistamines, antiparkinson drugs, and OTC cold and hay fever drugs increase anticholinergic side effects, which can include paralytic ileus and urinary retention. Phenothiazines and methylphenidate (Ritalin) can cause increased serum levels of TCAs, and sympathomimetics should be used cautiously. These combinations can lead to tachycardia, arrhythmias, and hypertension. When combined with TCAs, CNS depressants cause increased CNS depression.

Tricyclic antidepressants. The PDR does not recommend any TCA for use in children under 12 years old for the treatment of depression. The use of antidepressants not approved for pediatric use in the PDR must be carefully discussed with the parent and may require informed consent. Imipramine is not

Table 16–1   Relative Sedation and Anticholinergic Side Effects of TCAs

Drug	Sedation	Anticholinergic
Imipramine (Tofranil)	2+	2+
Desipramine (Norpramin)	1+	1+
Amitriptyline (Elavil)	4+	4+

From Pomeroy J and Gadow KE: Adolescent psychiatric disorders. In Matson JL, editor: Handbook of treatment approaches in childhood psychopathology, New York, 1988, Plenum Publishing Corp.

recommended for children under 6 years of age and is recommended for children over 6 for the treatment of enuresis. Although the PDR does not recommend the use of imipramine for childhood depression, several clinicians use it and their research supports its effectiveness. Puig-Antich, Ryan, and Rabinovich (1985) recommend that dosage be "increased every fourth day from 1.5 to 3, to 4, and to 5 mg/kg/day." The maximum dose for desipramine and amitriptyline is 5 mg/kg per day. Puig-Antich, Ryan, and Rabinovich (1985) and Martin and Agran (1988) indicate that serum levels are the crucial variable for clinical effectiveness. Imipramine should have a serum level of 150 to 240 ng/ml, desipramine 115 ng/ml, and amitriptyline 100 to 300 ng/ml for a therapeutic effect. As with adults, a period of 3 to 4 weeks is required before clinical improvement is noted.

NURSING IMPLICATIONS

Side effects. Nurses must assess for anticholinergic side effects, be prepared to treat them symptomatically, and be alert for anticholinergic toxicity. Dry mouth is alleviated by sugarless candies or sips of water, and good oral hygiene is important. Nurses should monitor for constipation and urinary hesitancy. A depressed child could develop serious complications from these anticholinergic effects. Since decreased sweating occurs, children should be guarded from overheating, particularly in hot weather. Nurses should evaluate high activity levels and anticipate a distended bladder or abdomen. Vital signs for elevated blood pressure and tachycardia are routine, and a blood pressure greater than 140/90 and a heart rate of greater than 130 are cause for alarm (Martin and Agran, 1988). Although hematologic disorders are uncommon, abnormal bruising and bleeding, fever, and sore throat warrant a CBC.

GI symptoms such as nausea, vomiting, abdominal pain, diarrhea, and anorexia occur if these drugs are withdrawn abruptly. Gradual withdrawal should be practiced. An acute onset of these symptoms along with headache and flu-like symptoms may indicate a lack of compliance to the drug.

Interactions. Nurses should be aware of the drug interactions with TCAs. Drugs that potentiate anticholinergic or sympathomimetic effects or that elevate TCA serum levels should be questioned if ordered by the physician.

Toxicity. Children are thought to be more sensitive to overdoses of imipramine than are adults. Although deaths of children prescribed TCAs have been reported, most TCA poisoning in children is due to their taking a parent's TCA. Imipramine pamoate (Tofranil-PM) is never given to children because the smallest available unit dose is 75 mg.

TCAs have a narrow therapeutic index: the difference between a therapeutic dose and a lethal dose is small. For this reason careful adherence to the prescribed dose is important, and the drug must be kept out of the child's control. Peripheral toxic effects include tachycardia and arrhythmias, and diarrhea or constipation can occur, as can urinary retention. Central toxic effects may include muscle rigidity, hyperactive reflex, sedation, ataxia, respiratory depression, and convulsions. If TCA overdose is suspected, hospitalization is *required*. Vomiting to rid the body of unabsorbed drug and activated charcoal to prevent further absorption are emergency treatment measures. Nurses should monitor vital signs for heart rate and rhythm and respirations.

Parent teaching. Parents should be taught that a clinical effect takes 3 to 4 weeks to develop. Measures to provide psychotherapeutic support for the parents during this lag time are important. Clinicians should instruct the parent to carefully administer the exact amount of drug, to keep the drug away from the affected child and the siblings, and to never give other drugs without approval from the physician or nurse. In addition, parents must be given an adequate amount of information about side effects so that they can recognize and report serious side effects.

ANTIMANIA DRUG

Lithium. Lithium was first reported for the treatment of mania by Cade in 1949. At that time, lithium was banned in the United States because of several deaths associated with it. Unaware of its low therapeutic index, many physicians ordered lithium salt as a salt substitute for cardiac clients, and some died from lithium toxicity. When the ban on lithium was lifted in the late 1960s, it was used successfully in the treatment of adult manic-depressive patients. Research on its effectiveness in child manic-depression is not as substantial.

Lithium has serious side effects in adults, but children tolerate the drug well. Lithium decreases free thyroxine and triiodothyronine, but increased thyroid-releasing hormone compensates in euthyroid patients. Children should have baseline thyroid hormone levels taken (Puig-Antich, Ryan, and Rabinovich, 1985). After stabilization occurs, monthly serum levels are adequate. There is a concern among clinicians that long-term use of lithium may cause renal damage, but research does not support this concern (Khandelwal, Vijoy, and Murphy, 1984). Lithium causes sodium diuresis, and the excretion of lithium is tied to sodium excretion. A decrease in sodium intake can lead to lithium toxicity (> 1.5 mEq/l). Other side effects include weakness, tremor, weight gain, stomachache, and blurred vision. Nausea and vomiting, slurring of speech, and drowsiness may be early indications of toxicity (Puig-Antich, Ryan, and Rabinovich, 1985).

Lithium interacts with several other drugs. Some drugs increase serum lithium levels (most diuretics, salt substitutes); some drugs decrease lithium serum levels (alcohol, aminophylline, antacids, caffeine, sodium bicarbonate); and lithium decreases the serum levels of some drugs (antipsychotic drugs). Lithium and haloperidol reportedly cause neurotoxicity when used together.

Lithium has been used in children under 12 years of age who were diagnosed as manic, but it is not PDR-approved for this use. Therefore, use of this drug should be carefully discussed with parents. Dosage of 30 mg/kg to 40 mg/kg per day have been reported. The effectiveness of lithium is not clear. Weller, Weller, and Fristad (1986) suggest 900 mg/day in divided doses for children 25 to 40 kg, 1200 mg/day in divided doses for children 40 to 50 kg, and 1500 mg/day in divided doses for children 50 to 60 kg. The effective serum level range is 0.6 to 1.2 mEq/L mEg/L.

NURSING IMPLICATIONS

Side effects. Nurses act as facilitators, help clients deal with minor side effects, and closely observe effects that might indicate toxicity. Many side effects can be treated symptomatically. Clinicians should take and record vital signs at least daily and, if the child experiences tachycardia, contact the physician. They can minimize nausea by giving lithium with meals, and relieve thirst by instructing clients to drink adequate amounts of water daily. If diarrhea occurs, the child should be observed closely because loss of sodium through extra-urinary routes can lead to lithium toxicity.

Interactions. The most serious interactions are those that increase lithium serum levels. Salt substitutes that reduce the amount of sodium ingested lead to increased levels of lithium. Other drugs decrease the serum level and should be avoided to gain a consistent therapeutic plasma level. Nurses should therefore monitor all drugs to decrease drug interactions.

Toxicity. Lithium has a low therapeutic index, and frequent serum levels are thus indicated. Children may require daily blood levels. Lithium levels are at their most accurate in the morning, 10 to 12 hours after the last dose. Toxicity can be precipitated by common conditions that affect fluid and electrolyte balance such as excessive sweating, diarrhea, vomiting, and decreased salt intake. There is no pharmacologic antidote for lithium poisoning. If toxicity is suspected, nurses should halt its use and the use of any drug that slows lithium excretion and notify the physician. Hastening lithium excretion by using mannitol or acetazolamine is an appropriate treatment plan.

Parent teaching. Parents should be instructed about the signs of lithium toxicity and told to withhold the drug and call the physician if toxic symptoms appear. Parents living with a manic child should know that Lithium has a lag period of up to 10 days. They should give medications on time and should use the accurate prescribed dose. Parents also need to prepare and serve meals consistently and understand the basic information about sodium-lithium excretion, for example, that depleted sodium will lead to excessive lithium levels and that increased sodium will lead to decreased lithium levels.

Special Issues

ENURESIS

Enuresis is a developmental eliminative disorder in children 5 years and older, manifested by involuntary urination during sleep. Enuresis is more common in males, and approximately 20% of these children have psychiatric symptoms. A number of approaches have been used. Behavioral approaches (for example, buzzer pads) have proven effective for some children, and for others a pharmacologic approach has been beneficial. Imipramine (Tofranil) is approved for enuresis in children 6 years old and older. It is believed that the same anticholinergic effect causing urinary hesitancy and retention in adults is responsible for imipramine's therapeutic effect in enuretic children.

Imipramine (Tofranil). Clients are given 25 mg daily, one hour before bedtime. After 1 week the dosage can be increased to 50 mg in children 6 to 12 years of age. For enuretic children who wet the bed early in the night, it may be more effective to give imipramine earlier and in divided doses. Side effects are relatively unimportant at these dosages. Children should not be given more than 2.5 mg/kg per day. Imipramine pamoate (Tofranil-PM) is contraindicated in children because the smallest unit dose is 75 mg.

TOURETTE'S SYNDROME

Tourette's Syndrome (TS) is characterized by involuntary, repetitive, purposeless muscle movements, such as gyrating, hopping, clapping, and kicking, accompanied by multiple verbal tics including screaming and coprolalia (Adkins, 1989). Coprolalia, the utterance of filthy, obscene language, causes numerous social problems for the client and family and occurs in approximately 40% of clients with TS. It can progress to phrases that are filled with cursing and sexually offensive language. Some clients utter profanities as soon as the thought comes into their minds without the usual social restraint. Haloperidol is the drug of choice for TS.

Haloperidol (Haldol). The recommended dosage of haloperidol for TS is 0.05 mg/kg to 0.075 mg/kg per day. The child should not be given more than 6 mg daily, and EPS are significant. Young and others (1985) recommended an initial dose of 0.5 mg/day, slowly increased to 3 to 4 mg/day. The drug is effective for approximately 80% of clients (Young and others, 1985).

Clonidine (Catapres). Clonidine is an antihypertensive drug that is used by many clinicians although it is not FDA approved for use in TS. It is a alpha-adrenergic agonist that should be initiated at low doses of 0.05 mg/day and slowly increased for several weeks to 0.15 to 0.30 mg/day. Dosages of over 0.4 to 0.5 mg/day lead to side effects (Gallico, Burns, and Grob, 1988). Clonidine has a slower onset of action than haloperidol, taking up to 3 weeks or more before a therapeutic improvement is noted (Young and others, 1985). Side effects include sedation, dry mouth, and hypotension.

Pimozide (Orap). Pimozide is an antipsychotic drug indicated for managing severe motor or vocal tics in clients with TS. It is not recommended for use in children under 12 years of age. Clinical experience with children is limited, but favorable results have been reported (Adkins, 1989).

SEPARATION ANXIETY

Separation anxiety is common and psychiatric professionals are often consulted when children refuse to attend school (school phobia). The adult equivalent is agoraphobia. When coupled with appropriate psychotherapeutic intervention, imipramine (Tofranil) is recommended for these children. Gittelman-Klein (1975) studied 100 children and stated, "This is one of the few psychiatric treatments that, when successful, induces complete remission." Jaffe and Magnuson (1985) recommend 1.0 to 5.0 mg/kg/day for children suffering from separation anxiety. The dosage should not exceed 200 mg/day (Gittelman-Klein, 1975).

Miscellaneous Drugs

Carbamazepine (Tegretol). An anticonvulsant, carbamazepine is used in a variety of psychiatric diagnoses. It has been effective in the treatment of mania and impulsive behavior. The drug has been used in the treatment of organic mental disease, depression, catatonia, schizophrenia, panic disorder, borderline personality, obsessive compulsive disorder, hypochondriacal psychosis, explosive disorder, and stuttering.

Benzodiazepines. These antianxiety agents have been used in the treatment of separation anxiety. Common benzodiazepines used in children are diazepam

(Valium), chlordiazepoxide (Librium), and alprazolam (Xanax). Side effects include sedation and paradoxical agitation or excitement. Reactions occur if these drugs are withdrawn too quickly and may include severe anxiety and seizures.

The recommended dosage of diazepam for children with anxiety is 1 to 2.5 mg three to four times per day. The dosage can be increased as needed and tolerated. Diazepam should not be used in children under 6 months of age.

The recommended dosage of chlordiazepoxide for childhood anxiety is 5 mg two to four times per day. Therapy with chlordiazepoxide should be initiated at the lowest dose and increased as required. It should not be used in children under 6 years of age.

The recommended dosage for alprazolam is 0.25 to 3 mg per day (Gallico, Burns, and Grob, 1988). Withdrawal reactions appear to be especially significant with this drug.

Summary

Child psychopharmacology has evolved over the past 50 years to the point where greater specificity of treatment is available. Research is finding a pharmacologic response to many of the disturbing disorders encountered in children. This avenue of intervention holds much promise, but associated risks are apparent. Child psychiatric nurses must be careful in the administration of these drugs, understand the side effects of these drugs, be aware of drug interactions and toxic reactions, and teach parents.

REFERENCES

Adkins AS: Helping your patient cope with Tourette syndrome, Pediatr Nurs 15:135, 1989.

Bradley C: The behavior of children receiving Benzedrine, Am J Psychiatry, 94:577, 1937.

Campbell M: Schizophrenic disorders and pervasive developmental disorders/infantile autism. In Wiener JM, editor: Diagnosis and psychopharmacology of childhood and adolescent disorders, New York, 1985, John Wiley & Sons, Inc.

Campbell M and Pali M: Measurement of tardive dyskinesia, Psychopharmacol Bull 21:106, 1985.

Engelhardt DM and Polizos P: Adverse effects of pharmacotherapy in childhood psychosis. In Lipton MA, DiMascio A, and Killam KF, editors: Psychopharmacology: a generation of progress, New York, 1978, Raven Press.

Gadow KE: Children on medication, vol 1, San Diego, 1986, College-Hill Press.

Gallico RP, Burns TJ, and Grob CS: Emotional and behavioral problems in children with learning disabilities, Boston, 1988, College-Hill Press.

Gittelman-Klein R: Pharmacotherapy and management of pathological separation anxiety. In Gittelman-Klein R, editor: Recent advances in child psychopharmacology, New York, 1975, Human Sciences Press, Inc.

Jaffe SL and Magnuson JV: Anxiety disorders. In Weiner J, editor: Diagnosis and psychopharmacology of childhood and adolescent disorders, New York, 1985, John Wiley & Sons, Inc.

Joshi PT, Capozzoli JA, and Coyle JT: Low-dose neuroleptic therapy for children with childhood onset pervasive developmental disorder, Am J Psychiatry, 145:335, 1988.

Keltner NL: Antipsychotic drugs. In Shlafer M and Marieb EN, editors: The nurse, pharmacology, and drug therapy, Menlo Park, Calif, 1989a, Addison-Wesley Publishing Co, Inc.

Keltner NL: Drugs for the treatment of depression and mania. In Shlafer M and Marieb EN, editors: The nurse, pharmacology, and drug therapy, Menlo Park, Calif, 1989b, Addison-Wesley Publishing Co, Inc.

Keltner NL and McIntyre C: Neuroleptic malignant syndrome, Neurosurg Nurs 17:362, 1985.

Khandelwal SK, Vijoy KV, and Murphy RS: Renal function in children receiving long-term lithium prophylaxis, Am J Psychiatry 141:278, 1984.

LaGreca AM and Quay HC: Behavior disorders in children. In Ender NS and Hunt J, editors: Personality and the behavior disorders, ed 2, New York, 1984, Wiley & Sons, Inc.

Martin JE and Agran M: Pharmacotherapy. In Matson JL, editor: Handbook of treatment approaches in childhood psychopathology, New York, 1988, Plenum Publishing Corp.

Physician's desk reference, Oradell, NJ, 1990, Medical Economic Co, Inc.

Pomeroy J and Gadow KE: Adolescent psychiatric disorders. In Matson JL, editor: Handbook of treatment approaches in childhood psychopathology, New York, 1988, Plenum Publishing Corp.

Puig-Antich J: Affective disorder. In Kaplan SI and Sadock BJ, editors: Comprehensive textbook of psychiatry IV, Baltimore, 1985, Williams & Wilkins.

Puig-Antich J, Ryan ND, and Rabinovich H: Affective disorders in childhood and adolescence. In Wiener JM, editor: Diagnosis and psychopharmacology for childhood and adolescent disorder, New York, 1985, John Wiley & Sons, Inc.

Rutter M and others: Research report: Isle of Wight studies, 1964–1974, Psychol Med 6:313, 1976.

Weller EB, Weller RA, and Fristad MA: Lithium dosage guide for prepubertal children: a preliminary report, J Am Acad Child Psychiatry 25:92, 1986.

Werry J: Pediatric psychopharmacology, New York, 1978, Brunner/Mazel, Inc.

Wiener JM: Psychopharmacology in childhood and adolescence, New York, 1977, Basic Books, Inc, Publishers.

Wiener JM and Jaffe SL: Historical overview of childhood and adolescent psychopharmacology. In Wiener JM, editor: Diagnosis and psychopharmacology of childhood and adolescent disorders, New York, 1985, John Wiley & Sons, Inc.

Young JG and others: Tourette's syndrome and tic disorders. In Wiener JM, editor: Diagnosis and psychopharmacology of childhood and adolescent disorders, New York, 1985, John Wiley & Sons, Inc.

Chapter 17

Child Psychotherapy
and Play Therapy

Child psychotherapy comprises the direct intervention methods used to promote behavioral changes. Play therapy, direct counseling, cognitive therapy, and behavior modification are all treatment methods that help change the children's undesirable behaviors, ease their psychic pain, and improve their relationships with others. The goal of therapy is the resolution of children's emotional, behavioral, and interpersonal problems.

During the last few decades the focus has changed, from the individual treatment focus that characterized the beginning years of child psychiatry, to the parental involvement focus that is currently emphasized. This changing perspective is partly due to the growth of family theories and therapies that stress the dynamic relationship between symptoms and the interpersonal context in which they occur. The behavior of children is more dependent on environmental forces and changes than the actions of adults; children tend to react rather than initiate change. Children lack the power to take action when confronted with environmental stressors, such as divorce, school, peer pressure, and dysfunctional parents. Family therapy teaches parents to be therapeutic agents (Guerney, 1983; Bonnard, 1978). Because their problems may be normal responses to a stressful environment and because they are dependent on it, incorporating this environment into treatment is important. Individual therapy is often indicated to help them cope with a stressful environmental situation (Brown and Prout, 1990).

At this time, there are three schools of family systems therapy—structural, strategic and systemic—and clinical research confirms that it is more effective to promote healthy family relationships by involving and educating parents and others who affect the child (Casey and Berman, 1985).

The role of parents and children's state of dependency exert a powerful impact on therapy. Determining the parent-child relationship is a central part of the diagnostic process; Modifying problems in this relationship is a central part of the treatment process. A good working alliance between therapists and parents is essential and often the basis of successful treatment.

Most contemporary child clinicians use many techniques simultaneously: child and family interventions, behavior management techniques, and school personnel consultation (Golden, 1983). Traditional models emphasized adherence to the principles and practices of one specific school or theory of therapy. Current treatment approaches are based on the assumption that child psychiatric disorders are multifaceted and require the concurrent use of a variety of approaches (Barker, 1990).

An example of these eclectic therapies is Keats' multimodal approach (1979). Expanding on Lazarus' multimodal adult therapy concept with its acronym, BASIC ID, Keats added three additional interactive modalities on which assessment and intervention decisions are based. BASIC ID (behavior, affect, sensation, imagery, cognition, interpersonal relationships, and drugs and diet [Lazarus, 1976]) became BASIC IDEAL in Keats' child treatment model, with the addition of educational pursuits, adults in children's life, and learning their culture.

The major assumptions of these eclectic approaches are consistent with the standards of child and adolescent psychiatric mental health nursing (ANA, 1982); however, they differ from some earlier child therapy assumptions. The assumptions of the new approaches are that interdisciplinary, collaborative, coordinated interventions are essential and involve professionals with expertise in different areas and that the person does not have to be a professional psychotherapist to have a therapeutic impact: parents, peers, and nonprofessionals can play significant roles (Brown and Prout, 1990).

A core of therapeutic intervention principles are applied wherever treatment occurs. Many established adult therapy models (such as psychoanalytic, cognitive, person-centered, reality, rational-emotive, behavioral, and systemic psychotherapies) are used in child interventions — the theoretic and clinical tenets and the explanations of etiology are used for all ages. Treatment takes place in many settings: the home, the classroom, the clinic playroom, the community agency, and the hospital. Although settings vary, the therapeutic model selected and implemented does not.

Child Client and Child Interventions

Psychotherapeutic interventions with children differ from interventions with adults and adolescents; the younger the child, the greater these differences (Barker, 1990). The child client is one whose "defenses are fragile, cognitive capacity poor, anxiety easily stimulated, superego limited, and for whom magic and omnipotence prevail" (Chetnik, 1990). The child is in the process of developing new personality structures, and symptoms and actions are often expressions of this. Thus, therapists not only work with the problem that has brought the child to therapy, but also serves as a developmental facilitator to help the child learn to deal with the stresses of normal development and maturation.

Children are more labile, have broader mood swings in emotions, and usually exhibit a wider range of normal emotional and behavioral responses and behaviors during the course of treatment than adults. However, once a relationship is established, they are more pliable and amenable to therapeutic influences than adults.

Children perceive, conceptualize, and react to interpersonal events in characteristic ways that depend on their level of development. Regardless of the model of psychotherapy used, clinicians need to consider that children's "ability to conceptualize the motivations, feelings and behaviors of themselves and others changes dramatically over time, along with their understanding of social causality and their ability to infer predictable patterns in their social worlds" (Bierman and Schwartz, 1986).

Two types of knowledge and skills are required for child counseling and effective implementation of psychotherapeutic techniques: (1) understanding and application of developmental stage theories, especially the theories of Freud, Piaget, Kohlberg, and Erikson, and (2) knowledge and understanding of specific variables that are developmental in nature, such as children's unique personality factors (Thomas, Chess, and Birch, 1968). The specific personality variables that most often present problems during childhood are dependency, anxiety, insecurity, aggressiveness, and achievement motivation. Some factors that influence the implementation of therapy with children are listed in the box.

Verbal Abilities and Communication Skills

The developmental level of children's verbal abilities and communication skills is important in child psychotherapy. These are markers of the developmental status of their cognitive structures. Evaluation of language use in social communication and of their ability to interact is based on norms that describe the relationship between the brain's maturity and children's thought processes. Thus, careful assessment of the four verbal areas — speech, voice, vocabulary and message — and of age-appropriate language use and thought processes is crucial.

Most children find it difficult to express themselves verbally. Their immature language development level and limited vocabularies restrict their ability to identify feelings and concerns. Children are in the process of developing their secondary process — thinking and their capacity for symbol formation, and most children think in concrete terms because abstract thinking has not yet developed.

Sometimes a communication disorder is the major diagnosis and the focus of therapy — seldom true of psychotherapy with adults. Communication problems present in disorders such as mental retardation, autism, stuttering, developmental language disorders, and childhood schizophrenia. If present in adults, these communication disorders have more severe disease implications (Barker, 1990).

Evaluation of children's expressive and receptive capacities influences and directs all contacts with them, from initial assessment to therapy termination. Most children express themselves most effectively through less direct, nonverbal means. Clinicians can use *diagnostic free play,* a combination play and verbal interview, to assess appropriate communication methods.

Language of Play

Developmentally, children progressively express feelings and needs using action, fantasy, and lastly language. They talk more freely in the language of play, because they preconsciously regard this special realm as once removed from the pressures and demands of everyday life (Anthony, 1986).

Factors in Therapeutic Relationships

Involuntary status and motivation

Children do not recognize that there is a problem and lack fundamental motivation for treatment (Tyson and Tyson, 1986). Seldom do children come to therapy voluntarily; usually they enter because of coercion or persuasion and harbor resentment toward parents and even clinicians (Barker, 1990).

Implications. Clinicians need to establish measures of motivation and cooperation.

Lack of understanding of psychotherapy

Usually adolescents and adults have preconceived notions of client behavior consisting of talking, thinking, and responding to the clinicians' questions. In contrast, children are unfamiliar with verbal therapy and are often incapable of participating in it.

Implications. Young children expect social transactions with the clinician to be similar to those with parents. School-aged children harbor distorted stereotypes about mental health clinicians and care. Clinicians should initially focus on educating children about therapy and the procedures that will occur.

Reinforcement of treatment goals

Children, especially those with problems, tend to forget, avoid, or deny the therapeutic process.

Implications. Clinicians need to focus on the therapeutic tasks to be achieved, renegotiate frequently, and continually monitor children's perceptions of treatment.

Fear of punishment

Unlike adults, children are usually seen in therapy for alleged misdeeds, based on something someone says they did. Thus, they fear that treatment will pass judgment on them and that they are bad, defective, or crazy. They have limited understanding of verbal explanations and no frame of reference of future changes and improvements. Developmental limitations intensify children's self-doubts, fears, and sense of inadequacy.

Implications. Clinicians should reassure children that therapy is not punishment.

Clinician reaction

Strong countertransference reactions and feelings of confusion, bewilderment, frustration, anger, helplessness, and rescue fantasies are common among child clinicians.

Implications. Clinicians need to analyze the treatment process objectively, obtain peer consultation, and recognize that feelings are more intense when working with children.

Therapists need to capitalize on this kind of communication, which is between primitive behavior and sophisticated verbalization. Therapists' office needs to be a playground in which children's world can be projected—an unstructured setting with paper, toys and drawing materials, a place where the internal characters can come to life. Therapists' task is to provide a structure that facilitates the emergence of these stories.

Play alters the raw, overwhelming emotions that arise in children in times of anxiety, and it provides a natural vehicle for expression of these emotions. Play emerges from children's internal life, and it typically expresses their major internal issues. The use of play is the difference between child and adult intervention, and evaluation using play is a major procedural difference between the adult and child MSE (see Chapter 3).

ATTITUDES TOWARD PLAY AND FANTASY

Before the seventeenth century, religious views on children's activities were strict and controlling, and play was discouraged and viewed as dangerous. Perceptions of play as harmful continue and explain the reason many modern parents and professionals distrust it.

Play is unplanned, thus unpredictable, and this causes uneasiness in adults. The make-believe aspects and their capacity to change reality used to be considered the elements of mental illness at the extreme, and of dishonesty at best. Thus early religious leaders were concerned that excessive play and fantasy in childhood would damage later adult relationships. It was thought that pretending and childhood games would create habits and attitudes that would characterize adult social interactions if continued into adult life (Berne, 1978).

Even when the child labor laws were passed and compulsory education in America was instituted, the strong Puritan work ethic was not sympathetic to free play or school time spent ungainfully. Children moved from the serious work in the field, to the serious work in the factory, and then to serious school work. Thus, religious, economic, and social factors demanded an official political declaration to convince Americans that the childhood years are a time of trial, set aside so that children can use play to find out about themselves and their world.

Although the words of the proclamation dignified *play* synonymously with *work*, they illustrate the usual way play is defined; that is, its contrast to what is *not play*. Play continues to be characterized as frivolous, spontaneous, and lacking in purpose. The lack of productivity and seriousness that characterizes play may be why little play research has been conducted by pragmatic traditional scientists.

Only recently have scientists begun the serious study of imagination and fantasy, activities that have gained respectability and scientific credibility with the discovery of split-brain theory. The contribution of fun, humor, and fantasy to development is only now gaining credence. At the same time, many right-brain interventions (such as relaxation, visualization, and imagination) offer valuable and essential coping skills. Popular best-sellers, such as *Anatomy of an Illness* (Cousins, 1980), have exerted a powerful influence, changing many traditional, negative attitudes about play, fantasy, and imagery.

POWER OF PLAY AND FANTASY

Despite adult efforts to control children's play, children have defended it against adult intrusion, building their own play culture. For centuries, children of all cultures have played the same kinds of games, with rules uniformly transmitted from one generation to the next. The existence and transmission of children's play culture is an extraordinary finding: play is transmitted through nursery rhymes, fairy tales, parables, and songs. Most rules and styles of games are taught by older to younger children; these rules remain inviolate over time.

The play peer culture, with its discounting of adult lifestyles and values, is characteristic of youth's counterculture that begins in early childhood and evolves to adolescent rebellion and alienation from adult social roles (Bronfenbrenner, 1976). In the extreme, children participate in counterculture *deep play* in which stakes are high and the culture, as well as the childrens lives, can be damaged or destroyed. Bruner (1972) cites membership in youth gangs and certain games such as Russian roulette as examples of deep play that have serious outcomes.

Those who support the therapeutic use of play and fantasy emphasize its multidimensional values. In physical development, play facilitates mastery by strengthening the integration of the physical and neurologic process. Play facilitates cognitive learning, and some maintain that fantasy and imagination are building-blocks for problem solving, divergent thinking, and creativity (Piaget, 1962). Children make contact with one another, practice communication, and interpersonal skills through play and fantasy. Game rules are important in moral development. Play also contributes to the development of self-concept by providing a private reality that protects their egocentric world from the real world they must accommodate every day.

Enhancing self-control through play and fantasy helps children with problems ranging from fear to attention span deficits and reality distortions, regardless of the problem's etiology. Play is used in primary prevention in children at risk of developing mental illness and in secondary prevention at the first sign of mental health problems. Normal development is supported by using play with teaching, anticipatory guidance, support for age-appropriate behaviors, developmental and situational crisis counseling, and coping and competency fostering. Tertiary prevention involves teaching parents age-appropriate play behaviors and activities for children.

PLAY, FANTASY, AND IMAGINATION

Fantasy is a component of play and is defined as *unrestrained* imagination. *Fantasy play* refers to imaginative play, and *dramatic play* refers to the dramas and theatrics that children generate spontaneously. These elaborate fantasies may resemble fairy tales, but they may also be projections of experiences in their life.

Imagery has been defined as a mental picture of something that is not actually present. *Imagination* is the capacity to daydream or fantasize, to relive the past, or to probe the future through pictures in the mind's eye.

Singer and Switzer (1980) claim imagination is one of the greatest resources humans possess and is "wired to the natural functioning of the brain and is a powerful resource for healthy escape, self-entertainment and for fuller or more effective living, coping through the effective use of the imaginative powers." The ability to recall the past and relive important moments enriches the present and prevents children from repeating mistakes or destructive patterns. Imagination is used to explore and experience the future before it happens, to plan constructive, creative problem-solving strategies, and to play with impossibilities.

In reality, play and fantasy are important for mental health and are not the same as hallucinations or delusions (Manosevitz, Fling, and Prentice, 1989). Unlike the mentally disturbed child, the child who plays and daydreams knows the boundaries between fantasy and reality. Fantasy helps the normal child test the boundaries between what is real and what is imagined. Repetition characteristic of child's play facilitates means consolidation and adeptness in managing hurts, misunderstandings and traumas — not obsessions or compulsions. As in dramatic play, repetition in games is essential, because once the basics are mastered and become habits, the mind is free to be creative.

Play moves the child toward the more sophisticated expressions of general intelligence. Research indicates that children exhibiting greater spontaneous fantasy activities differ from those exhibiting lower amounts. High fantasizers had more parental interactions that involved fantasy and more contact with their parents than with their siblings. Children of parents who create complicated imaginary situations have higher levels of verbal intelligence and academic achievement. Close parental relationships foster the development of intelligence and a fantasy-promoting family background is advocated.

Studies that identify imaginative children by using the ambiguous Rorschach tests indicate that children who associate the inkblots with active human figures are more imaginative and controlled than those who see the inkblots as inanimate objects. Rorschach proposed that people who see lively human activities in the blots tend to heed the movements and imaginings of their inner eye. In contrast, those who perceive inanimate objects tend not to organize inkblots into their personal images and respond only to obvious characteristics. These children are more likely to be impulsive and dependent on the external environment. Researchers reported that hyperactive retarded children are less likely to see movement in inkblots than more relaxed retarded children, and observations of kindergarten classes found that children who show little imagination in inkblot readings are unable to sit still. Children as young as 3 or 4 years of age were likely to be more restless if their Rorschach responses are unimaginative. This becomes more pronounced with age, and these children tend to become more aggressive (Singer and Switzer, 1980). Children that show limited imagination in their play should be reevaluated, because psychologic tests may explain the child's imagination and fantasy life is impoverished.

Children of equal intelligence but unequal imaginations also differ in sensitivity to reality. Children whose play lacks make-believe are likely to have trouble recalling and integrating details of events they hear about, thus the imaginative children do better in those school tasks that involve more than rote memory. In addition, research suggests that the richer and greater the child's fantasy experiences, the less likely the child will act out.

Most children have vivid and active imaginations, and often their mind is filled with lively and frightening imagery of ghosts, goblins, and monsters. By using coping imagery, clinicians and parents can relate stories that help instill basic psychologic realities.

NORMAL PLAY

Changes in a child's characteristic play is a major behavioral change — the chief complaint parents state when they seek professional help. Children need to engage in age-appropriate play, and parents should be taught the kind of games that are usually played by their child's age group. When used in therapy, children's play is evaluated and included in assessment data. Nurse clinicians working with children also need a clear concept of the behaviors and activities that constitute normal age-appropriate play for children of different social and cultural groups. These norms are the baseline for play assessment and the frame of reference from which psychopathologic evaluations are conducted. The criterion for classification of age-appropriate play activities and toys is the *physical action* of the child on nonhuman and human objects (parents, peers, and self).

Developmental Theories

Child developmental theorists, such as Piaget and Kohlberg (Piers, 1972), defined play as conflict-free activities. They used play as a framework for theory development in other areas of child development. Most conflict-free theories define play as requiring a nonliteral frame of mind that buffers the players from the normal consequences of their actions. Thus play is also insulation from the consequences of risk-taking and is essential for development of adult problem-solving skills and coping strategies (Bruner, 1972).

Piaget stated that the meaning and structure of play of normal preschoolers is different from that of normal school-aged children. Preschool children engage in *symbolic play* and are preoccupied with giants, heroes, and powerful figures. In play, they bring the powerful significant others in their lives under control. The construction of play symbols were *distorting assimilations,* similar to the mental constructions found in dreams that are characterized by displacement and condensation. Spontaneous verbalizations during play are comparable to adult free associations. At 6 or 7 years of age, normal children attain the concrete operational thinking that enables them to construct a lawful world and to reason about that world. Personal needs are socialized through play and through the sharing of victories and defeats. As these cognitive structures emerge, children prefer games that involve peers, such as baseball, football, and collaborative dramatic doll play. While some school-aged children's play seems symbolic, it includes social and collective elements of the immediate environment and lacks the highly personal quality of the symbolic play of preschoolers.

Erikson (1940) viewed play as conflict-laden. His widely used frameworks identify intrinsic psychologic reasons that normal children use specific toys and games at various ages and stages:

1. Children aged 1 to 3 are in the anal-muscular stage with the developmental tasks of resolving the conflict of autonomy versus shame and doubt, and they prefer parallel play.
2. Children aged 3 to 6 are in the genital-locomotor stage with the developmental tasks of resolving the conflict of initiative versus guilt, and they enjoy cooperative play, fantasy, and elaborate dramatic scenes through which they symbolically resolve conflicts by fantasy and by imitation of adults.
3. Children aged 6 to 12 are in the genital-locomotive stage with the developmental tasks of resolving the conflict of industry versus inferiority, and they prefer games governed by complex rules and regulations such as chess.

Allen (1970) grouped age, central themes, fantasies, play materials, and secondary gains to be considered:

Group I: Central theme of anxieties concern the body. Feelings of helplessness may be denied by compensatory fantasies of grandeur. Preferred play materials relate to body functions and body parts.

Group II: Central theme relates to pre-Oedipal relationships and fear of loss of love objects. Repetition, mirroring play, and maternal play with dolls and stuffed animals occur. Play focuses on learning to delay gratification.

Group III: Oedipal relations and defenses begin at about 3 years of age. Spontaneous dramatic play occurs with a wide variety of emotions, roles, and plots, with fantasies of a social, creative nature. Coplay helps child prepare for adult roles.

Group IV: Sibling relations and fear of the superego begin at approximately 6 years of age. The importance of rules, codes, and rituals in board games such as chess and checkers are common. Organized coplay to learn cooperation with siblings, peers, and parents predominates.

ASSESSMENT OF PSYCHOPATHOLOGY

Signs and symptoms of dysfunctional uses of fantasy and play. Play has been used as an intervention, but no cohesive theory of normal or abnormal play yet exists. Baseline normal play formats are used to evaluate psychopathology. Excessive uses of play, fantasy, and daydreaming may have negative implications, especially when children use imagination as a defense. Fantasy play is dangerous when used habitually to escape from problems. Excessive daydreaming to avoid competition with contemporaries or to compensate for a deficiency may lead to serious maladjustments. Fantasies are harmful if children are dominated by persistent fantasies of violence, blood, or hurting others; daydreams become more real and pleasant than real life; and children pattern their life after a fairy tale in which their identity is different from reality.

ASSESSMENT OF SYMBOLIC DEVELOPMENT

In recent decades, transactional and interactional research has moved from viewing play as a vehicle for theory generation in a specific area of development to studying play as it develops and interacts with other developing aspects. Research findings indicate a common developmental sequence of object use that precedes the emergence of symbolic play (Sroufe, 1979). Clinicians can expand diagnostic assessment to include the development of symbology, and they can initiate the activities that foster symbolic activities.

Children's symbolic systems are intact when their levels of cognitive development, play, language, and self-knowledge are organized meaningfully. Language and play begin with decentration, progress to decontextualization, and merge to integration of objects and social play (Bretherton and Waters, 1985).

Children's ability to share information with clinicians conveying intentions, cognition, and feelings depends on their developmental age and stage. During the first 8 to 9 months, play is primarily visual-tactile object exploration and manipulation. Near the end of the first year, infants begin to manipulate objects in relational and combinational ways. By the start of the second year, true symbolic use of objects emerges and elaborates. However, it is only after mastering verbal internal-state labels that children can communicate about past or anticipated feelings, goals, intentions, and cognition.

IMAGINARY COMPANIONS

An imaginary companion is an invisible character, usually the same age as the child, named and referred to in conversation with other persons or played with directly for at least several months that has "an air of reality for the child but no apparent objective basis" (Svendsen, 1934). The difference between imaginary companions and other forms of fantasy is that imaginary companions occupy physical space in the actual world (to the child) and other fantasies are contained in the imagination and do not have a quasiphysical presence. Imaginary companions are the chief complaint when they interfere with daily life and annoy parents who must deal with them.

There currently are no generally accepted criteria of what constitutes an imaginary companion; however, it is estimated that 13% to 30% of all children have them (Nagera, 1981). Viewed as a transitory phenomenon, the existence of an imaginary companion usually warrants a normal diagnosis that merits careful assessment.

The imaginary companion phenomenon is a special type of fantasy that shares the characteristics of daydreams and other imaginary experiences. Psychoanalytic theory holds that this phenomenon is ruled by the pleasure principle, that it is an attempt at wish fulfillment that ignores reality, and that it is not usually reality adapted. Children fantasizing imaginary companions are aware of their fantasy's unreality—their reality testing remains unimpaired.

In adults an intense fantasy life usually implies withdrawal from an unpleasant real world to a more satisfactory inner world. However, children bring their imaginary companion into their real life and try to have it accepted by others. Children with an unhealthy imagination abandon the real world and are unable to establish meaningful relationships. In contrast, children with a healthy imagination employ fantasy to solve problems while maintaining human ties (Fraiberg, 1959).

Imaginary companions differ from other types of imaginative personification (Svendsen, 1934). Young children's imaginary companions reflect their animistic concept of the world and their strong belief in magic and omnipotence of thought. Older post-Oedipal children refrain from free disclosure of imaginary friends.

Psychoanalysts claim that imaginary companions are latency-age phenomena similar to latency children's fantasy of having a twin, which results from disappointment in parents during earlier Oedipal situations, and emerges as children search for a partner who will give them love, attention, and companionship and provide an escape from loneliness (Burlingham 1945). Once that role is fulfilled, the companion tends to disappear (Nagera, 1981).

Others believe that imaginary companions help satisfy children's need for social interaction. Children create imaginary playmates when real ones are lacking, unlike many adults who find great satisfaction in being alone. Often children have more than one imaginary companion (Belcher, 1987). Imaginary companions may have positive value and be positively correlated with mental health. Children who have imaginary

---

Functions of Imaginary Companions

1. Superego auxiliaries: Imaginary companions act as external controls needed before the superego is established in younger children and as a prop for an established superego in older children.
2. Discharge of unacceptable impulses: Children attribute their misbehavior to companions because of their misunderstanding of parental prohibitions or their fear of parental response.
3. Aide in mastery of stressful situations: Children personify their imaginary companion as someone who is competent, enabling them to conquer stressful situations vicariously.
4. Prolongation of feelings of omnipotence and control: Imaginary playmates ease the gradual, painful shifting of children's belief in their omnipotence to belief in parents.
5. Personification of ego ideals: Children endow their companion with the characteristic of being a good, clever, strong, lovable child, attributes children feel they lack. The companion is a weapon for defiance and a channel for the negative aspects of young children's ambivalence.
6. Management of loneliness, neglect, and rejection: Imaginary companions may be the result of children's unsatisfied instinct for gregariousness that disappears once their loneliness is fulfilled by schoolmates and friendships.
7. Adjustment to the birth of a sibling: Children create a more faithful, reliable companion and form a relationship with this fantasy because of their mother's limited withdrawal of attention. Companions help deal with painful realities, provide a denial mechanism, alleviate loneliness, and lighten guilt.
8. Management of changes: Imaginary companions may provide a coping mechanism for children's reaction to sudden change and losses.
9. Protection against regression and symptom formation: Imaginary companions act as a temporary measure that compensates for a frustrating, difficult external reality and prevents the development of neurosis.
10. Transitional object: Imaginary companions are personified as others on whom children depend but are not present in situations of special stress such as the first day of school.

Modified from Nagera H: The developmental approach to childhood psychopathology, New York, 1981, Jason Aronson, Inc.

---

companions are more intelligent and creative and have a greater waiting ability than those who do not (Manosevitz, 1977). Functions attributed to imaginary companions, depending on the needs of the child who creates them, are presented in the box.

THERAPEUTIC USE OF PLAY AND FANTASY

Not all experts agree that play is an effective therapeutic medium. Some professionals place a high value on verbal interventions and negate the therapeutic use of play and imagination:

1. Psychoanalytic ego psychology: These clinicians focus on material that gives insight into the level of psychosexual development, predominant modality,

sexual-aggressive drive, guilt, object relations and range, strength, and modulation of defenses.

2. Phenomenologic or humanistic-existential theory: Clinicians focus on children's phenomenologic interpretation of their world and their self-concept. Play examination is of little value in this therapeutic model (Axline, 1969; Moustakas, 1959).
3. Behavioral psychology: These clinicians focus on children in real-life situations to identify environmental stimuli and reinforce target behaviors. Diagnostic play evaluations are seldom used (Sattler, 1988).
4. Cognitive theory: Clinicians use play if nonverbal, special equipment is needed to ascertain cognitive constructs. A structured task-oriented interview is used for diagnostic evaluation (Dobbs, 1985).

Play Assessment and Therapy

Play assessment and play therapy is used to discover and resolve problems and is best suited for nonpsychotic children with mental disorders. Play analysis is based on psychoanalytic theories and interprets children's behavior to discover deeply repressed feelings and fixations. Structured or directive play is frequently used in anticipatory play therapy before traumatic hospital procedures and with mentally retarded children. It is used to develop children's ability to learn and understand experience. It is based on learning and communication theories. Unstructured or nondirective play therapy is based on nondirective systems and communication theories and the premise that the less the intrusion, the more children will reveal. Unstructured and structured play are nonthreatening therapeutic methods that encourage emotional expression without the anxiety caused by the inability to verbalize discriptively. The goal of play therapy is to promote separation of fantasy from reality and to help children assimilate reality into their world. Therapists uncover illogical manifestations of play and provide a corrective environment.

GENERAL APPEARANCE

Children's general appearance is evaluated initially and in subsequent sessions. Those with an angry facial expression and body stance may have destructive play behaviors. Apathetic children may display helpless play behavior and require nurses to assist them. Children with a sad, lethargic appearance may lack enthusiasm or interest in play, and hyperactive children will initiate but not complete activities and be easily distracted.

Children using dolls often name them for significant others in their life, and one doll may become a child's projected self. Stressful past, present, or anticipated threatening situations may be played out and children sometimes ask the clinician to play the doll's role. This is an opportunity for the therapists to reflect children's feelings and show empathy, clarify their feelings, and provide insight.

PATTERNS OF RELATEDNESS

Children's patterns of relatedness provide other critical baseline data and may vary in subsequent play session. These patterns occur in play and in informal contacts

before the play session. Examples of patterns of relatedness include the following:
1. Impersonal styles, such as treating others as objects or toys
2. Mechanical, dehumanized patterns
3. Detached, aloof demeanor
4. Maintenance of a safe distance from others
5. Demonstration of a need to control and dominate others, shown in giving others orders during unstructured play
6. Demonstrations of seductiveness and promiscuous behavior

AFFECTS AND ANXIETY

The range and degrees of emotions that children demonstrate are compared with normal age- and stage-appropriate behaviors. Affects include anger, competitiveness, envy, rage, compassion, empathy, affection, warmth, and emotional hunger.

Anxiety is related to emotions, and although it usually is not directly observed, it can be inferred from distress signs and abrupt theme disruptions. Children's anxiety may be due to bodily damage, separation, loss of sense of self or love of another, abandonment, or earlier infant global anxiety.

Assessment of anxiety is based on theme and disruption sequences and formulation of hypotheses about the disruption's precipitating factors. During unstructured play, disruption occurs when children are in a troublesome anxiety-producing situation. They show disorganized thinking or loss of control. They may throw things or may exhibit clinging or dependency behaviors. They may switch activities and carry out the same theme in a less frightening manner. For example, a boy playing a doll family theme may abruptly stop, run to get a toy gun, and then resume the original theme. The child has introduced a new theme—one of violence. Armed, he resumes family play. This disruption and sequence suggests that something has caused the boy to perceive some danger in the play family's activities, because he seemed to feel less anxiety when he was armed and protected. Theme disruption frequently occurs in children whose parents are abusive or are violently argumentative.

PLAY AND SPACE

Children's use of space provides information on the degree of organization of their personality and on the ways in which they experience events—prototaxic, parataxic, or syntaxic. Ideally, children initially observe the environment, move in broad exploration, develop areas of play, and finally synthesize different areas in play themes.

Children who experience events in the prototaxic mode are in the mode of infancy. The environment is experienced globally as a series of events having only momentary meaning—no connections are made between past, present, and future; relationships of cause and effect, and spatial dimensions (Lazaroff, 1962). Severely anxious children exhibit prototaxic behavior, initiating sequential activities unrelated to themes initiated previously. Their use of space is similar to verbalizations of adults in panic states who express unrelated ideas or ideas whose relationship the listener cannot grasp. Psychotic children have involuntary access to a greater parts of their own inner space and that of other persons, and they have diffuse, undifferentiated body boundaries. Their intense anxiety limits their perceptions, and they focus on specific, unrelated details. As anxiety progresses, they disconnect themselves and create autistic worlds (Forrest, 1978). Children with organic deficits display activities that are momentary and lack differentiation. Repetitive actions, blocking, flight of ideas and scattering are common. An example of prototaxis is when children repeatedly ask to be taken to the playroom, though in the playroom. Phobic children may limit their use of space, staying in one corner of the room for the entire session, and hyperactive, distracted children move about the room, impulsively touching everything yet unable to develop or structure spontaneous play.

HELP-SEEKING BEHAVIORS

Many nurses look for connections between words and ideas and between actions and thoughts. When these connections are missing, nurses may become anxious and dismiss their observations as meaningless, thereby denying their importance. Sometimes they assume that they understand the behavior without further exploration.

Often when disruptions occur, nurses respond to tensions with soothing comments and actions. These empathetic responses may limit their ability to objectively assess play behavior. For diagnostic purposes, it is important to note disrupting themes, sequences, degree of disorganization created, and children's ability to reorganize *without* comfort and help (Greenspan and Greenspan, 1981). When children are unable to deal with anxiety, they need to know that the nurse was not upset and that the nurse will listen to them in later sessions.

The assessment of play behavior may suggest that additional psychologic evaluations are necessary to rule out central nervous system immaturity, minimal dysfunctional disorders, or more serious thought disorders. The Bender visual motor gestalt test may verify that children are functioning at an immature level, despite intact physical and neurologic integrity.

Psychotherapeutic Inverventions

NONDIRECTIVE SYSTEMS OF PSYCHOTHERAPY

The assumptions of relationship therapies are that children have currently restrained or unavailable resources within them for growth. The goal is to help children use these resources for healthy growth instead of for self-defeating activities and behaviors. Tenets in the philosophy of relationship therapy include the following (Pothier, 1976):

1. The relationship is the determining aspect of the therapeutic process.
2. The emphasis is on experiencing emotional dynamics not on employing insight or interpretations.
3. The focus is on the dynamics of the here-and-now relationship not past relationships.
4. The creative positive aspects of children's personality are strengthened.
5. Therapy is adapted to individual needs and to changes in children.
6. A major goal is to help children in the constructive management of themselves in therapy and in life situations.

7. Resistance is seen as a positive statement of will striving for independence and as a force to be encouraged, strengthened, and directed.
8. Children are recognized as a social being needing another person or persons for self-realization and development.

DIRECTIVE SYSTEMS OF PSYCHOTHERAPY

Both relationship therapy and directive therapy focus on verbal and nonverbal communication. In directive therapy, however, clinicians use more intrusive direct actions, and confronting interventions are based on Gestalt concepts such as those developed by Perls (1969) to break through defenses. These interventions are done with great care when working with withdrawn or severely disturbed children. Directive methods are best suited for short-term interventions with children who are experiencing developmental or situations problems. Techniques emphasize the use of media or activities that help children become aware of their feelings.

BEHAVIORAL MODIFICATION ADAPTATIONS

Theraplay differs from most forms of child treatment because it uses active physical contact and control. It grew from DesLauriers and Carlson's work (1969) with severely disturbed autistic and psychotic children. Children were forced to acknowledge the presence of the therapist, who, in these interactions, insisted on eye contact and who spoke loudly when ignored. Theraplay techniques have been adapted for use in children with less severe psychologic conditions, psychosocial problems, and retardation and are similar to some infant stimulation techniques.

Brody (1978) adapted DesLauriers' method to children with milder disturbances, renaming it *developmental play*. Both theraplay and developmental play treat children at their developmental rather than chronologic age level. Therapists plan and structure each session, define problems, do not consider clients' opinions, and often act against children's wishes.

While not indicated for all children, these interventions are of special value when working with children with psychosocial problems, early deprivation, and low self-confidence. Parents can easily be taught the structured exercises and activities, thus the approach is useful when training parents to be their child's therapists.

The principles of theraplay assume that a reciprocal interaction fosters children's development and is based on the mother-infant model in which attachment promotes autonomy and each child requires a supportive and stimulating environment to develop normally. The corrective therapeutic experience involves a reexperiencing of the initial environmental context with remediation. Four types of maternal behaviors are used:

1. Structuring: Established limits foster children's learning of body boundaries. Maternal behaviors include defining, forbidding, outlining, reassuring, speaking firmly, clarifying, holding, restraining, and taking charge and responsibility.
2. Challenging: Teasing, daring, encouraging, vocalizing, and encouraging initiation of action foster autonomy and separateness.
3. Intruding: Tickling, bouncing, swinging, and surprising are sensitively controlled so that children are not overstimulated and withdraw.

4. Nurturing: Cuddling, catering, pampering, rocking, feeding, hugging convey acceptance, appreciation, and love through touch, sound, and body contact.

BEHAVIORAL INTERVENTIONS

Split-brain theory. Before split-brain theory was developed by Sperry in 1973, scientists believed that the two hemispheres functioned similarly. Surgical procedures separating the hemispheres have shown that their function and processing works in fundamentally different ways (Ornstein, 1978). Each hemisphere has separate sensations, perceptions, concepts, and impulses to act, with related volitional, cognitive, and learning experiences. The left hemisphere deals with rational material, receptive and expressive language, mathematics, and cognitive data. It processes and arranges all information and places them in the correct order. The right hemisphere perceives the total picture of the puzzle that the left has organized. Right-brain functioning is imagistic, implicative, contextual, and fluid—the home of metaphoric language. It deals with visual and auditory imagery, spatial representation, melodic thought, fantasy, and what scientists call the "emotional components of ongoing thought," that is, the ability to think in images and sounds rather than in words (Edwards, 1979).

Split-brain theory has had a profound impact on many traditional concepts of child development in general and on therapies with children specifically. It isnow suggested that there are many kinds of intelligence, and this may provide many new options for all children, especially those whose IQs are considered biologically limited. Split-brain theory has prompted exploration of new instructional methods and has expanded the focus and rationale for cognitive and behavioral therapies.

Metaphors and hypnotherapy. Erickson developed techniques using indirect forms of communication, which found theoretic rationale in split-brain theory decades after their wide-spread acceptance and clinical application. Erickson noticed that therapy was often impeded by the clients' unwillingness to accept ideas communicated directly by therapists. Indirect methods, he found, were beneficial to clients who were resistant to therapy, and his techniques are widely used.

The metaphor is a symbolic representation that is used to convey an idea indirectly yet more meaningfully. Metaphor's special power with children is that they can intuitively relate to an experience through stories.

Symbols also suggest the presence of meaning beyond the surface appearance. Jung posited that symbols mediated the "entire landscape of psychic life" and are *archetypes,* the inherited elements of human psyche that reflect common patterns of experience throughout history. Archetypes are metaphoric prototypes representing milestones in mankind's evolution and, according to Jung, are expressed in dreams, myths, fairy tales, and stories. They are powerful evokers of emotional responses, awe, and inspiration. Without emotional valences, symbols are meaningless.

Metaphors, anecdotes, and other indirect approaches are essential when dealing with resistance to therapy. Metaphors stimulate the interest of bored children or of those whose concentration lapses. Anecdotes and short stories illustrate important aspects of experiences, suggest solutions to problems, help people recognize themselves and their characteristics, seed ideas and create motivation, and can be used by clinicians to control the therapeutic relationship. They also embed directives, decrease resistance, redefine problems, build the ego, act as a model for communication, remind clients of their own resources, and desensitize people from fears (Barker, 1985).

Neurolinguistic communication theory. When Erickson and Rossi (1980) developed a theoretic explanation for Erickson's use of metaphors, an important link between metaphor, symptoms, physiology, and therapeutic interventions that include play was identified. The theory related the use of the metaphor with brain physiology, specifically, the right brain, which is activated in processing metaphoric types of communication. The right hemisphere is more involved in mediating emotional and imagistic processes, and psychosomatic symptoms are processed by predominantly right-brain functions (Laria, 1973). The neurolinguistic (NPL) theory of communication held that the right-hemispheric mediation of both symptom and metaphorical meaning explained why metaphoric approaches to therapy were less time-consuming than psychoanalytically oriented approaches.

Later, linguists Bandler and Grinder (1975) joined Rossi, and these scientists identified a linguistically-oriented framework to explain the dynamics of Erickson's metaphor use. They claim that the metaphor operates on a triadic principle: The metaphor presents a surface structure of meaning in the actual words of the story; which activates an associated deep structure of meaning that is *indirectly* relevant to the listener; which in turn activates a recovered deep structure of meaning that is *directly* relevant to the listener.

When listeners arrive at the third step, a transderivational search is activated in which they relate the metaphor to themselves, generating the maximally relevant meaning (Bandler and Grinder, 1975).

Application of Erickson's approaches to therapeutic work with children emphasizes creative reframing and unconscious learning. This is a shift in emphasis from traditional psychology of pathology to a psychology and perspective of potential initiated by the therapeutic use of metaphors. Therapeutic metaphors most often used in therapeutic communication with children are listed in the box, and directions for constructing metaphors in child treatment can be found in *Therapeutic Metaphors* (Gordon, 1978), with suggestions for combining the use of metaphors and paradox with traditional therapies. The case example illustrates the use of metaphors in the psychotherapy of a schizophrenic child whose parents were involved in the psychotic process.

Case Example

Yvette was a 12-year-old girl. She was said always to have been shy and quiet, and she had few friends. She was referred for psychiatric assessment at the suggestion of her teacher at school, where Yvette was in a special class. Yvette's academic progress was poor, she had become almost completely socially isolated, and her behavior was becoming increasingly bizarre.

Because of diagnostic uncertainty, Yvette was admitted to a children's psychiatric inpatient unit for assessment. It became clear that she was auditorily hallucinated and also held a number of delusional beliefs. A diagnosis of juvenile schizophrenia was made.

Therapeutic Metaphors

1. Metaphoric stories: Carefully planned stories are developed to achieve major therapeutic goals.
2. Anecdotes and short stories: These are used to make a point or achieve specific goals, and the careful preparation of metaphoric stories is not required. They are not isomorphic with real life situations.
3. Analogies and similes: Common figures of speech, these are useful alternatives to the direct statement of ideas, especially ideas the person being addressed may be reluctant to accept if communicated directly. Knowledge of the person's interest or occupation is useful.
4. Relationship metaphors: The use of one relationship for another through role modeling.
5. Metaphor tasks: These include rituals that help children and families negotiate developmental stages and accomplishes the following:
   a. Removes discrepancies by using behavior in one context that is appropriate and useful in another situation but not in the one being used.
   b. Establishes stability by prescribing rituals to carry out alone, conveying the message that order can replace chaos.
   c. Relabels or reframes by providing a framework in which symptoms are seen as valuable.
   d. Permits symbolic expressions of feelings.
   e. Produces change in family and structures family members' behavior in new ways.
6. Metaphoric objects: Used in play therapy, children express themselves and work though feelings about others.
7. Artistic metaphors: These are productions representing a feeling state or significant experience.

Modified from Barker P: Using metaphors in psychotherapy, New York, 1985, Brunner/Mazel, Inc.

Assessment of the family indicated that the relationship between Yvette and her mother was close and that there was much emotional distance between Yvette and her 10-year-old sister Zoe. The father seemed to play little part in Yvette's life, though he agreed passively with his wife's views about Yvette. Yvette's mother treated her as a very special child who required much care and who could not be expected to do most of the things a normal 12-year-old would do. Yvette was receiving conflicting messages about whether or not she should grow up and become more independent of the parents. They said that she should but demanded little of her and accepted her quiet, withdrawn ways.

Family therapy was recommended, and the parents agreed to this. Progress was at first slow. The parents, led by the mother, seemed reluctant to accept that there was anything wrong with Yvette. They were particularly upset by the suggestion that Yvette was hallucinated. Although they admitted that she had some imaginary friends, the parents insisted that this was not unusual—lots of children had imaginary friends, and Yvette's had just stayed around a little longer than most other children's.

In view of the family's reluctance to accept that Yvette was either hallucinated or deluded, the therapist and team decided to accept the family's view and agreed that Yvette had imaginary friends with whom she talked and who were sometimes a help and a comfort to her. The clinical situation was thus reframed in developmental terms.

Once the view of Yvette's symptoms had been agreed on, a mass of information about Yvette's delusional world emerged. The therapy team also discovered that the mother seemed to know almost as much about the imaginary world as Yvette.

While the parents had been reluctant to accept that Yvette was hallucinated or psychotic, they found it impossible to deny that it would be better for her to have more real friends and fewer imaginary ones. Achieving this therefore became an agreed aim of treatment. A program was developed whereby Yvette was allowed to talk out loud to her imaginary friends only at certain times, and the times when she could discuss them with her mother or other family members were also restricted. These regulations were presented as being a response to Yvette's gradual acquisition of friends at school and a way of encouraging her to make more friends.

Symptoms can themselves be represented metaphorically. This can be helpful when a family or a client refuse to accept the treating professional's view of certain symptomatic behavior. In a sense the parents were involved in the psychotic process. The process of having imaginary friends and then giving them up for real ones became a metaphor for being in a psychotic, delusional world and coming out of it.

Treating psychotic behavior by initially accepting clients' delusional beliefs and then reframing them metaphorically (as when Yvette's symptoms were reframed in developmental terms) may be a therapeutic approach that holds promise. The therapist who wishes to treat a psychotic person using psychotherapy should first obtain a clear mental picture of the client's delusional world. It may then be possible to create a metaphor for the psychotic situation that can be used therapeutically.

Modified from Barker P: Using metaphors in psychotherapy. New York, 1985, Brunner/Mazel, Inc.

Bioinformational theory of imagery.   Clinical imagery studies and imagery research has been based on the assumption that the mind and body are inextricably linked through images and that imagination links the psyche and soma. Many clinical studies are grounded in earlier theories that attributed a neurobiologic basis for fantasy and imagination.

Imagery interventions address the biologic linkage in the brain that integrates physiologic, cognitive, affective, and behavioral responses. Images are defined as "internally constructed perceptual descriptions generated by sensory detection of a stimulus" (Langs, 1980). This definition holds that image formation causes simultaneous physiologic arousal that is coincidental with the context of the image, an assumption also used in NPL programming interventions. Imagery techniques are used to treat disease processes and to promote both physical and mental health. Therapists believe that the millions of scenes, events, conversations, and stories each individual has lived through, read about, heard, or witnessed secondhand are replayed by the brain in daydreams, night dreams, and fantasy.

Therapeutic values of play and imagery emerging from the recent research findings in this area include the following:

1. Imagery helps reduce stress, and when imaging techniques are used in relaxation interventions, there is an organized system of daydreaming and fantasy that usually occurs that is highly therapeutic.
2. Daydreams help children plan a more effective future. If they rehearse actions that they wish to take and review actions taken in the past, they can learn to understand constructive and creative behaviors and develop impulse control.
3. Imagery helps children gain control over undesirable habits. Using relationship therapy and controlled fantasy exercises, problems with overeating, nail-biting, temper tantrums, and other childhood habits have been extinguished.
4. Fantasies help children to be more sensitive to moods and needs of others, and thus are useful in enhancing social skills. The development of empathy requires a trained and active imagination.
5. Imagery and fantasies help children learn more about themselves, and thus enhance self-concepts, body images, and ego.
6. Daydreaming and reminiscing help children to deal effectively with loneliness and boredom. Past accomplishments and experiences can be comforting during periods of challenge, distress, and pain.

Research is being conducted on relaxation and imagery techniques that alleviate medical problems, such as stress, high blood pressure, sleep disorders, and the control of intractable pain. This use has resulted in child mental health clinicians being consulted to apply their knowledge of current split-brain techniques to relieve children's pain through biofeedback, imagery, and fantasy (Zeltzer, LeBaron, and Zeltzer, 1984; Kuttner, 1987). Clinicians need to consider the parameters for ethical decision-making when using new therapies (Busch, 1988; Miller, 1985).

Imagery, daydreams, and imagination are also seen as techniques for solving problems. They free the mind and provide individuals with the opportunity to move back or forward in imagination. Most authorities currently view adult daydreams and fantasy as extensions of children's ability to play and fantasize.

Associated imagery and step-up techniques. Associated imagery is analogous to free association and uses children's stream of consciousness to identify elements of the on-going thought processes. It draws on the unexplained contradictions between irrational thought and fantasy. Fantasy is used in evaluating productive thinking, examining the values and consequences of ideas.

The step-up technique is another intervention that uses imagery for diagnostic purposes, addressing the natural human tendency to resist or deny unpleasant thoughts, images, feelings, and events. With this technique, children transcend situations, face reality, view the stress-creating situation more dispassionately, and deal with it.

THERAPEUTIC INTERVENTIONS WITH PSYCHOTIC CHILDREN

Play therapy with psychotic children is seldom advised. When used, it differs from play therapy in emotionally troubled children because of the former's tendency to withdraw. Psychotic children vacillate between symbiotic and autistic states and often use primary processes employing the creative, imaginary reverie period during which time and space have no impact (Ekstein, 1966). The metaphor is used with psychotic children to facilitate contact with the outer world. Interpretations of the behavior or activities of the clinician may increase psychotic children's need to retreat to their inner world of sameness.

PREVENTIVE PLAY TECHNIQUES

Play therapy techniques have been adapted to classroom and school setting by teachers, and many parents have learned to be *filial* therapists for their child. Therapists have extended self-help concepts so that the children themselves can be taught to become their own play therapist.

Sculpting techniques with children in pediatric units provides nurses an initial experience for developing the skills of play interaction essential for working with children with mental disorders. Play therapy provides children the opportunitiy to integrate physical, emotional, cognitive, and social development and helps them strengthen developmental changes. Children usually terminate their therapy sessions once emotions and feelings are resolved positively.

REFERENCES

Allen FL: Therapy as a living experience. In Moustakas E, editor: Psychotherapy with children, New York, 1970, Ballantine/Del Rey/Fawcett Books.

American Nurses' Association: Standards of child and adolescent psychiatric mental health nursing, Kansas City, Mo, 1982, The Association.

Anthony J: The contributions of child psychoanalysis to psychoanalysis, Psychoanal Study Child 41:61, 1986.

Axline V: Play therapy, New York, 1969, Ballantine/Del Rey /Fawcett Books.

Bandler R and Grinder J: The patterns of the hypnotic techniques of Milton H. Erickson, MD, vol 1, Palo Alto, Calif, 1975, Behavior & Science Books.

Barker P: Using metaphors in psychotherapy, New York, 1985, Brunner/Mazel, Inc.

Barker P: Clinical interviews with children and adolescents, New York, 1990, WW Norton & Co, Inc.

Berne E: Games people play, New York, 1978, Anchor Books.

Bierman KL and Schwartz LA: Clinical child interviews: approaches and developmental considerations, J Child Adolesc Psychother 3:267, 1986.

Bonnard A: A mother as therapist for her obsessive child. In Schaefer CE and Millman HL, editors: Therapies for children, San Francisco, 1978, Jossey-Bass, Inc, Publishers.

Bretherton I and Waters E, editors: Growing points of attachment theory and research, Monographs for the Society for Research in Child Development, No. 209, 1985.

Brody V: Developmental play: a relationship focused program for children, J Child Welfare 57:591, 1978.

Bronfenbrenner V: The ecology of human development, Cambridge, Mass, 1976, Harvard University Press.

Brown DT and Prout HT, editors: Counseling and psychotherapy with children and adolescents, ed 2, Brandon, Vt, 1990, Clinical Psychology Publishing Co, Inc.

Bruner J: Nature and the uses of human development, Am Psychologist 8:687, 1972.

Burlingham D: The fantasy of having a twin, Psychoanal Study Child 1:205, 1945.

Busch D: Ethical decision-making in paradoxical intervention, J Child Adolescent Psychia Ment Health Nurs 1:58, 1988.

Casey RJ and Berman JS: The outcome of psychotherapy with children, Psychol Bull 98:388, 1985.

Chethik M: Techniques of child therapy, New York, 1990, The Guilford Press.

Cousins N: Anatomy of an illness, New York, 1980, Harper & Row Publishers, Inc.

DesLauriers AM and Carlson CE: Your child is asleep: early infantile autism, Homewood, Ill, 1969, The Dorsey Press.

Dobbs JB: A child psychotherapy primer, New York, 1985, Human Sciences Press, Inc.

Edwards B: Drawing on the right side of the brain, Los Angeles, 1979, Jeremy P Tarcher, Inc.

Ekstein R: Children of time, space, of action and impulse, New York, 1966, Appleton-Century-Crofts.

Erikson E: Studies in the interpretation of play, Genetic Psychology Monographs, No.22, 1940.

Erickson M and Rossi E: Two-level commmunication and the microdynamics of trance and suggestion. In Rossi E, editor: The collected papers of Milton H. Erickson on hypnosis, vol 1, New York, 1980, Irvington.

Forrest DV: Spatial play, Psychiatry 41:1, 1978.

Fraiberg S: The magic years, New York, 1959, Scribner Book Co, Inc.

Golden LB: A critical case study of play therapy, J Child Adolesc Psychotherapy 2:286, 1983.

Greenspan S and Greenspan N: The clinical interview of the child, New York, 1981, Basic Books, Inc, Publishers.

Guerney L: Client centered (non-directive) play therapy. In Schaefer CE and O'Conner KJ, editors: Handbook of play therapy, New York, 1983, John Wiley & Son, Inc.

Keats DB: Multimodal therapy with children, New York, 1979, Pergamon Press, Inc.

Kuttner L: Favorite stories: a hypnotic pain reduction technique for children in acute pain, Am J Clin Hypn 6:12, 1987

Laria A: The working brain, New York, 1973, Basic Books, Inc, Publishers.

Lazarus AA: Multimodal behavior therapy, New York, 1976, Springer Publishing Co, Inc.

Manosevitz M, Fling S, and Prentice NM: Imaginary companions in young children: relationhips with intelligence, creativity and waiting ability, J Child Psychol Psychiatry 18:73, 1989.

Miller NE: Some professonal and scientific problems and opportunities for biofeedback, Biofeedback Self-Regulation 10:3, 1985.

Moustakas CE: Psychotherapy with children: the living relationship, New York, 1959, Harper & Row, Publishers, Inc.

Nagera H: The developmental approach to childhood psychopathology, New York, 1981, Jason Aronson, Inc.

Ornstein R: The split and whole brain, Human Nature 1:76, 1978.

Perls F: Gestalt therapy verbatim, Lafayette, Calif, 1969, Real People Press.

Piers MW, editor: Play and development, New York, 1972, WW Norton & Co, Inc.

Pothier PC: Mental health counseling with children, Boston, Mass, 1976, Little, Brown & Co, Inc.

Sattler JM: Assessment of children, ed 3, San Diego, 1988, Jerome M Sattler, Publisher.

Singer JL and Switzer H: Mind-play: the creative use of fantasy, Englewood Cliffs, NJ, 1980, Prentice-Hall, Inc.

Sperry R: Lateral specialization of cerebral function in surgically separated hemispheres. In McGuigan FJ and Schoonover RA, editors: The psychophysiology of thinking, New York, 1973, Academic Press, Inc.

Sroufe LA: The coherence of individual development, Am Psychol 34:834, 1979.

Svendsen M: Children's imaginary companions, Arch Neurol Psychiatry 2:985, 1934.

Thomas A, Chess S, and Birch HG: Temperament and behavior disorders in children, New York, 1968, New York University Press.

Tyson R and Tyson P: The concept of transference in child psychoanalysis, J Am Acad Child Psychiatry 25:30, 1986.

Zeltzer L, LeBaron S, and Zeltzer PM: The effectiveness of behavioral intervention for reducing nausea and vomiting in children and adolescents receiving chemotherapy, J Clin Oncol 2:683, 1984.

Chapter 18

Interventions with Sibling, Peer, and Group Therapies

Patricia Whisonant Brown

Intrapsychic processes and interpersonal experiences are significant factors in psychiatric care. The theories and techniques discussed in this chapter draw on the second group of experiences, the interpersonal experience. Interpersonal experiences move beyond the individual to consider the social environment and its impact on children. The following interventions focus on sibling and peer experiences in individual and group situations.

Theoretic Considerations

Children with ego deficits are delayed in their development, because of the separation-individuation process. This process begins with children's differentiation from their mother and progresses to the development of independent object relations. The degree of developmental delay, their age, and their stage of development must be considered when choosing a treatment technique.

OBJECT RELATIONS THEORY

Object relations theory focuses on the individuation process between the emerging self and the object or significant other. Good object relations are important in the development of a clear sense of self, and each stage of development has an important function (Kohut, 1977; Mahler, 1966; Winnicott, 1964). Interventions that focus on the correction of problems grounded in the first three stages are best when they are one-to-one and when they concentrate on fulfilling object consistency needs.

In the first phase, from birth to 4 months, the *autistic* and *symbiotic* subphases occur, and a part-object relationship with the mother exists. That is, children lack a boundary concept of their mother. They bond with a part of the mother, such as her face, and believe they can recreate the partial object, by simply desiring it. In the first phase, therapists' task is to provide constancy and to be present and supportive to facilitate bonding and, through the therapeutic alliance, to help them progress to the second phase.

The symbiotic subphase occurs between 4 and 6 months of age. During this differentiation, children's body image shifts from an introspective focus to a sense of body periphery awareness. This new awareness is a requirement for body-ego formation and a full sense of self (Mahler, 1966). The therapeutic task is to help establish boundaries and diminish children's fears of loss.

The next phase is the separation-individuation phase, which is life's major conflict — the longing for autonomy versus the urge to stay fused with the mother. The degree to which the child (or client with the therapist) resolves the conflict determines the extent to which they can go through life without pathologic consequences.

Once anxiety has been mastered, the basis for the next stage of ego development, the interpersonal interaction stage, can occur. At this point of the normal developmental sequence, the mother's role becomes less prominent, and object relations expand to include the father and siblings if present. If there are no siblings in the home, then peers take on a greater role. Children's relationships with parents and siblings are called *primary object relationships,* and relationships to peers are referred to as *secondary transference relationships*.

The relationship with siblings provides a bridging relationship between the family and the world. At this point, therapists' role is less dominant. If children are receiving inpatient therapy, peer interactions become primary group peer therapy is the treatment of choice. If receiving outpatient therapy, children participate in group and individual psychotherapy, with peer interaction processing included in the group's discussions.

After the age of 5 to 6, people outside the family are increasingly important and gradually become central to children. This decade-long shift in relationships should be well underway by the age of 20. The way in which individuals relate to other people is a central personality characteristic, and peer interaction therapy is an essential component of a comprehensive treatment plan. Children are especially receptive to the group and peer intervention techniques that restructure their inadequate and immature object constancy.

Sibling Therapy

Sibling therapy is an innovative therapeutic technique that draws on family subsystem theory. Child psychiatry has historically emphasized the mother-child bond and only recently has the sibling bond been viewed as a contributing factor that provides a special influential relationship within the family.

The first egalitarian relationship that children encounter involves a sibling. In a culture that is increasingly peer oriented and less hierarchical, sibling relationships are the most powerful and enduring intimate connections experienced (Kahn and Lewis, 1988). The enduring sibling bond emphasizes the pervasive roles siblings play in individual personality development (Furman and Buhrmester, 1985).

Research and clinical studies. Analysts have relegated sibling relationships to a secondary role and have given them only a cursory discussion. Some psychoanalysts have included siblings in their theories, stressing their roles as rivals for the mother's love or as parent surrogates (Raser, 1985). Mahler (1966) was one of the first child psychoanalysts to highlight instances of pathologic mother-child relationships in which siblings gained support from each other, and he also made important distinctions between sibling envy, rivalry, and jealousy that are used in contemporary sibling therapy. These three emotions exist on a continuum: *Sibling envy,* which is normal, occurs between two in the dyad and usually when the younger child wishes for the older child's genetically determined traits (such as brown eyes or blond hair) or developmentally different traits (such as achievement in athletics or body [breast] development). *Sibling rivalry,* in contrast, involves three people and is the competition of two siblings for the attention of the preferred parent. Sibling rivalry is also an expected healthy reaction. When one sibling perceives that the other has attained the special love of the parent permanently, *pathologic jealousy* develops.

The importance of sibling roles in personality development was reintroduced into psychoanalytic theory with the Yale longitudinal studies (Solnit, 1983). The conclusions indicated that excluding the role of siblings in psychoanalysis was a serious omission and that sibling roles were significant in personality development. The inclusion of sibling relations broadens and extends the psychoanalytic perspective and provides a new perspective on family subsystems' effect on personality development.

Several developmentalists have studied the effect of sibling relationships on life change adjustment and mate selection. Linton (1967) stressed that sibling relationships affected the choice of marital partner, and Wallerstein (1985) found that children with siblings adjusted better to divorce than children without siblings.

The seminal work of Adler, Toman, and Perlmutter (1988) on birth order's influence on personality development stimulated initial research interest in sibling relationships. These influences are referred to as *structural variables* (Furman, 1982). Alfred Adler (1920) was one of the earliest family constellation researchers to observe family roles. These initial observations were further expanded and systematized by Toman (1969). Toman's research focused on the influence of birth order on the personality structure of the developing child within the family system. His theory correlates the personality characteristics of children to birth order, marriage compatibility, and success in later parent and family constellations.

Incorporating Eric Erikson's psychosocial model of development, Perlmutter (1988) used a theoretic perspective based on birth order dynamics. His findings challenged many popular accepted misconceptions, such as behaviors attributed to the first or last children (Hoopes and Harper, 1987).

After studies of structural variables, another hypothesis was introduced, which held that the qualities of sibling relationships are probably not exclusively—or even primarily determined by the structural variables (Furman and Buhrmester, 1985).

Characteristics of a Healthy Sibling Relationship

Dominance by/of sibling	Affection
Nurture by/of sibling	Admiration by/of sibling
Aggression/antagonism	Companionship
Intimacy	Competition
Similarity	Prosocial behavior
Parental partiality	Quarreling

Modified from Furman W and Buhrmester D: Children's perception of the qualities of sibling relationships, Child Dev 56:2, 1985.

Scientists supporting this hypothesis focused on studying the quality instead of the structure of sibling relationships. They felt it incorrect to explain family constellation effects solely in terms of their impact on the qualities of sibling relationships. Structural or constellation variables affect the sibling relationship as do parent-child relations and marital relations.

Nursing Interventions

ASSESSMENT

Brothers and sisters can be a source of frequent companionship, help, or emotional support. In some instances, older siblings can compensate somewhat for absent or distant parents. In their many interactions with each other, siblings may acquire many of the social and cognitive skills important to healthy development. The specific influence varies considerably because of diversity in the qualities or characteristics of sibling relationships. Characteristics of a healthy sibling relationship found by Furman and Buhrmester are shown in the box, and a model of normal sibling relationships is shown in Figure 18-1.

INDICATIONS FOR SIBLING THERAPY

Lewis's description (1988) of situations may be helpful to nurse clinicians working with siblings in joint sessions. When there is a problem between the siblings or when parents and siblings have shared the experience of a crisis, Lewis recommends that clinicians interview the siblings separately for the identified problem and then resume family therapy. With a family that has no structure, she recommends that only the siblings be counseled because of the parents' inability to relate to the family system emotionally.

Problems that arise from the relationship between siblings range from severe sibling antagonism to pseudotogetherness. This reaction may be a response to family dynamics. However, the siblings' problem needs to be dealt with first to alleviate the symptoms before further progress can be achieved.

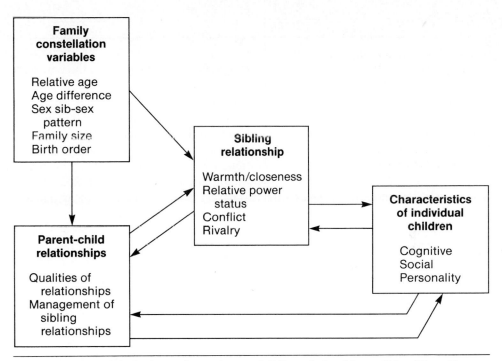

Figure 18-1   Model of primary determinants of sibling relationship qualities. (From Furman W and Buhrmester D: Children's perception of the qualities of sibling relationships, Child Dev 56:2, 1985.)

Lewis also discusses the use of sibling therapy when the family does not directly express concern over sibling interactions but is concerned with the children's failure at productive peer relationships. If a sibling is not being accepted by peers and is fighting at school, sibling sessions can draw on the strengths of the better adjusted sibling to provide role modeling and feedback of more appropriate peer inter-actions.

When a family is in crisis, the members are initially seen together, and later each subsystem is seen until the crisis is alleviated. For example, in a divorce, siblings usually benefit from discussing their conflict together without the parents' presence.

When there is no stable family structure, children need a sense of family belonging, even if they are separated and in foster homes. For example, when a severely depressed and dysfunctional mother is emotionally unavailable to the siblings, they can bond through the therapeutic process and supply the family attachment needed for healthy survival. When a sibling is in crisis, such as one caused by a diagnosis of a life-threatening illness or when a sibling has a severe problem, such as depression or substance abuse, sibling therapy can help provide the necessary support. The case example illustrates the dynamics of a dysfunctional family producing pathologic jealousy.

Case Example

Mr. and Mrs. Frank brought 10-year-old Paul and 12-year-old Bruce for admission to an inpatient psychiatric unit. The parents' major complaint was that the boys were out of control. Mrs. Frank, who had been discharged from her second psychiatric hospitalization (for attempting suicide 2 weeks earlier), reported that Mr. Frank could hardly manage the boys during her absence. Mr. Frank said that he had expected things to calm down after his wife's return home; however, the boys' acting out and fighting became progressively worse. The decision to request hospitalization of their sons was made when Mr. Frank caught his sons in homoerotic activity.

Bruce had been in another short-term inpatient psychiatric facility, with a diagnosis of adjustment disorder with psychoses. This was Paul's first psychiatric hospitalization. The parents reported that Bruce's self-care had deteriorated since the mother was hospitalized. He was neglecting to bathe and was passively expressing his defiance in other self-negating behaviors. Paul's reaction, in contrast, was a serious bicycle accident that resulted in an inguinal hernia. Paul had a history of bicycle accidents in which he acted out his self-destructive impulses, and he was being more defiant and direct in expressing his anger toward his parents.

Initial psychologic screening showed that Paul and Bruce were in a sadomasochistic relationship and that the patterns indicated increased enmeshing with the parents, particularly to gain attention from them. The psychologist's impression was that Paul maintained a superficial facade of adequate function that masked an intense affective disturbance emerging covertly in his responses to projective tests in the psychologic testing protocol. Bruce's psychologic tests indicated an underlying primary thought-process disorder.

The parents also had psychologic problems. The mother had recently been hospitalized, there was a history of alcohol addiction, and the father was on medication to control his temper.

Bruce and Paul were both admitted to the unit, and each was assigned to a different team and to different primary therapists. It was expected that different primary therapists would alleviate their intense rivalry and promote treatment.

Paul had difficulty adjusting to the unit, and although he expressed concern about his brother, he also manipulated Bruce and evoked his anger, creating yet another situation in which Bruce would receive negative attention and Paul would be the innocent victim and elicit positive responses from the staff. When the boys were admitted, marital sessions were initiated, and during this time, the parents were more concerned about Bruce than Paul. When asked about this, both boys said that their parents had been more concerned about Bruce for some time. This parental preference further intensified the rivalry and became a serious staff concern.

The staff decided to transfer Bruce to another treatment setting after considerable efforts failed to dilute the disruptive rivalry. Since Paul was the younger of the two brothers, had not been previously treated, and was functioning more congruently with the other clients, he remained.

After Bruce left the unit, Paul identified more with his male primary therapist and became engaged in that therapeutic alliance. Bruce completed the 3-month short-term treatment and returned to live with his parents, stabilized on medications.

The marital sessions changed slowly, and after about 6 months of weekly sessions, the parents revealed that Bruce was their preferred child. They attributed this preference to Mr. Frank's hesitancy about having a second child. When Paul was born, Mr. Frank distanced himself from Paul and became aligned with Bruce. In response, Mrs. Frank became more protective of Paul to compensate. As the parents' treatment progressed and as they became aware of the implications of their preferences, the nurse identified the need for Paul to have sibling sessions with Bruce before joining the family sessions to strengthen the sibling subsystem and bonds and to decrease the sibling rivalry.

During the sibling sessions, the boys were able to discuss their awareness of the parental preferences and the ways they used it against each other. After several months of sibling therapy, they were able to discuss the extreme jealousy that each experienced. As the nature of their relationship changed from rivalry to supportive bonding, they could actively cooperate in activities. They completed play tasks by interacting, they collaboratively built card houses, they communicated while watching sports on television together, and they discussed different points of view without violent outbursts.

Once these bonds had strengthened, Bruce became more angry with his parents and seemed to bond intensely with Paul. Back at home, he was reluctant to participate with his parents without his brother being present. He seemed to co-exist with his parents at home and developed several satisfactory peer relationships as he entered adolescence.

The first step toward involving the total family in joint therapy was to place Paul and his mother in dydactic therapy. During these sessions, Paul expressed his guilty feelings for being preferred and overprotected by his mother, his fear of losing her from her attempted suicide and her alcohol abuse, and his concern that his mother had intensified her protective and unconscious persistent physical stimulation — hugging, touching, and kissing — which had become more distressing to him as he neared puberty.

Several months later, Paul began sessions with his father. In these sessions he expressed his feelings of estrangement and pain. After this issue was resolved, Bruce joined these sessions — but was no longer seen as the preferred child. At first, Bruce was distressed by the displacement, but Paul was delighted to be preferred by his father. However, after several sessions of preferential treatment, Paul realigned with Bruce.

Finally, the sessions included the mother. The reunion of the family was based on the careful reconstruction of the family constellation, with the parental system and sibling subsystem revised. To solidify this reconstructed family, therapists held a family session in which family members discussed their view of the interactive process within the total system and within the subsystem.

MANAGEMENT

When more than one child in a family requires psychiatric hospitalization, siblings should ideally be treated in the same treatment setting. This allows clinicians to use the presence and participation of the other sibling(s) for whom these dynamics apply and who are important to another's ego development. Sibling relationships have powerful dynamics since siblings are important transference objects. When these relationships are tapped into and guided as the children progress in their developmental course, their influence can result in remarkable therapeutic changes in individual, sibling, and family dynamics. However, these powerful dynamics can interfere with earlier developmental problems that must be resolved first before the sibling or peer issues can be dealt with therapeutically.

The priorities in sibling treatment are to provide each child with necessary individual treatment in the milieu, and to have a milieu that can control and manipulate the primary transference sibling dynamic. The therapeutic goal is to implement age-appropriate and individualized care that allows each sibling to work on unique separation-individuation issues.

When siblings are treated in the same milieu, the major concern is to ensure that the staff does not separate out and show preferences. One clinician needs to be responsible for the overall case management. However, each child needs to have a different therapist to reenact earlier developmental transferences and distortions. Each has such intensified jealousy that no one therapist could perceive the distortions correctly. Supervision of the therapists to monitor transference and countertransference is essential.

The initiation of martial sessions allows the bond between parents to be explored and strengthened so that they do not need to draw a sibling into their dynamics. The triangle is the basic unit of an emotional system, that is, a twosome and an outsider. When tension is experienced, each person will try to include the outsider (the Bowen System Theory).

NURSING DIAGNOSIS

The case example clearly illustrates the nursing diagnosis of *altered family process*. NANDA has also listed *altered role performance* and *altered growth and development* as diagnoses that may be appropriate for dysfunctional sibling relationships.

Examples of cases where altered role performance may be the appropriate nursing diagnosis would include situations in which a sibling is attempting or has taken over a parental (pseudoadult) role in the family, or where the younger sibling is upstaging the older sibling's position. The role confusion and family subsystem problems will need to be addressed if the family becomes dysfunctional or if a family member cannot tolerate this family system dynamic. Role changes and confusion are frequently seen in families of alcoholics when *enabling* by different family members occurs.

The altered growth and development diagnosis applies when the sibling and child roles are replaced by a parental role. It may also be appropriate when excessive sibling rivalry and aggression prevents the child's maturation and independence development or prevents the child's learning to control aggressive impulses.

Sibling incest. Aggression in the family often takes the form of sexual abuse. While father-daughter incest is the most studied and reported, sibling incest is considered to be more common (though also more underreported) (Gilbert, 1989). While some experts view it as nonabusive and not serious, sibling incest can prevent normal sexual and emotional maturation (Russell, 1986).

Bank and Kahn (1982) stated that the high accessibility of siblings to each other and the parents' inability to meet the needs of the children are preconditions for incestuous sibling relationships. Although the specific motivation underlying sibling incest is not clear and the duration and configuration of the incestuous relationship can vary, they have described two general types of sibling incest: *power-oriented, aggressive incest* and *nurturing, loving incest.*

Sibling therapy involves reinstatement of the incest barrier by reorganizing the family structure, reducing unsupervised sibling access, fostering the parent-child bond, helping the victimized sibling resolve feelings involved, and teaching the offending sibling other ways to fulfill needs and impulses. As the sibling relationship is reestablished, they can move forward in their development.

SUMMARY

As the theoretic writings and the case study illustrate, families whose constellations include more than a single offspring add specific and different dynamics to the family system. The sibling relationship begins in early childhood, aids in personality growth, and may be one of the most enduring, powerful, and available therapeutic bonds.

Peer Therapy

For many years the prevailing source of theory building to explain the etiology and dynamics of mental illness was the study of parent-child relationships. This continued for several decades after Freud's work. The significance of the association between childhood peer relationships and later mental health first appeared as unexpected findings in studies in which many possible variables were viewed. Cowen and others (1973) showed that other children could identify peers who would later become mentally ill better than adults. They also showed that children's perceptions of ways in which others viewed them were accurate.

Interactions of withdrawn and aggressive children and other peer interaction patterns have been studied. These studies suggest that specific difficulties in peer relationships during childhood may be associated with specific diagnoses for mental illness during adulthood, but the exact relationship is still unclear (Crockett, 1984). In general, it is thought that the long-term prognosis for children who have antisocial behavior was much worse than that for children who were shy, withdrawn, or overanxious and that children with close stable friendships had higher self-esteem than their classmates who did not have such friendships.

Mental health professionals, child care workers, teachers, and other professionals who are responsible for assessing the normal development of children have the primary task of evaluating and fostering age-appropriate peer-peer interaction (Grunebaum and Solomon, 1980). Asher, Hymel, and Renshaw (1984) developed an assessment tool to measure loneliness as compared to popularity with peers (see box).

PEER RELATIONSHIPS

Throughout life humans tend to seek out companionship with peers of the same generation and sex. Friendship, one of the most sought after experiences, is frequently more enduring than marital or sexual relationships.

Asher Assessment Tool

1. It is easy for me to make friends at school.
2. I like to read.*
3. I have nobody to talk to in class.
4. I am good at working with other children in my class.
5. I watch television a lot.*
6. It is hard for me to make friends at school.†
7. I like school.*
8. I have lots of friends in my class.
9. I feel alone at school.†
10. I can find a friend in my class when I need one.
11. I play sports a lot.†
12. It is hard to get kids in school to like me.†
13. I like science.*
14. I do not have anyone to play with at school.†
15. I like music.*
16. I get along with my classmates.
17. I feel left out of things at school.†
18. There are no other kids I can go to when I need help in school.†
19. I am lonely at school.†
20. I am well liked by the kids in my class.
21. I like playing board games a lot.*
22. I do not have any friends in class.†

Modified from Asher SR, Hymel S, and Renshaw PD: Loneliness in children, Child Dev 55:1457, 1984.
* Items classified as hobby or interest items.
† Items for which response order was reversed for scoring.

Peer relationships occur in a developmental sequence, and play interaction is the primary peer activity. In comparison, sibling friendships frequently overlap in this area, but sibling relationships show a more intense bonding, and their significance ranges beyond peer interaction to the interlocking roles within a dynamic family system.

However, peers do add dynamics to children's growth and development. They foster the ability to know friend from foe, find and maintain position in social hierarchies, handle aggression, conduct adult heterosexual relationships, and finally, cooperate with others in tasks necessary for survival (Grunebaum and Solomon, 1980).

To evaluate the quality and age appropriateness of peer relationships, clinicians must be aware of developmental milestones. Some questions that should be considered when assessing the individual child include the following (Stuart and Sundeen, 1987):

1. Are relationships formed with children whose ages are near the child's age?
2. Are these relationships with the same sex or opposite sex children?
3. What is the child's position in the power structure of the group?

4. How easily does the child approach other children and get along with them?
5. Does the child have a best friend?
6. Is the child able to interact at the age-appropriate development phase?

Developmental Sequence

Toddlerhood. The steps identified as the developmental sequence involved in toddlers' peer interactions are: (1) simple object-centered contacts (age 10 to 14 months), (2) peer-oriented contacts (ages 12 to 20 months), and (3) complex sustained interactions (ages 18 to 30 months). The advance to the second step occurs when children maintain interactions in the absence of toys. In the third step the advancement of skills centers around children's abilities to take complementary roles; for example, throwing a ball to one another (Mueller and Lucas, 1975).

Grunebaum and Solomon (1982) emphasized the following aspects of these early peer relationships: First, peer relationships are fostered by good parental relationships. Second, objects, toys, food, music, and social settings can facilitate peer relationships. Third, friendships at this stage are formed on the basis of shared interest in particular objects and near-equal skill level. At this age, they also cannot distinguish between the subjective and objective aspects of behavior, that is, intentional versus accidental behavior.

Preschool children. The play of preschool children builds on the skills developed during the toddler years. The beginnings of friendships established in the toddler period is marked by ambivalence at age 3 to 4 years. Children's resentment of siblings is contrasted by feelings of tenderness and protection. Best friends can also become worst enemies and return to best friends overnight.

Garvey and Hogan (1973) described the next developmental sequence that occurs when children reach the age of 4. This phase is characterized by mutual response to peers and the ability to adapt words and actions to those of playmates. It is during this time that children begin to view playmates as individuals instead of objects. This finding further increases children's wish to bond with peers. When able to choose interactional activities, they tend to be more interested in dramatic play rather than art, music, or table games. It is also during this time that aggression becomes modulated and socialized.

At approximately age 3 to 4, imaginary companions are frequently verbalized. It is interesting to note, however, that the use of imaginary friends is most frequently seen in the oldest child or the only child (Manosevitz, Prentice, and Wilson, 1973).

These two stages in which peer relationships are being established are characterized by the supervision of adults. Children are learning to differentiate their feelings from those of others. However, they will still define a close friend as someone who performs the activities that they want to do (Grunebaum and Solomon, 1982). Perhaps the most striking characteristic of this period is that children are rarely involved in solitary play (Garvey, 1977).

Middle childhood. By the age of 5 to 6 years, communication ability increases and egocentrism decreases. This allows children to develop social skills and interactions quickly.

By this time, children do not choose friends by availability alone but instead are seeking out peer experiences. They wish to understand others and have others understand them. Frequently in this age group, two children link up as best friends, leaving out a third friend.

Latency-age friendships are also laced with difficulties. Friendship pairing can change frequently, and scapegoating or aggressive attacks are seen. This particular peer dynamic occurs because morality and values are emerging. The superego's development of strict limit guidelines produces anxiety and guilt, and projection onto peers is a way of managing these feelings.

Cognitive ability has matured so that children can manage a series of purposive activities, and the superego development allows acceptance of the rules of structured games. Children gain reassurance from the friendship obtained from sharing this purposeful activity with others.

By the age of 8 to 9 years, children perceive school's main purpose as an opportunity to contact with friends. A shift from activity sharing to interest in friends' personalities occurs during this time. Friendships are generally made between children of the same sex, and there is much overt verbal hostility between boys and girls. By 9 to 10 years of age, each child has developed a strong sense of the attributes of fairness in a companionship.

Preadolescents. Cliques and gangs are ways this age group shows its profound need for peer relationships and acceptance. Parents will frequently see their child defending a peer against parental criticism, an important growth step for a child.

Children greatly fear rejection by the group and long for acceptance into a peer circle. They learn to defend themselves from the anxiety of rejection and from actual peer attack to form peer relationships. Friends often give each other presents and may join secret societies or clubs.

Perhaps the most significant developmental milestone during this time, is the attainment of a best friend. This usually occurs at 10 or 11 years of age. A best friend is defined as a friend of the same sex who shares innermost feelings and fantasies. Although this best friendship is less transient than prior developmental phases, it also may end abruptly. However, the exclusiveness and sharing that this relationship provides is an important rehearsal for the more permanent and enduring intimacy to be shared with others later in life (Weiner and Elkind, 1972).

Group Therapies

Play therapy groups of five or six members are useful for children with behavior problems such as impulse control, expressions of aggression, autonomy, regression, and sibling rivalry. Using a group of children who are heterogeneous or homogeneous depends on the developmental task and stage.

The group process that occurs with child participants has been compared to projective tests: the material is alive and multidimensional, and each child actively participates. The more the members participate in the process, the more likely the therapeutic changes. The process requires involvement, and interactions ideally accomplish the following:

1. Develop more positive self-concepts
2. Increase frustration tolerance
3. Delay gratification
4. Promote verbalization rather than acting-out of feelings
5. Develop acceptable outlets for aggression expression
6. Help children become comfortable in the structure of a group
7. Improve peer relationships

Other members of the group act as models and suggest alternatives to present behaviors. Nurses may point out a child's behavior to the other children, asking for better ways of problem solving. The group grows and shares as it learns. The group also helps the child apply new learning in a peer interaction setting, and provides guidance during the accommodation process.

The way children interact within a group plays a powerful role in forming and influencing societal behaviors of individuals, and in shaping individuals' identities. Peer relationships have been shown to be the most important prognostic factor in the long-term outcome of children and adolescents with emotional disorders (Sundby and Keyberg, 1969).

Yalom (1985) has studied the importance of member-to-member cohesion for successful group therapy, and his research suggests that member-to-member comments are often the most important and most helpful, according to group members' feedback. Children are often referred for group therapy because of their inability to relate to others.

In Grunebaum and Solomon's (1980) peer paradigm, the group facilitator's task is to foster sequential growth in peer relationship and group formation. The group leader should show the group the way individual fantasies, multiple transferences, defenses against trust or intimacy, and choice of a particular role in the group relate to social development. This peer theory then would suggest that while transference to the group facilitator may be dealt with in the early stages of the group process for the individual, in the later stages the facilitator should treat it as a form of resistance to group formation.

The DSM-III-R does not reflect a developmental paradigm that emphasizes peer socialization. Grunebaum and Solomon (1980) state that if they did, referral to groups would be more effective and practitioners would ask more frequently about childhood and adult peer relationships, important friendships, and the influence of siblings. Once an assessment is completed, group techniques can be attempted to improve peer interactions.

DANCE/MOVEMENT THERAPY

Dance may be the most fundamental way to directly express self through body movements. Dance/movement therapy is based on the assumption that the body and the mind are interrelated. The technique is appropriate for group and individual sessions. Therapists work directly on a body level with individuals who are unable to relate to their environment or communicate in a normal manner.

Emotional disturbance is often observable in movement behavior. For example, schizophrenia is reflected in clients' fragmented gestures and postures. Depressed clients may display flaccidity and immobility. Therapists work directly with clients, connecting the body movement with internal feelings and defenses. Emphasis is placed on safety so that charged emotions can be expressed and clients can reintegrate at a higher level.

By linking children's movement patterns to developmental levels, clinicians can determine the fixation or regression point when growth was first inhibited.* Attributes of tension flow, shape flow, directional shaping, and other body movement can be interpreted psychodynamically to show successful object-relationship attainment.

Infants, children, and adolescents share the phenomenon of a rapidly changing body with which to experience and understand the outside world. Because of dance/movement's emphasis on nonverbal body-level communication, it can treat Down's syndrome, blindness, deafness, and developmental delay. Therapists may include parents and siblings to create healthier interactions and therefore improve object relations.

Autistic children can also benefit greatly from this technique. Therapists can use body movement to make contact and form a relationship. Children with organic impairments or learning disabilities can benefit from the use of intact abilities.

OTHER PEER THERAPIES

Other therapies that involves the use of play and peer interactions are used to encourage children to develop satisfying recreational, normal peer interests, and skills. Activities can include athletics, dancing, arts and crafts, music, and camping. Major techniques include mutual drawing and painting, mutual storytelling, puppets, formal games, and music.

The use of drawing and painting allows interaction so that children can express inner reality and outer reality (DiLeo, 1973). In mutual drawing, therapists and children interact by means of the drawing, especially useful when verbal interaction is impossible.

Mutual storytelling can also be used to express children's feelings. The story is the vehicle for communication. Children tell a story, and the therapist privately interprets the psychodynamic meaning and reframes the story with healthier coping strategies or perceptions (Gardner, 1971). It is also useful to combine drawings and storytelling.

Puppets can be useful, especially with children who feel they are too old to play with toys. Through make-believe characters, thoughts that clients cannot state directly can be expressed.

Formal games are themselves expressions of communication. The type of game Therapists schedule, the rules that are given and followed, and the process by which clients win or lose initiate important peer interactions. Formal games are divided into games of physical skills (basketball), games of chance (card games or bingo), and games of strategies (chess).

---

* American Dance Therapy Association brochure, 2000 Century Plaza, Suite 108, Columbia, Md, 21044.

SUMMARY

Interventions in psychiatric care frequently draw on the interactional, interpersonal process of an individual. This chapter has attempted to outline the theoretic considerations and application to interventions using sibling therapy and peer therapy, including group, dance/movement, recreational, and creative therapies.

REFERENCES

Adler A: The practice and theory of individual psychology, ed 2, Totowa, NJ, 1973, Littlefield (originally published in 1920; translated by P Radin).

Asher SR, Hymel S, and Renshaw PD: Loneliness in children, Child Dev 55:1457, 1984.

Bank SP and Kahn MD: The sibling bond, New York, 1982, Basic Books, Inc, Publishers.

Cowen EL and others: Long-term follow-up of early detected vulnerable children, J Consult Clin Psychol 41:438, 1973.

Crockett MS: Exploring peer relationships, J Psychosoc Nurs Ment Health Serv 10:18, 1984.

DiLeo JH: Children's drawings as diagnostic aids, New York, 1973, Brunner/Mazel, Inc.

Dunn J: Sibling relationships in early childhood, Child Dev 4:79, 1983.

Furman W and Buhrmester D: Children's perception of the qualities of sibling relationships, Child Dev 56:2, 1985.

Gardner R: Therapeutic communication with children: the mutual storytelling technique, New York, 1971, Science House.

Garvey C: The developing child, Cambridge, Mass, 1977, Harvard University Press.

Garvey C and Hogan R: Social speech and social interaction: ego-centrism revisited, Child Dev 44:562, 1973.

Grunebaum H and Solomon L: Toward a peer theory of group psychotherapy I: on the developmental significance of peers and play, Int J Group Psychother 30:23, 1980.

Grunebaum H and Solomon L: Toward a theory of peer relationships, II: on the stages of social development and their relationship to group psychotherapy, Group Psychother 3:32, 1982.

Hoopes M and Harper J: Birth order roles and sibling patterns in individual and family therapy, Rockville, Md, 1987, Aspen Publishers, Inc.

Kahn M and Lewis K: Siblings in therapy: lifespan and clinical issues, New York, 1988, WW Norton & Co, Inc.

Kohut H: The restoration of the self, New York, 1977, International Press.

Lewis CR: Listening to children, New York, 1985, Jason Aronson, Inc.

Lewis K: Young siblings in brief therapy. In Kahn M and Lewis K, editors: Sibling in therapy, New York, 1988, WW Norton and Co, Inc.

Linton JA: A psychoanalytic view of the family, Psychoanal Forum 3:10, 1967.

Mahler MS: Notes on the development of basic moods, New York, 1966, International Universities Press.

Manasevitz M, Prentice NM, and Wilson F: Individual and family correlates of imaginary companions in preschool children, Dev Psychol 82:72, 1973.

Mueller E and Lucas J: Developmental analyses of peer interaction among toddlers. In Lewis M and Rosenblum A, editors: Friendships and peer relations, New York, 1973, John Wiley & Sons, Inc.

Perlmutter M: Enchantment of siblings: effects of birth order and trance on family myth. In Kahn M and Lewis K, editors: Sibling in therapy, New York, 1988, WW Norton and Co Inc.

Raser S: On the place of siblings in psychoanalysis, Psychol Rev 72:3, 1985.

Russell DSH: The secret trauma, New York, 1986, Basic Books, Inc, Publishers.

Solnit A: The sibling experience, Psychoanal Study Child 38:281, 1983.

Stuart G and Sundeen S: Principles and practice of psychiatric nursing, ed 3, St Louis, 1987, The CV Mosby Co.

Sundby H and Keyberg P: Prognosis in child psychiatry, Baltimore, 1969, William & Wilkins.

Toman W: Family constellation: theory and practice of a psychological game, New York, 1969, Springer Publishing Co, Inc.

Wallerstein J: Children of divorce: preliminary report of a ten year follow-up of older children and adolescents, J Am Acad Child Psych 245:545, 1985.

Weiner I and Elkind D: Child development: a core approach, New York, 1972, John Wiley & Sons, Inc.

Winnicott DW: The child, the family and the outside world, New York, 1964, Penguin Books.

Yalom I: The theory and practice of group psychotherapy, New York, 1985, Basic Books, Inc, Publishers.

Chapter 19

Psychiatric Hospitals, Milieu, and Hospital Treatment Programs

Patricia Whisonant Brown
Patricia Clunn

Statistics indicate that children currently have the highest rate increases in mental disorders. The Institute of Medicine (1988) estimates that 7.5 million children (12% of the 63 million children under the age of 18) suffer from one or more mental disorders. Other studies estimate that 70% to 80% of the children that require mental health services do not receive them (U.S. Office of Technology Assessment, 1986). It is projected that between 1980 and 2005, an increase in child mental health disorders is likely. The absence of effective prevention techniques will result in these disorders continuing into adulthood (Chamberlain, 1988).

The NIMH reports that since World War II, the age of onset of mental disorders has continued to decrease, and the 1980 census reflected this trend. In addition, these forecasts were made before the reversal in birth rate trends that occurred in the 1980s. At that time, the steady birthrate decline of the 1960s suddenly stopped, and the birth rate has increased annually. In 1988, the National Center for Health Statistics reported that every day, 10,721 babies were born, of which 10% to 15% will require mental health services in the next 5 to 10 years (Chamberlain, 1988).

The increased incidence of children's mental disorders could be due to the social and cultural turmoil of the past few decades that has been characterized by a loss of traditional family values, economic austerity, and diminishing public support of many institutions such as medicine and psychiatry. Experts cite the federal fiscal cutbacks in money to mental health; the shift from federal to state funding of psychiatric facilities and training; and the changes in health care reimbursement policies, such as the implementation of DRGs to explain the diminishing preventative focus and resultant increase in serious psychiatric problems (English and others, 1986). Others emphasize more biologic reasons—from the increased viral infections and the prevalence of poor nutrition to the mental and physical health epidemics such as AIDS and drug abuse.

Child psychiatric hospitals have been overextended for decades. Many states with insufficient available hospital beds have sent children elsewhere for inpatient treatment. The National Mental Health Association (1989) reported that there were

22,472 children in state hospitals and 4,098 children in out-of-state private residential treatment facilities in 1986.

The lack of child psychiatric facilities emphasizes the deficiency in human and physical resources. The limited number of community-based out-of-home services for children contribute to the demand for hospitals, and children do not have the variety of treatment options that are provided to adolescents and adults.

Treatment programs in child psychiatric hospitals must concentrate on (1) meeting the developmental age- and stage-specific needs of the child and (2) intervening in the child's psychopathology through individual, peer group, and milieu activities and through educational and family therapies. Quality assurance is critical.

Child Psychiatric Hospitals and Treatment Programs

It is often assumed that hospitals are uniform in their pattern of organization, administration, staffing, and programs. However, child psychopathology requires different treatment programs from those of psychiatric hospitals designed for adolescents, adults, and the aging.

The physical structure of the child psychiatric hospital should be based on the age group it serves. Recreational activity programs require play areas, and different play materials, and equipment appropriate for the preschool and school-aged child. School-aged children need areas and classrooms within the unit, or the hospital must arrange for children to attend community schools.

The evolution of child psychiatric hospitals initiated staffing patterns and treatment perspectives that contribute to many current conflicts and problems. There are also physical and theoretic differences between publicly and privately funded child treatment facilities.

MODEL TREATMENT PROGRAMS

Most model hospital treatment programs developed as child psychiatry evolved, and many of the prototypes are supported privately and administered by pioneering child psychiatric theorists. Treatment concepts may be biased by the theoretic orientation of the founding psychiatrists, and the different ideologies produce different philosophies, administrative structures, staff utilization, and treatment regimes (Strauss and others, 1964).

Some child psychiatric hospitals are *residential treatment centers,* a term that distinguishes long-term settings from hospitals. Model treatment centers continue to be ground-breaking, innovative settings with original, sometimes controversial, therapeutic regimes. Several model centers have national reputations for treatment of specific psychopathologies or age-specific concerns.

PUBLIC AND PRIVATE FUNDED CHILD PSYCHIATRIC HOSPITALS

Private and public child treatment delivery models are not uniform in their organization, administration, staffing, and programs. Private settings are usually accessible only to children of families with substantial resources. They have highly trained professionals who almost exclusively focus on child dyadic or small-group relationships. Administration, paperwork, scheduling, telephoning and other functions are generally relegated to nonprofessional staff. In most large community mental health centers and state hospitals, adjunct staff and paraprofessionals have the major responsibilities for client care, and the highly trained professional staff are responsible for administration, paperwork, and supervision of nonprofessional child-care workers (O'Connor, Klassen, and O'Connor, 1979).

CURRENT NURSING ROLES

Current roles of child psychiatric nurses emerged from roles designed in earlier treatment settings. Until the ANA child psychiatric nursing standards were developed, the roles, functions, and competencies of these nurses varied remarkably between settings, depending on the continuing in-service education provided by the hospital.

Current variations in child psychiatric treatment and roles are the result of two different patterns of philosophy. One is rooted in the social and welfare needs of children, and the other in the medical model, emphasizing long-term care, maintenance of impaired children, and psychiatric treatments for children with behavioral problems unresponsive to environmental change and community intervention. These two patterns also influence organization, staffing, and programs in child psychiatric hospitals and have led to the establishment of the kinds of hospitals shown in the box that are seen today (Sonis, 1972).

COMMUNITY MENTAL HEALTH ACT

During the emphasis on civil rights in the 1960s, child advocates wanted to eliminate, reform, or supplement existing child psychiatric inpatient facilities in remote state institutions. They believed in treatment's inclusion of children's family and the use of special school facilities, if needed. The Community Mental Health Act required new children services. Changes have included the shift from large state institutions to smaller public general hospitals closer to home, which has encouraged program development in community services for children.

The move from remote hospitals resulted in publicly supported community mental health centers dedicated to furnishing patients more community-oriented services, such as family, outpatient, and partial care and crisis intervention. Psychiatric consultation to the public schools was important because children's mental problems often surfaced upon entry into school. Early identification and treatment could avert later serious problems.

The relocation of psychiatric services educational and research facilities improved opportunities of community based institutions to recruit better-trained child mental health professionals and promoted a closer liaison with pediatric and neurologic services. This fostered an interdisciplinary team approach that has become the hallmark of psychiatric care for the developing child.

The Community Mental Health Act's major limitation and on-going problem is the failure of the continuum of mental health services set forth in the act and the Least Restrictive Principle for children. Children who need other than inpatient hospital care have limited available alternative forms of public-supported

---

Classification of Hospital Care

Placement units

These units are private facilities, indirectly supported through contracts for service with city, county, and state welfare departments. They treat children with unmanageable behavior in the community that brought them to the attention of courts and child welfare services and provide emergency, crisis, and acute services.

Residential center units

These units are primarily private or financially supported through federated charities and public sources. They use community resources for education, socialization, and recreation with a community and family focus. Most children housed in them are less disturbed, with needs for long-term care because of social factors such as dysfunctional families.

Psychiatric inpatient units

These centers are under private, public, or university medical center auspices and integrate with other child psychiatric services offered. They focus on clinical training using psychiatric diagnoses and treatment regimes. They are self-sufficient physical plants with programs providing for most needs. Children housed in these programs are usually more disturbed than those found in most other treatment centers. Services include emergency, crisis, acute, and long-term programs.

State hospital units

Supported by the mental health system, these facilities provide long-term care of children with chronic psychiatric disabilities such as schizophrenia, severe behavior disorders, and social pathology. They usually offer acute and long-term care, day care, and partial hospitalization. They are self-sufficient units providing for total physical needs. Limited professional staff members manage long-term care and rehabilitation programs.

---

placements. Alternative agencies that provide other forms of rehabilitation are needed (Pothier, 1989).

The effect of psychiatric disorders in children on future cognitive ability, social skills, and effective relationships has been acknowledged by society; however, social policies have not been consistent in providing supportive health care funding or facilities. The forging of any health care policy is fraught with conflict and competition, which may account for the intensification of existing problems.

The National Mental Health Association's invisible children project reported that 91% of the placement in out-of-state agencies were initiated by state nonmental health agencies and strongly suggested that because of historical schisms, the mental health care of children is affected by overlapping between the social, legal, and mental health systems. The findings of this project are shown in the box.

Invisible Children Project Findings

1. A total of 22,472 children were in state hospitals and another 4,098 were in out-of-state placements, primarily private residential treatment facilities, with 91% of the placements initiated by state agencies other than mental health.
   a. Child welfare agencies placed 46%, educational agencies 28%, justice agencies 17%, and mental health state agencies 9%.
   b. More than 14,000 children and adolescents were placed in mental health facilities (other than state hospitals) within the state in 16 states. Almost 58% were placed more than 100 miles from home in 5 states.
2. A total of 81% of the children in out-of-state placements were sent to private residential treatment facilities, with an average cost of $52,300 per episode and an average length of stay in out-of-state facilities of 15.4 months.
3. The average length of stay in state hospitals was 4.2 months, with an average per diem rate of $299.16 and an average hospital cost of $38,218 per episode. The total cost for 22,472 children in state hospitals was $858.8 million.
4. A total of 70% of funds for children with mental disorders were spent on residential facilities, even though admission facility in many instances was unnecessary and inappropriate and many children could have been treated effectively in the home or community. Policy makers also falsely assumed that intensive services were synonymous only with residential care.
5. State mental health officials and local mental health associations surveyed advocated the following chronologic priorities:
   a. Intensive in-home crisis counseling services
   b. Early identification and intervention
   c. Day treatment
   d. Outpatient treatment
   e. Therapeutic foster care
   f. Prevention services
   g. Residential treatment centers and inpatient hospitalization

Modified from State hospitals and out-of-state placements widely used for children. NMHA survey finds, Hosp Community Psychiatry p 861, Aug 1989.

Based on the findings of this survey, the National Mental Health Association recommended that child advocates work aggressively to increase children's mental health services in local communities and states and to do the following:

1. Adopt a children's bill of rights to protect them from inappropriate placements.
2. Identify all children in institutional placements and plan for their return home.
3. Prohibit placements outside the state's jurisdiction and the admission of children to adult wards of state hospitals.
4. Establish a gatekeeper system to ensure appropriateness of placement of children in out-of-home treatment facilities.

The 1960s' relocation and establishment of treatment facilities in community general hospitals supported insurance coverage of clients with psychiatric diagnoses. The inclusion of child and adolescent diagnoses in the official DSM-III in 1980 provided further possibilities of DRGs. Third-party insurers have become increasingly involved in reimbursement for child psychiatric hospital expenditures, and state and federal funds have steadily diminished. At this time, most insurance agancies are not willing to cover more than a relatively short hospital stay, a requirement that limits continuity of care for children needing long-term residential hospital care. Care providers and insurance carriers are involved in a heated debate over DRGs (Christ, Andrews, and Tsemberis, 1989).

The majority of children with serious mental disorders are from families with limited financial resources and have no health insurance. Thus, the growth of private psychiatric care facilities for children and adolescents has become a major area of controversy. Although professionals hold that privately funded agencies provide opportunities for creative and innovative programs, others express strong concerns for quality assurance, noting that there are more quality assurance regulations for services paid for by the state (Pothier, 1989). Many private inpatient agencies strongly support the medical model, thus nurses' role focuses on implementing medical regimens rather than on developing nursing interventions.

Another problem is that the medical hospital format reinforces adherence to traditional interventions and concepts aimed at the identified client. For example, the innovative child treatment programs at the Philadelphia Child Guidance Clinic is structured on a family system approach with apartment therapy. The child and family are hospitalized as a group in an apartment for treatment. This unique hospital structure is designed to create desirable changes in the child and family system, to support family members' strengths, and to prevent the disruption of parents and sibling separation from the child at the time of admission (Goren, 1979).

The hospitalization of the identified child also limits the use of many systems methods for treating the family as a whole. With the relocation of psychiatry to the community, the problems have expanded to include many social issues not previously part of the psychiatric care system: substance abuse, child and spouse abuse, children of divorce, maintenance of successful marital relations, and prevention of adolescent pregnancies. The plethora of social problems that the staff of community mental health centers address reflects the public acceptance of psychiatric therapies, although it simultaneously strains existing resources. The need is growing to develop and expand intervention modes to encompass ecounits larger than the child and family unit. There are limits to the number and kinds of services mental health facilities can provide. The role and purpose of the child psychiatric hospital and other community institutions needs to be realistically reassessed so that child psychiatric hospitals are not continually overtaxed.

ADVANCES IN CHILD PSYCHIATRIC HOSPITAL CARE

The most significant outcome of the Community Mental Health Act for child psychiatric hospitals has been the remarkable scientific advances in the field of child psychiatry. During the past few decades there has been an extraordinary growth in child theories and related therapeutic interventions. The relocation of child psychiatric hospitals—from isolated settings to the mainstream of society, adult psychiatry, and medicine—has contributed largely to this phenomena. Mental disorders in children have always been a difficult concept for society, health professions, and even adult psychiatrists to recognize and appreciate. Exposure to children with mental disorders has not only contributed to consciousness-raising but has recruited many excellent scientists and clinicians into the field.

During the 1940s and 1950s, psychoanalysis and psychodynamic therapies, reported to be the most developed of treatments, were of limited application in child psychiatric hospitals, especially publicly supported state hospitals. Psychopharmacology was in its infancy, and behavior modification had not yet emerged as a treatment modality.

In contrast, by 1975 more than 130 therapeutic modalities were listed, and adult and child psychiatry was characterized and described as a specialty area that had been revolutionized. Commenting on the proliferation of possible therapeutic interventions and the remarkable changes, one expert clinician has stated (Harrison, 1977):

Thus it was no great challenge 25 years ago to be a versatile, all encompassing psychiatric practitioner. Today such an accomplishment is barely within the reach of even the most knowledgeable and gifted child psychiatrists. It would not be a rash prediction to assert that soon it will be utterly impossible for any one person to be a Renaissance practitioner of child psychiatry capable of mastering all reasonable therapeutic interventions.

As the field of child psychiatry has evolved and therapeutic interventions have multiplied, concerns have appeared in the literature about the proliferation and diversity in the child psychiatric theories as they distinguished different hospital treatment milieus. Some uncertainties were expressed, stressing that the multiplicity of theories and unique treatment programs described in the literature tended to weaken the focus and evolution of a strong clinical science in child psychiatry. However, certain principles appear to be basic to all child psychotherapy and most of the stated differences in theoretic frameworks faded in actual clinical practice (Group for the Advancement of Psychiatry, 1982).

During the past decade, the trend in child therapy techniques has been to move away from the earlier narrow focus of implementing one theory in a specific treatment setting, and to move toward an eclecticism, defined as the "process of selecting concepts, methods and strategies from a variety of current theories that work" (Schaefer, 1988). Most child psychiatric professionals now use multiple procedures and interventions and no longer restrict treatment environments to a single theory or treatment method. This trend has gradually evolved with the realization that no one therapeutic approach or method is equally effective with all psychological disorders. Most treatment settings now follow a prescriptive approach and adapt individual and milieu interventions to the particular case, rather than force a child into one all-purpose treatment mode. This prescriptive stance, called *differential therapeutics,* includes behavioral, cognitive, and dynamic approaches. Another therapeutic approach that combines techniques and adds therapeutic power is *multimodal therapy,* which uses therapeutic interventions to alter the behavioral, affective, sensate, imagery, and cognitive modalities in the context of interpersonal relationships.

Issues in Hospital Treatment Programs

ADMISSION

Admission to a psychiatric facility is serious and anxiety-producing to a child. Parents are distraught and family life is disrupted. For a facility to provide good care to this child, resources must be in place to care for the child, educate the child and parents, and help parents cope with the implications of their child's mental disorder. Therefore, the main goal of any treatment facility should be the creation of a treatment environment that maximizes the opportunity for the release of psychopathology so that the child and the family can pursue healthy, age-appropriate developmental tasks. Therapeutic attention must be on the following areas (National Association of Private Psychiatric Hospitals, 1984):

1. Skills of daily living
2. Psychoeducational and/or vocational remediation and development
3. Opportunities to develop interpersonal skills within the group setting
4. Restoration of family functioning
5. Enhanced use of community support systems

Admission to an inpatient unit is considered only when outpatient treatment is not feasible due to previous failure, nature of illness, need of a restrictive environment, suicidal or homicidal acts, fire setting, sexual promiscuity, running away, or the child's inability to function within the family, school, and community. The child's developmental stage, the child's family, and the availability of community treatment resources and support systems are important considerations when a child is hospitalized.

In many states, interagency panels review all requests for admission to publicly supported hospitals by state review panels that examine the information on the child and make recommendations for the most appropriate level of care. Usually the information needed includes the outpatient psychiatric and medical review, diagnostic interview impressions, psychologic tests, developmental scales, and baseline data concerning the family's level of functioning. While public-supported institutions' criteria for inpatient admission may vary from state to state, the National Association of Private Psychiatric Hospitals has proposed the checklist shown in the box.

LENGTH OF STAY

As more sophisticated treatment approaches have developed and more positive attitudes toward these children have emerged, the length of stay is variable. The young child's developmental stage influences the decision because attachment to the primary caregiver plays a crucial role in personality development and symptom reduction (Rowe, 1988). As a general rule, the length of stay is based on the disorganization and incapacitation experienced in family, school, and community.

THERAPEUTIC MILIEU

The milieu is the child's therapeutic environment within the hospital setting. Age-specific adjustments are made in the milieu in accord with the child's developmental needs.

Requirements for Inpatient Admission

___ 1. Client presents danger or potential danger to self.

___ 2. Client presents danger or potential danger to others.

___ 3. Client presents antisystems or bizarre behavior that is destructive to the community.

___ 4. Client is unable to attend to age-appropriate responsibilities.

___ 5. Client demonstrates significantly impaired reality testing.

___ 6. Client exhibits impaired judgment and logical thinking.

___ 7. Client is unable to function in native environment.

___ 8. Client's pathologic behavior has persisted or escalated in spite of outpatient treatment.

___ 9. Client exhibits pronounced affective behavior disturbance.

___ 10. Client demonstrates impending loss of control.

___ 11. Client needs high dose, unusual medication, or somatic and psychologic treatment with potentially serious side effects.

___ 12. Client's support system is so disturbed by behavior that treatment is jeopardized.

___ 13. A noxious native environment exists that jeopardized the client's outpatient treatment, and a lesser level of care is not appropriate or available.

___ 14. The client cannot function without extensive coordinated help from others in present state.

___ 15. The client requires 24-hour, skilled comprehensive and intensive observation.

___ 16. The clinical need for an intensive inpatient evaluation exists.

Modified from The National Association of Private Psychiatric Hospitals, Guidelines for psychiatric hospital programs: children and adolescents, Mar 1984.

The milieu for preschool children must be structured and satisfy their developmental needs through an exclusive primary relationship between each child and a staff member, and remission partly depends on this attachment. The length of time required to develop this relationship varies and is influenced by children's temperament and psychopathology. Usually it is longer than insurance standards and hospital resources allow.

For school-aged children the milieu includes all aspects of the usual environment: school, peers, staff, family, and play and recreational activities. The treatment program requires active participation and includes interactions with a variety of people and experiences. These constant interactions become therapeutically corrective learning experiences when used in individual or group therapy experiences and establishes a feedback system for children within the milieu. Families need to be involved in individual, group, sibling, and family sessions throughout the hospital stay.

The milieu should have an established *child privilege system*. Overall privileges are earned and maintained by cooperation and working in the therapeutic community, groups, and schools. Each increase in privileges should have a concurrent rise in responsibility. The system should be structured so that new privileges are granted through the concurrence of the individual therapist and the treatment team. This reduces splitting and ensures a collective approach to treatment.

The inpatient privilege structure should be based on children's developmental level and the developmental tasks to be accomplished. It includes an introductory level in which severely disturbed children are monitored for suicidal, homicidal, and elopement risks. All members of the community should be aware of children's status and the imposed limitations in movement and activities. It can be explained to children as a level designed for those who are having difficulty feeling safe or trusting others.

The second privilege level usually occurs when staff are relatively comfortable with children's impulse control and believe that they are benefitting from the treatment program. The highest privilege levels are usually designed to enable movement within the facility, and then later in the community for the purpose of practicing new interactions and using new skills in different settings.

Administrative staffing should include a medical director who is a certified child psychiatrist with both clinical and administrative experience, a program director who is a psychiatrist, and a psychologist. Ideally, nurses and social workers should both hold master's or doctoral degrees.

Staffing depends on the size of the unit and the child to staff ratio needed to implement the milieu philosophy. The age and needs of the clients are important considerations, as well as the severity of psychopathology. In hospital units housing preschool-aged children, the staff to child ratios are usually higher because preschoolers require close supervision. The clinical staff should include psychotherapists and family therapists from the four mental health professions — psychiatry, nursing specialty, psychology and social work.

Privileging for child psychiatric nurses. The psychiatric nurses' privileging process has been adopted by several hospitals for all nurses as part of quality assurance programs, with revisions to fit the particular specialty service. Privileging is the authorization of selected advanced nursing tasks through peer review of the clinical expertise and education. The purpose of privileging is to acknowledge nurses' education and skill level and to prevent nurses from receiving assignments for which they are not prepared. The policy and procedure guidelines for nurse privileging are shown in the box, and privileging criteria are shown in Table 19-1.

Milieu activity therapies. In comparison to adolescent and adult units, activity therapies in child psychiatric units are crucial. Activity therapies include games to enhance development level, recreational group activities to foster peer interactions, and arts to foster creativity.

School-aged children need to attend school, if possible, and occupational and recreational activities are structured so that they can exercise normally. The kind of teachers necessary varies, since many hospitalized school-aged children are in community schools' special educational programs that are based on cognitive deficits and delays and not on psychopathology.

The nursing staff is usually composed of a nursing care coordinator, registered nurses, licensed practical nurses, and paraprofessionals. All staff have major influences, and all members of the multidisciplinary team are responsible for the

Policy on Credentialing and Privileging

Nursing credentials and privileging committee

Purpose. To develop, implement, and evaluate policies that govern the assigning of clinical privileges to nursing staff.

Functions. Plan and evaluate criteria that serve as the basis for the granting of clinical privileges; review each candidate's application for clinical privileges; recommend to the Director of Nursing assignment of clinical privileges to the nursing staff according to education, training, and demonstrated ability; review individual nursing staff's clinical privileges no less often than every 2 years and recommend continuation or modification; and provide clinical privileging documentation for personnel records.

Membership. Representation from clinical areas and levels of professional nursing staff includes the Assistant Director of Nursing, Director of Nursing Education, Nurse Clinical Specialist, Nurse Recruiter, Nurse Supervisor, and Coordinator or Head Nurse.

Meetings. Meetings are held monthly or more often if needed. If data is received indicating the need for an immediate review of a nurse's privileges, the chairperson shall call a special meeting within one week to conduct this review.

Procedures

Credential review.
1. A registered nurse applicant's credentials will be reviewed in accordance with the state personnel job specifications and the specific criteria of the position.
2. During orientation, a clear statement of position requirements shall be made available to the applicant, as well as the standards of Psychiatric and Mental Health Nursing Practice of the American Nurses' Association and the Nursing Department Policy Statement on Level of Preparation and Level of Practice.
3. During orientation, the nurse will sign a form indicating that all elements are understood and agreed on. This form will be retained by the Nurse Recruiter and available for review by the Privileging Committee.

Special privileges.
1. Special privileges may be requested by a registered nurse. The request is initiated by means of an application to the Nursing Credentials and Privileging Committee.
2. The application must state the privilege requested and the relevant qualifications.
3. This application is then reviewed in accordance with the stated criteria specified in the Policy Statement on Level of Preparation and Level of Practice and the document "Nursing Department Privileging Criteria."

Application submission.
1. Each registered nurse may submit a clinical privileging application at such time as the nurse feels prepared to meet the relevant criteria.
2. Application submission is encouraged at the time of annual performance appraisals.

Status review.
1. The privileging status of each registered nurse is reviewed every 2 years in accordance with the policy on credentials and privileging of clinical staff, defined in the medical staff bylaws.
2. A record of all privileges granted shall be kept on file.

Modified from Rowland HS and Rowland BL: The manual of nursing quality assurance, Psychiatric Mental Health Nursing, vol 1, Rockville, Md, 1988, Aspen Publishers, Inc.

Table 19–1 Nursing Department Privileging Criteria

Activity privileged	Level 1 (with supervision)	Level 2 (independently)	Level 3 (supervise)	Level 4 (teach)
Leadership of information sharing and social skills client groups	Knowledge of content area and basic group dynamics	20 hours supervised experience Documentation of performance by clinical supervisor[*]	Completion of graduate level course in modality and 40 hours supervised experience Documentation of continuing education every 2 years[†]	Completion of graduate level course in group dynamics and 40 hours supervised experience Documentation of continuing education every 2 years
Individual psychotherapy	Completion of graduate level courses in modality	Masters in nursing or closely related field and/or ANA certification in adult mental health nursing	Masters in nursing or closely related field and/or ANA certification in adult psychiatric mental health nursing	
Group psychotherapy	Documentation of performance by clinical supervisor	20 hours supervised experience in modality	40 hours supervised experience in modality	
Family therapy		Documentation of continuing education every 2 years	Documentation of continuing education every 2 years	

Preceptorship for nurse internship program in conjunction with nursing education	Completion of workshop for preceptors; 3 years psychiatric nursing experience
	Letters of recommendation from immediate supervisor, or ADN, or NCS, and director of nursing education
	2 years psychiatric nursing experience
Nursing coordination of electroconvulsive treatment	Completion of training program as defined by nursing education
	CPR certified (yearly); completion of emergency medication review (yearly), Flynn resuscitator and emergency cart review (yearly)

From Rowland HS and Rowland BL: The manual of nursing quality assurance, Psychiatric Mental Health Nursing, vol 1, Rockville, Md, 1988, Aspen Publishers, Inc.

*Clinical supervision: Supervision by clinician privileged to supervise in modality.
†Continuing education: Formal education offering in modality.

community structure's consistency. Staff must be willing to act as role models for the children; to use attachment, authority, confrontation, and limit setting; to provide experiences to help children master age-appropriate developmental tasks; and to give emotional support. Staff continuously establish, maintain, and terminate therapeutic relationships, and within these relationships they provide for normal developmental needs of the children they serve. Therapeutic relationships with children from 6 to 12 years of age are established through individual play therapy, drawing, and mutual play activities.

Both preschool and school-aged children are encouraged to participate in peer activities to enhance their social development through activities and games with rules and routines. Play serves as a vehicle for growth and maturation and is thus a major tool in psychotherapeutic work with children (Lego, 1984). Its use in the therapeutic milieu has many developmental and therapeutic purposes, includine working out problematic experiences, such as abuse; learning about interpersonal relationships; learning to compete, cooperate, and collaborate with peers and adults; mastering unpleasant and new experiences; and acting out uncomfortable emotions symbolically or gradually, so that ultimately they can be felt (Lego, 1984).

In the therapeutic milieu, games and game strategies foster communication, problem solving, ego enhancement and socialization. Play activities and games are also used as vehicles to enhance children's relationship to the individual therapist.

There is a need for staff working in child treatment facilities to be aware of the relationship between pathologic excitement in children and staff disagreements. Symptoms initially interpreted as pathologic may later be found to be the child's acting out of the therapist's poorly suppressed impulses or of the staff's interpersonal conflicts. The unknowing misuse of the therapeutic process can be recognized. Although awareness may not resolve the professional conflict, it can mitigate or even eliminate a client's participation (Giffin, 1954).

EVALUATION OF THE MILIEU

Quality assurance in psychiatric units or hospitals should be part of the hospital's overall quality assurance program. These criteria must address the care issues specific to standards of psychiatric nursing in general and to child psychiatric nursing specifically. The departmental quality assurance program can be a tool for the attainment of high quality, cost-effective child care. A problem-focused approach has been recommended by the Joint Commission to improve the care being rendered, to streamline procedures, and to free staff time from repetitious activities (Evans and Lewis, 1985).

The quality assurance program in child psychiatric hospitals should relate care to established standards, such as the American Nurses' Association's *Standards of Psychiatric Mental Health Nursing Practice* (1984) and the *Standards of Child Psychiatric Mental Health Nursing Practice* (1985), which provide guidelines for developing practice standards that are specific to the unit's needs. These standards were written to provide process and outcome criteria. The knowledge needed by nurses to function at the different privileging levels and in other areas handled by quality assurance programs can be assessed by using the published ANA knowledge, comprehension, and skill taxonomy descriptions published in credentialing materials (see Chapters 2 and 3).

Quality assurance standards should include a hospital-wide endeavor including assessment of client care rendered and the correction of identified problems. The program should include a list of specific problems unique to child psychiatric hospitals. Quality assurance methods involve utilization review, monitoring of identified standards of care, infection control, client care monitoring, facility evaluation, safety specific to the child's developmental age and stage, RN license and advanced practice credentials, and staff development programs. Policy-and-procedure manuals should be developed to assure staff are provided effective administrative leadership and guidelines, and to assure overall program evaluation.

PARTIAL HOSPITALIZATION

Partial hospitalization is defined by the National Association of Private Psychiatric Hospitals (1984) as follows:

Partial hospitalization is a generic term embracing day, evening and weekend treatment programs that employ an integrated and comprehensive schedule of recognized psychiatric treatment. It may be a free standing unit or a component of a mental health center, serving as a link in the continuum of therapeutic modalities to comprise a full comprehensive mental health service for that community.

There is strong evidence that many psychiatric clients benefit from partial hospitalization as well as they do from traditional hospitalization. These programs are less expensive and less intensive methods of treatment, and they implement the principle of the *least restrictive alternative*. A range of services usually found in comprehensive psychiatric hospital programs are provided, such as diagnostic, medical, psychiatric, psychosocial, and prevocational treatment. Partial hospitalization is designed for clients who require coordinated intensive, comprehensive, and multidisciplinary treatment that is not provided in an outpatient clinic setting. It is appropriate for individuals who are emotionally impaired but who function minimally and presents no imminent potential for harm to themselves or others. This professionally supervised alternative to inpatient care provides a more flexible form of treatment. Therapeutic modalities in a structured environment may include group, family, and individual therapy and pharmacologic psychodrama, and occupational/recreational therapies.

Children who would benefit from partial hospitalization have many disabilities that are not easily categorized. Some types of patient subgroups that appear appropriate for this treatment approach include children in acute crisis, children in transition from an inpatient facility to outpatient facility, and children in need of extended care that is not as intensive as inpatient treatment.

Lengths of treatment in partial hospitalization differ. As an overall guideline, the following lengths of stay have been suggested: Acutely ill clients will need to attend the program 3 hours daily for 5 to 7 days a week for 2 weeks to 3 months, depending on the severity and duration of symptoms. They should have a 6-hour orientation period (especially children). Children in transition from the hospital to the community may attend full or part-time, depending on their need and the duration of inpatient status. Flexibility is important in these programs to enable clients to resume their life at a tolerable rate. The speed at which individuals can handle the transition depends on their pathology and their social support.

Some patients with severe pathology require extended intensive care in partial hospitalization programs, which reduces the need for prolonged inpatient treatment. During partial hospitalization, the goal is more independent living. Inpatient treatment may regress or suppress independent functioning.

During treatment planning, clinicians should consider the strengths of the individual and emphasize clients assuming responsibility and decision making. During orientation, pathologic reactions to separation from the hospital unit must be diagnosed and dealt with therapeutically.

Disadvantages to partial hospitalization treatment include staff discouragement because of clients' home situations, testing of staff by clients desiring inpatient status, ease of discontinuation of day programs by clients, transportation concerns to fulfill scheduled therapies, and the greater expense of the programs compared to outpatient care.

Staffing of these programs varies. The program should address psychologic, psychopharmacologic, interpersonal, and vocational educational areas. Appropriate staffing consists of an administrator with a master's degree and administrative experience, a clinical specialist, a psychiatrist, a social worker, two case workers, a recreational therapist, an occupational therapist, three or four paraprofessionals, and a teaching staff if children do not attend community schools (Lego, 1984).

Discharge criteria include symptom and behavioral problem relief so that significant interference with social, vocational, and educational functioning is absent and observation and protection is no longer required; age-appropriate self-care; existence of appropriate support resources in the community; and attainment of partial hospitalization goals.

OUTPATIENT TREATMENT

Outpatient treatment consists of individual psychotherapy, group psychotherapy and family therapy. Depending on age and personality, children usually interpret outpatient treatment as a way to discuss and solve problems with help from others.

A playroom is the normal environment for play or talk sessions, although economic and spacing problems have caused some individual therapists to use offices. Periodic assessments and peer review should be made of children's progress in treatment. When termination is appropriate, treatment is most often tapered off on a timetable that is primarily set by each child. Continued contact may occur a few times a year until the child no longer desires it (Lego, 1984).

REFERENCES

Chamberlain JG: Challenges for child psychiatric nursing, J Child Adolesc Psychia Ment Health Nurs 1:2, 1988 (editorial).

Christ AE, Andrews H, and Tsemberis S: Fiscal implications of a childhood disorder DRG, J Am Acad Child Adolesc Psychiatry 5:729, 1989.

English JT and others: Diagnostic related groups and general hospital psychiatry: the APA study, Am J Psychiatry 143:131, 1986.

Evans CLS and Lewis SK: Nursing administration of psychiatric mental health care, Baltimore, 1985, Aspen Publishers, Inc.

Giffin ME: Specific factors determining antisocial acting out, Am J Orthopsychiatry 24:668, 1954.

Goren S: A systems approach to emotional disorders of children, Nurs Clin North Am 14:457, 1979.

Group for the Advancement of Psychiatry: The process of child therapy, New York, 1982, Brunner/Mazel, Inc.

Harrison SI: Reassessment of eclecticism in child psychiatric treatment. In McMillan MF and Henao S, editors: Child psychiatry: treatment and research, New York, 1977, Brunner/Mazel, Inc.

Institute of Medicine: Research on children and adolescents with mental, behavioral and developmental disorders, Washington, DC, 1988, National Academy Press.

Lego S: The American handbook of psychiatric nursing, Philadelphia, 1984, JB Lippincott Co.

National Association of Private Psychiatric Hospitals: Guidelines for psychiatric hospital programs: children and adolescents, Mar 1984.

National Association of Private Psychiatric Hospitals: Guidelines for psychiatric hospital programs: partial hospitalization, Mar 1984.

National Mental Health Association: Invisible child project—1986–1987, Alexandria, Va, 1989, The National Mental Health Association.

O'Connor WA, Klassen D, and O'Connor KS: Evaluating human service programs: psychosocial methods. In Abmed P and Coelho G, editors: Toward a new definition of health, New York, 1979, Plenum Publishing Corp.

Pothier P: The impact of privatization of psychiatric care on children and adolescents, Arch Psychiatr Nurs 3:123, 1989.

Rowe J: Attachment theory and the milieu treatment of children, J Child Adolesc Psychia Ment Health Nurs 1:66, 1988.

Rowland HS and Rowland BL: The manual of nursing quality assurance, Psychiatric Mental Health Nursing, vol 1, Rockville, Md, 1988, Aspen Publishers, Inc.

Schaefer CE, editor: Innovative intervention in child and adolescent therapy, New York, 1988, John Wiley & Sons, Inc.

Sonis M: Residential treatment. In Freedman AM and Kaplan HI, editors: The child: his psychological and cultural development, vol 2, New York, 1972, Atheneum.

State hospitals and out-of-state placements widely used for children. NMHA survey finds, Hosp Community Psychiatry p 861, Aug 1989.

Strauss A and others: Psychiatric ideologies and institutions, London, 1964, Free Press of Glencoe.

US Congress Office of Technology Assessment: Children's mental health: problems and services background paper, Pub No OTA-BP-H-23, Washington, DC, 1986, US Government Printing Office.

Chapter 20

Care for the Caregiver

Judy A. Rollins

We drain ourselves. We dip into our buckets — ladling kindness, concern, knowledge, helpfulness, that which is our goodness, our best — to fill the buckets of others, most of the time without a second thought. After all, it is our job; it is what we do. But our buckets are not bottomless. When we hear the clanging of the ladle in the bucket, we know we are getting empty.

Nursing Practice and Stress

Nursing can be physically and emotionally demanding, particularly in the hospital setting where the impact of the current nursing shortage is felt most acutely:

> I just can't keep going at this pace — never having lunch breaks, always working overtime, and still leaving before everything is done. I love nursing, but it demands tremendous energy every day (Huey and Hartley, 1988).

Many nurses work well beyond a traditional 8-hour day. The extra time is often not a conscious choice but an unwelcome necessity. Nurses are also expected to work odd hours, often rotating shifts that disrupt their natural circadian rhythm (Monk, 1986). Because new graduates are typically assigned to off-shift work, the lack of seasoned personnel to help them make critical decisions causes a stressful and potentially dangerous situation. In many instances, stress results from nurses' inability to meet personal expectations of the professional role, for example, when unable to give the care they believe their clients need (Huey and Hartley, 1988).

A report issued by the National Institute of Occupational Safety and Health (NIOSH) identified the health care profession as one of the most stressful occupations. The reason cited was that workers have a great deal of responsibility for the welfare of their clients without the authority to have complete control over that welfare (Daleo, 1986). Frustrations also result from societal expectations and the difficulty in combining family and career.

High levels of stress can produce psychosomatic disorders, poor mental health, alcoholism, and drug abuse. It is also costly to the hospital because of increased absenteeism, tardiness, and sabotage. A recent report estimates that stress annually costs hospitals an average of $1003 per employee. The total stress-related expense for large hospitals can be as high as $1.5 million or 3% of a hospital's operating budget annually (Hospitals, 1988). Stress may produce *burnout*, a gradually

---

Stressors of Psychiatric Nursing

1. Not being notified of changes before they occur
2. Dealing with people in key management positions who are unable to make decisions
3. Lack of support from administration
4. Having excessive paperwork
5. Working for an administration that believes in change for the sake of change
6. Being responsible for too many widely divergent things
7. Not having suggestions acted on in a timely fashion
8. Trying to do the job in spite of no one listening or caring
9. Receiving no recognition for a job well done
10. Having administrative work interfere with client care

---

developing syndrome in which previously committed workers disengage from their work and lose respect for their clients, jeopardizing nurses' ability to provide high-quality care.

Co-workers will be affected not only by their own job stress but by the behavior of other members of the health care team. A burned-out team member creates discord and often extra work for co-workers, adding a new source of stress to the team system. Furthermore, job stress may be introduced into nurses' family system.

PSYCHIATRIC NURSING AND STRESS

Psychiatric nurses work with a population of clients that are often highly resistant or show little progress or change. There may be little or no immediate gratification for time and energy expended. In some instances, psychiatric nurses' role and those of other treatment team members are not clearly defined, resulting in conflict and tension among staff, an absence of support from colleagues, and an abundance of criticism. Violence constitutes another real, if unacknowledged, occupational hazard in the mental health treatment setting (Soloff, 1987). In a recent study of staff injuries from inpatient violence at a state hospital, Carmel and Hunter (1989) found that 121 staff members sustained 135 injuries. Nursing staff sustained 120 of these injuries, for a rate of 16 injuries per 100 staff members.

Although certain stressors are associated with psychiatric nursing, research indicates that experiences such as a physical threat by a client are not the dominant item perceived as stressful. Only 11 of the 78 items identified as stressors were specific to the mental health treatment setting (see box). Approximately 50% of the high-stress items related to organizational management.

Child psychiatric nursing. In a general pediatric or a psychiatric pediatric setting, certain common ideas may influence nurses' feelings and actions. People generally believe that childhood is a happy time, that children should not suffer, and that being born in America guarantees a happy, healthy life (Hall, Hardin and Conatser, 1982). Reality can be overwhelmingly painful for new graduate nurses and seasoned professionals. Nurses are frustrated because children often must return to the unhealthy environment that cultivated their mental health problems.

A lack of education and clinical experience in psychiatric nursing may result in feelings of insecurity for new nurses. With the integrated model commonly used in nursing education, many schools of nursing do not offer the psychiatric nursing theory course (Arnswald, 1987). Many nursing students graduate without any appreciable experience in the care of mentally ill clients (Dumas, 1983). Psychiatric nursing care of children also requires an in-depth knowledge of child development, which some clinicians lack.

Sources of Support for the Caregiver

There are three primary resources for support for nurses working in child psychiatry: administration, colleagues, and the nurses themselves. All share responsibility for preventative as well as remedial efforts to ameliorate the negative effects of stress.

ADMINISTRATIVE SUPPORT

Administrators are increasingly aware of the importance of retaining experienced nurses rather than recruiting new ones. The American Organization for Nurse Executives (AONE) postulated that it takes 60 to 90 days to recruit a nurse. During this time, hospitals typically hire a temporary nurse who is paid time and a half and remains during the new employee's orientation period, with an approximate cost of $20,000. This amount excludes costs for advertising, nurse recruiter salary, travel expenses, literature, and public relations activities. Furthermore, it may take 6 to 9 months for the new nurse to achieve the same effectiveness of an experienced nurse (Hospitals, 1987). Stress caused by poor communication or a shortage of workers can reduce productivity by 20% to 30%. Administrators may find it more economical to provide support, leading to satisfied employees who are committed to the hospital and are highly productive (Patterson and Eppich, 1987).

A commitment to quality care for clients and staff begins with hospital leadership. The leadership process involves pathfinding, decision making, and implementation. Effective leaders are concerned with abstract and daily activities. Attention to everyday events instills enthusiasm in staff members and facilitates implementation of ideas. To positively influence hospitals' organization, supervisors must help subordinates solve problems and promote independence and responsibility without feeling threatened. They need to implicitly trust their employees' judgment and act as a role model (Metzger, 1987).

In a recent study, head nurses and staff nurses indicated that they seldom met formally with the clinical directors. Virtually all communication was informal and constant, and much of it was initiated by the staff nurse. Clinicians were pleased with this format because they could devote their energy to their clients.

Research further reveals that hospitals can promote excellence by hiring nurses who are skilled at assessing emotional, developmental, and academic needs of children and who can communicate with and foster the involvement of clients and their families. The box on p. 455 details the guidelines to change and support nursing staff members.

Supportive Hiring Practices

1. Hire new and experienced nurses.
   a. New graduates offer enthusiasm, book knowledge, and creativity.
   b. Experienced nurses offer working knowledge.
2. Select nurses carefully.
   a. Determine if nurses' client care philosophy is consistent with nursing depart-
      ment's.
      (1) Ask about their philosophy of client care.
      (2) Offer hypothetic situations and ask their opinion.
   b. Look for creativity to introduce new ideas into the unit.
   c. Make expectations clear.
3. Leave a position open rather than fill it with an inappropriate person.
4. Provide effective orientation.
5. Counsel the nurse to seek other employment if conflicts are seen during orientation.

Nurse participation in the planning process is important in creating a less stressful work environment. Planning should be linked with strategic management and human resource planning and needs the commitment of trustees, top management, physicians, and nursing staff. Nurses participate more effectively in planning if decision making is decentralized. Limited administrative and supervisory personnel are effective because a stable, educated staff markedly decreases the need for supervision and increases the span of control. Innovative hospitals also allow individual head nurses to determine unit-based standards and policies while following the general outlines of the hospital.

Hospital environments should enhance feelings of self-esteem and comfort and promote competent performance. Their design should allow staff members to communicate easily with families and provide private areas away from clients and families. Nurses should be involved in the development of the hospital environment.

Hospitals can be supportive of nurses by providing opportunities for creativity and growth (see box on p. 456). Most offer either partial or total tuition reimbursement for work-related college courses. Many hospitals send staff nurses to conferences, workshops, meetings, and seminars and pay the event's fee.

In-service education, a Joint Commission on Accreditation of Health Care Organizations (JCAHO) requirement, provides another opportunity for creative expression and professional growth. In one magnet hospital, each unit has its own in-service coordinator, and staff nurses rotate through the position, with a new coordinator every quarter. The in-service coordinator assess the needs of the staff, chooses topics, selects presenters, and works with coordinators from other units. Coordinators also develop creative methods to present information, such as posters, videos, games, or puzzles. Recognition by administrators indicates that these efforts are supported and appreciated and promotes self-esteem.

Support groups are helpful for nurses who work in high stress areas such as psychiatry. They may be formal or informal but should provide flexibility and be encouraged by administrators. The most effective type of support group involves

---

Practices to Encourage Creativity and Growth

1. Provide pay and resources to find solutions to problems.
2. Allow library research to develop care plans for difficult clients.
3. Encourage development of planning committees, project groups, research committees, and pilot studies.
4. Allow staff nurses to attend committee meetings, conferences, and seminars in place
   of a department head.
5. Establish a recognition or reward system for new ideas (for example, employee of the
   month, routine press releases by public relations department, awards, and bonuses).
6. Promote regular meetings of nurses and staff members with the CEO.
7. Implement suggestion boxes.

---

self-help and is based on the helper-therapy principle in which each member serves as the agent and target of help (Riessman, 1965). Levy (1979) classified the processes that occur as either behaviorally oriented or cognitively oriented (see box on p. 457). In the *behaviorally oriented* process of social reinforcement, direct and vicarious reinforcements facilitate the development of desirable behaviors and the elimination of control of problematic behaviors. Members learn methods to control their feelings and thoughts, and modeling is provided. *Mastery modeling* is provided by clinicians who manage the realities of working in a psychiatric setting, and *coping modeling* is demonstrated by nurses who have not. *Demystification,* a cognitively oriented process, occurs when group members hear others speak of identical concerns and feelings. By sharing, advice giving, and self-disclosure with experienced staff, members can reconstruct a problem and discover alternative methods of action. Group members develop better analytic and discriminative abilities, support effective change, and reduce feelings of isolation. Because the self-help group develops its own norms and structure, members can build a new identity and increase their self-esteem (Levy, 1979).

An increasing number of hospitals have developed Employee Assistance Programs (EAPs) to provide support for nurses and other hospital employees. While originally intended to serve employees with a drug or alcohol problem, most have expanded their services to other mental health issues and family problems. EAPs provide understanding and confidential assistance to clinicians having difficulties, whether the problems are self-reported or brought to the EAP's attention by others. EAP representatives conduct or arrange interventions and treatment and smooth the transition to the working environment. A consistent and objective tool, such as the monitored treatment program with a return to work contract, monitors success and compliance with treatment (Robbins, 1987).

Hospitals have developed other supportive programs or policies to meet the unique needs of their nurses (see box on p. 457). A needs assessment questionnaire for nurses identifies individual and group needs and their priority. For example, a nurse may be covered under a spouse's medical insurance and would rather have a different benefit instead of additional insurance coverage. The *cafeteria approach* allowing employees to select benefit participation has been enthusiastically received.

Self-Help Group Process

Behaviorally oriented processes

1. Social reinforcement
2. Self-control behaviors
3. Modeling
4. Promoting change

Cognitively oriented processes

1. Demystification
2. Information and advice
3. Alternative perceptions of problems and solutions
4. Enhancement of discriminative abilities
5. Support for changes in attitude
6. Reduction of isolation
7. Alternative or substitute culture and social structure

Modified from Levy L: Processes and activities in groups. In Lieberman MA and others, editors: Self-help groups for coping with crisis: origins, members, process, and impact, San Francisco, 1979, Jossey-Bass, Inc, Publishers.

Supportive Nursing Programs

1. Maternity, paternity, and adoption leave
2. On-site child care facility
3. Sick-child care
4. Time off to care for sick child
5. Weekend work of 36 hours equals pay for 40 hours
6. Flex time
7. Flex pool
8. Patrolled parking lot
9. Escort to parking lot
10. On-site dry cleaning
11. Cafeteria approach to benefits
12. Health and fitness center
13. Contract with community fitness center
14. Free university tuition for nurse, spouse, and dependent children
15. Reimbursement for professional dues
16. On-site college courses

SUPPORT FROM COLLEAGUES

Many nurses mention their co-workers when asked about the positive aspects of their work. Colleagues are excellent support resources and can reduce job stress and lead to better health (House, 1981). To build positive working relationships, clinicians should view other staff members as collaborators (Zins, 1985). Individuals contribute

---

Coping: A Personal Test

1. Do you feel that you have a supportive family? If so, score 10 points.
2. Add 10 points if you actively pursue a hobby.
3. Do you belong to some social activity group that meets at least once a month (other than your family)? If so, score 10 points.
4. Are you within 5 lb of your ideal body weight, considering your health, age, and bone structure? If so, score 15 points.
5. Add 5 points for each time you exercise 30 minutes or longer during an average week.
6. Add 5 points for each nutritionally balanced and wholesome meal you consume during an average day.
7. Do you do something you really enjoy that is solely for yourself during the week? If so, score 5 points.
8. Do you have a place in your home to relax or be by yourself? If so, score 10 points.
9. Add 10 points if you practice time-management techniques daily.
10. Subtract 10 points for each pack of cigarettes you smoke in an average day.
11. Do you use any drugs or alcohol to help you sleep? If so, subtract 5 points for each evening during an average week that this occurs.
12. Do you take any drugs or alcohol to reduce anxiety or calm you down? If so, subtract 10 points for each time that this occurs during the course of an average week.
13. Do you ever bring work home in the evening? Subtract 5 points for each evening during an average week that this occurs.

Scoring

A perfect score is 115 points. The higher the score, the greater the ability to cope with stress. A score of 50 to 60 points indicates an adequate ablity to cope with the most common sources of stress.

Modified from Everly G: Coping: a personal test, Washington Post Health, Apr 6, 1986.

---

their areas of strength and seek assistance from colleagues skilled in other areas (Bernstein and Halaszyn, 1989). A good working relationship among colleagues undermines staff-splitting attempts by clients or staff members. Clinicians should also develop outside support systems to receive straight feedback, problem-solving help, and emotional support (Scharer, 1988).

Nurses should develop a sensitivity to co-workers' needs. They support others by acknowledging the difficulty of a particular client or by temporarily fulfilling the other nurse's duties. Sharing personal information such as a pending divorce or the serious illness of a relative draws understanding and practical assistance from fellow nurses. Support from co-workers is crucial when a colleague experiences a particularly stressful work situation, for example, when a client commits suicide. Although it is important for colleagues to help each other, assistance may border on enabling, and the EAP may help nurses recognize this effect and create a climate in which requesting assistance is promoted and supported.

SELF-CARE

The most common reaction to stress is to ignore its existence and effect. The human body learns to adjust to the cumulative, intensifying stressors and is conditioned to sustain greater pressure levels without alleviating it (Daleo, 1986).

Nurses need to examine their interactions with clients and learn to modify their expectations of rewards, providing self-reward when appropriate. They should maintain good physical health by eating nutritiously, and exercising regularly. Nurses can use relaxation techniques to promote renewal and regeneration, which increases productivity and creative thinking ability (Daleo, 1986). Creative expression also reduces stress, as does prioritizing activities. The coping test in the box identifies behaviors that promote or alleviate stress and aids in planning a strategy for stress reduction.

REFERENCES

Arnswald L: Not fade away: are psych nurses an endangered species? J Psychosoc Nurs Ment Health Serv 25:31, 1987.

Bernstein G and Halaszyn J: Human services? That must be so rewarding, Baltimore, 1989, Paul H Brookes Publishing Co.

Carmel H and Hunter M: Staff injuries from inpatient violence, Hosp Community Psychiatry 40:41, 1989.

Daleo R: Taking care of the caregiver, Am J Hospice Care, p 33, Sept/Oct 1986.

Dumas R: Social, economic, and political factors and mental illness, J Psychosoc Nurs Ment Health Serv 21:31, 1983.

Everly G: Coping: a personal test, Washington Post Health, Apr 6, 1986.

Hall M, Hardin K, and Conatser C: The challenges of psychological care: In Fochtman D and Foley G, editors: Nursing care of the child with cancer, Boston, 1982, Little, Brown & Co, Inc.

High price tag on nursing recruitment, Hospitals p 150, Oct 1987.

Hospitals not immune to high cost of stress, Hospitals p 69, Oct 1988.

House J: Work stress and social support, Reading, Mass, 1981, Addison-Wesley Publishing Co, Inc.

Huey F and Hartley S: What keeps nursing in nursing: 3500 nurses tell their stories, Am J Nurs 87:181, 1988.

Levy L: Processes and activities in groups. In Lieberman MA and others, editors: Self-help groups for coping with crisis: origins, members, process, and impact, San Francisco, 1979, Jossey-Bass, Inc, Publishers.

Metzger N: Beyond survival to excellence, Health Care Superv 5:37, 1987.

Monk T: Advantages and disadvantages of rapidly rotating shift schedules—a circadian viewpoint, Human Factors, 28:553, 1986.

Patterson D and Eppich N: Family-centered care: can we afford it? Child Health Care 15:245, 1987.

Riessman F: The "helper-therapy principle," Soc Work 10:27, 1965.

Robbins C: A monitored treatment program for impaired health care professionals, J Nurs Adm 17:17, 1987.

Scharer K: Care for the caregiver, JAPON 5:24, 1988.

Soloff P: Emergency management of violents. In Hales RE and Frances AJ, editors: Psychiatry update: American psychiatric association annual review, vol 6, Washington, DC, 1987, American Psychiatric Press, Inc.

Zins J: Work relations management. In Maher CA, editor: Professional self-management: techniques for special services providers, Baltimore, 1985, Paul H Brookes Publishing Co.

Appendix A

DSM-III-R Classification Axes I and II Categories and Codes

All official DSM-III-R codes are included in ICD-9-CM. Codes followed by a * are used for more than one DSM-III-R diagnosis or subtype in order to maintain compatibility with ICD-9-CM.

Numbers in parentheses are page numbers.

A long dash following a diagnostic term indicates the need for a fifth digit subtype or other qualifying term.

The term *specify* following the name of some diagnostic categories indicates qualifying terms that clinicians may wish to add in parentheses after the name of the disorder.

NOS = Not Otherwise Specified

The current severity of a disorder may be specified after the diagnosis as:

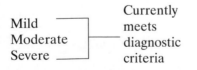

Mild ⎫
Moderate ⎬ Currently meets diagnostic criteria
Severe ⎭

- In partial remission (or residual state)
- In complete remission

Developmental Disorders

Note: These are coded on Axis II.

Mental retardation (28)

317.00	Mild mental retardation
318.00	Moderate mental retardation
318.10	Severe mental retardation
318.20	Profound mental retardation
319.00	Unspecified mental retardation

Pervasive developmental disorders (33)

299.00	Autistic disorder (38) Specify if childhood onset
299.80	Pervasive developmental disorder NOS

Specific developmental disorders (39)

Academic skills disorders.

315.10	Developmental arithmetic disorder (41)
315.80	Developmental expressive writing disorder (42)
315.00	Developmental reading disorder (43)

Language and speech disorders.

315.39	Developmental articulation disorder (44)
315.31*	Developmental expressive language disorder (45)
315.31*	Developmental receptive language disorder (47)

Motor skills disorder.

315.40	Developmental coordination disorder (48)
315.90*	Specific developmental disorder NOS

Other developmental disorders (49)

315.90*	Developmental disorder NOS

From American Psychiatric Association: Diagnostic and statistical manual of mental disorders, ed 3, rev, Washington, DC, 1987, American Psychiatric Association.

Disruptive Behavior Disorders (49)

314.01   Attention-deficit hyperactivity disorder (50)
         Conduct disorder (53)
312.20   group type
312.00   solitary aggressive type
312.90   undifferentiated type
313.81   Oppositional defiant disorder (56)

Anxiety Disorders of Childhood or Adolescence (58)

309.21   Separation anxiety disorder (58)
313.21   Avoidant disorder of childhood or adolescence (61)
313.00   Overanxious disorder (63)

Eating Disorders (65)

307.10   Anorexia nervosa (65)
307.51   Bulimia nervosa (67)
307.52   Pica (69)
307.53   Rumination disorder of infancy (70)
307.50   Eating disorder NOS

Gender Identity Disorders (71)

302.60   Gender identity disorder of childhood (71)
302.50   Transsexualism (74)
            Specify sexual history: asexual, homosexual, heterosexual, unspecified
302.85* Gender identity disorder of adolescence or adulthood, nontranssexual type (76)
            Specify sexual history: asexual, homosexual, heterosexual, unspecified
302.85* Gender identity disorder NOS

Tic Disorders (78)

307.23   Tourette's disorder (79)
307.22   Chronic motor or vocal tic disorder (81)

307.21   Transient tic disorder (81)
            Specify: single episode or recurrent
307.20   Tic disorder NOS

Elimination Disorders (82)

307.70   Functional encopresis (82)
            Specify: primary or secondary type
307.60   Functional enuresis (84)
            Specify: primary or secondary type
            Specify: nocturnal only, diurnal only, nocturnal and diurnal

Speech Disorders Not Elsewhere Classified (85)

307.00* Cluttering (85)
307.00* Stuttering (86)

Other Disorders of Infancy, Childhood, or Adolescence (88)

313.23   Elective mutism (88)
313.82   Identity disorder (89)
313.89   Reactive attachment disorder of infancy or early childhood (91)
307.30   Stereotype/habit disorder (93)
314.00   Undifferentiated attention-deficit disorder (95)

ORGANIC MENTAL DISORDERS (97)

Dementias Arising in the Senium and Presenium (119)

         Primary degenerative dementia of the Alzheimer type, senile onset (119)
290.30   with delirium
290.20   with delusions
290.21   with depression
290.00*   uncomplicated
            (Note: code 331.00 Alzheimer's disease on Axis III)

Code in fifth digit:
1 = with delirium, 2 = with
delusions, 3 = with depression,
0* = uncomplicated

290.1x   Primary degenerative de-
    mentia of the Alzheimer
    type, presenile onset,
    _____ (119) (Note: code
    331.00 Alzheimer's disease
    on Axis III)

290.4x   Multi-infarct dementia,
    _____ (121)

290.00*   Senile dementia NOS
    Specify etiology on Axis III
    if known

290.10*   Presenile dementia NOS
    Specify etiology on Axis III
    if known (Pick's disease,
    Jakob-Creutzfeldt disease)

Psychoactive Substance-Induced Organic Mental Disorders (123)

    Alcohol
303.00   intoxication (127)
291.40   idiosyncratic intoxication
    (128)
291.80   Uncomplicated alcohol
    withdrawal (129)
291.00   withdrawal delirium (131)
291.30   hallucinosis (131)
291.10   amnestic disorder (133)
291.20   Dementia associated with
    alcoholism (133)
    Amphetamine or similarly
    acting sympathomimetic
305.70*   intoxication (134)
292.00*   withdrawal (136)
292.81*   delirium (136)
292.11*   delusional disorder (137)
    Caffeine
305.90*   intoxication (138)
    Cannabis
305.20*   intoxication (139)
292.11*   delusional disorder (140)
    Cocaine
305.60*   intoxication (141)

292.00*   withdrawal (142)
292.81*   delirium (143)
292.11*   delusional disorder (143)
    Hallucinogen
305.30*   hallucinosis (144)
292.11*   delusional disorder (146)
292.84*   mood disorder (146)
292.89*   Posthallucinogen percep-
    tion disorder (147)
    Inhalant
305.90*   intoxication (148)
    Nicotine
292.00*   withdrawal (150)
    Opioid
305.50*   intoxication (151)
292.00*   withdrawal (152)
    Phencyclidine (PCP) or sim-
    ilarly acting arlcyclohexy-
    lamine
305.90*   intoxication (154)
292.81*   delirium (155)
292.11*   delusional disorder (156)
292.84*   mood disorder (156)
292.90*   organic mental disorder
    NOS
    Sedative, hypnotic, or anxi-
    olytic
305.40*   intoxication (158)
292.00*   Uncomplicated sedative,
    hypnotic, or anxiolytic
    withdrawal (159)
292.00*   withdrawal delirium (160)
292.83*   amnestic disorder (161)
    Other or unspecified psycho-
    active substance (162)
305.90*   intoxication
292.00*   withdrawal
292.81*   delirium
292.82*   dementia
292.83*   amnestic disorder
292.11*   delusional disorder
292.12*   hallucinosis
292.84*   mood disorder
292.89*   anxiety disorder
292.89*   personality disorder

292.90*   organic mental disorder
NOS

***Organic Mental Disorders Associated
with Axis III Physical Disorders or
Conditions, or Whose Etiology is
Unknown (162)***

293.00   Delirium (100)
294.10   Dementia (103)
294.00   Amnestic disorder (108)
293.81   Organic delusional disorder
(109)
293.82   Organic hallucinosis (110)
293.83   Organic mood disorder (111)
Specify: manic, depressed,
mixed
294.80*   Organic anxiety disorder
(113)
310.10   Organic personality disorder
(114)
Specify: if explosive type
294.80*   Organic mental disorder
NOS

**PSYCHOACTIVE SUBSTANCE USE
DISORDERS (165)**

Alcohol (173)
303.90   dependence
305.00   abuse
Amphetamine or similarly
acting sympathomimetic
(175)
304.40   dependence
305.70*   abuse
Cannabis (176)
304.30   dependence
305.20*   abuse
Cocaine (177)
304.20   dependence
305.60*   abuse
Hallucinogen (179)
304.50*   dependence
305.30*   abuse
Inhalant (180)
304.60   dependence
305.90*   abuse

Nicotine (181)
305.10   dependence
Opioid (182)
304.00   dependence
305.50*   abuse
Phencyclidine (PCP) or similarly acting arlcyclohexy-
lamine (183)
304.50*   dependence
305.90*   abuse
Sedative, hypnotic, or anxi-
olytic (184)
304.10   dependence
305.40*   abuse
304.90*   Polysubstance dependence
(185)
304.90*   Psychoactive substance dependence NOS
305.90*   Psychoactive substance
abuse NOS

SCHIZOPHRENIA (187)

Code in fifth digit; 1 = subchronic,
2 = chronic, 3 = subchronic with
acute exacerbation, 4 = chronic with
acute exacerbation, 5 = in remission,
0 = unspecified.
Schizophrenia,
295.2x   catatonic,_____
295.1x   disorganized,_____
295.3x   paranoid,_____
Specify if stable type
295.9x   undifferentiated,_____
295.6x   residual,_____
Specify if late onset

**DELUSIONAL (PARANOID) DISORDER
(199)**

297.10   Delusional (paranoid) disorder
Specify type: erotomanic
grandiose
jealous
persecutory
somatic
unspecified

PSYCHOTIC DISORDERS NOT ELSEWHERE CLASSIFIED (205)

298.80	Brief reactive psychosis (205)
295.40	Schizophreniform disorder (207)
	Specify: without good prognostic features or with good prognostic features
295.70	Schizoaffective disorder (208)
	Specify: bipolar type or depressive type
297.30	Induced psychotic disorder (210)
298.90	Psychotic disorder NOS (atypical psychosis) (211)

MOOD DISORDERS (213)

Code current state of major depression and bipolar disorder in fifth digit:

1 = mild
2 = moderate
3 = severe, without psychotic features
4 = with psychotic features (specify mood-congruent or mood-incongruent)
5 = in partial remission
6 = in full remission
0 = unspecified

For major depressive episodes, specify if chronic and specify if melancholic type.
For bipolar disorder, bipolar disorder NOS, recurrent major depression, and depressive disorder NOS, specify if seasonal pattern.

Bipolar Disorders

	Bipolar disorder, (225)
296.6x	mixed,_____
296.4x	manic,_____
296.5x	depressed,_____
301.13	Cyclothymia (226)
296.70	Bipolar disorder NOS

Depressive disorders

	Major depression, (228)
296.2x	single episode,_____
296.3x	recurrent,_____
300.40	Dysthymia (or depressive neurosis) (230)
	Specify: primary or secondary type
	Specify: early or late onset
311.00	Depressive disorder NOS

ANXIETY DISORDERS (OR ANXIETY AND PHOBIC NEUROSES) (235)

	Panic disorder (235)
300.21	with agoraphobia
	Specify: current severity of agoraphobic avoidance
	Specify: current severity of panic attacks
300.01	without agoraphobia
	Specify: current severity of panic attacks
300.22	Agoraphobia without history of panic disorder (240)
	Specify: with or without limited symptom attacks
300.23	Social phobia (241)
	Specify: if generalized type
300.29	Simple phobia (243)
300.30	Obsessive compulsive disorder (or obsessive compulsive neurosis) (245)
309.89	Post-traumatic stress disorder (247)
	Specify: if delayed onset
300.02	Generalized anxiety disorder (251)
300.00	Anxiety disorder NOS

SOMATOFORM DISORDERS (255)

300.70*	Body dysmorphic disorder (255)

300.11   Conversion disorder (or hysterical neurosis, conversion type) (257)
    Specify: single episode or recurrent
300.70*   Hypochondriasis (or hypochondriacal neurosis) (259)
300.81   Somatization disorder (261)
307.80   Somatoform pain disorder (264)
300.70   Undifferentiated somatoform disorder (266)
300.70*   Somatoform disorder NOS (267)

DISSOCIATIVE DISORDERS (OR HYSTERICAL NEUROSES, DISSOCIATIVE TYPE) (269)

300.14   Multiple personality disorder (269)
300.13   Psychogenic fugue (272)
300.12   Psychogenic amnesia (273)
300.60   Depersonalization disorder (or depersonalization neurosis) (275)
300.15   Dissociative disorder NOS

SEXUAL DISORDERS (279)

Paraphilias (279)

302.40   Exhibitionism (282)
302.81   Fetishism (282)
302.89   Frotteurism (283)
302.20   Pedophilia (284)
    Specify: same sex, opposite sex, same and opposite sex
    Specify: if limited to incest
    Specify: exclusive type or nonexclusive type
302.83   Sexual masochism (286)
302.84   Sexual sadism (287)
302.30   Transvestic fetishism (288)
302.82   Voyeurism (289)
302.90*   Paraphilia NOS (290)

Sexual Dysfunctions (290)

Specify: psychogenic only, or psychogenic and biogenic (Note: If biogenic only, code on Axis III)
Specify: lifelong or acquired
Specify: generalized or situational
    Sexual desire disorders (293)
302.71   Hypoactive sexual desire disorder
302.79   Sexual aversion disorder
    Sexual arousal disorders (294)
302.72*   Female sexual arousal disorder
302.72*   Male erectile disorder
    Orgasm disorders (294)
302.73   Inhibited female orgasm
302.74   Inhibited male orgasm
302.75   Premature ejaculation
    Sexual pain disorders (295)
302.76   Dyspareunia
306.51   Vaginismus
302.70   Sexual dysfunction NOS

Other Sexual Disorders

302.90*   Sexual disorder NOS

SLEEP DISORDERS (297)

Dyssomnias (298)

    Insomnia disorder
307.42*   related to another mental disorder (nonorganic) (300)
780.50*   related to known organic factor (300)
307.42*   Primary insomnia (301)
    Hypersomnia disorder
307.44   related to another mental disorder (nonorganic) (303)
780.50*   related to a known organic factor (303)
780.54   Primary hypersomnia (305)

307.45   Sleep-wake schedule disorder (305)
         Specify: advanced or delayed phase type, disorganized type, frequently changing type
         Other dyssomnias
307.40* Dyssomnia NOS

Parasomnias (308)

307.47   Dream anxiety disorder (nightmare disorder) (308)
307.46* Sleep terror disorder (310)
307.46* Sleepwalking disorder (311)
307.40* Parasomnia NOS (313)

FACTITIOUS DISORDERS (315)

         Factitious disorder
301.51   with physical symptoms (316)
300.16   with psychological symptoms (318)
300.19   Factitious disorder NOS (320)

IMPULSE CONTROL DISORDERS NOT ELSEWHERE CLASSIFIED (321)

312.34   Intermittent explosive disorder (321)
312.32   Kleptomania (322)
312.31   Pathological gambling (324)
312.33   Pyromania (325)
312.39* Trichotillomania (326)
312.39* Impulse control disorder NOS (328)

ADJUSTMENT DISORDER (329)

         Adjustment disorder
309.24   with anxious mood
309.00   with depressed mood
309.30   with disturbance of conduct
309.40   with mixed disturbance of emotions and conduct
309.28   with mixed emotional features

309.82   with physical complaints
209.83   with withdrawal
309.23   with work (or academic) inhibition
309.90   Adjustment disorder NOS

PSYCHOLOGICAL FACTORS AFFECTING PHYSICAL CONDITION (333)

316.00   Psychological factors affecting physical condition
         Specify physical condition on Axis III

Personality Disorders (335)

Note: These are coded on Axis II.

Cluster A

301.00   Paranoid (337)
301.20   Schizoid (339)
301.22   Schizotypal (340)

Cluster B

301.70   Antisocial (342)
301.83   Borderline (346)
301.50   Histrionic (348)
301.81   Narcissistic (349)

Cluster C

301.82   Avoidant (351)
301.60   Dependent (353)
301.40   Obsessive compulsive (354)
301.84   Passive aggressive (356)
301.90   Personality disorder NOS

V CODES FOR CONDITIONS NOT ATTRIBUTABLE TO A MENTAL DISORDER THAT ARE A FOCUS OF ATTENTION OR TREATMENT (359)

V62.30   Academic problem
V71.01   Adult antisocial behavior

V40.00   Borderline intellectual functioning (Note: This is coded on Axis II.)

V71.02	Childhood or adolescent antisocial behavior
V65.20	Malingering
V61.10	Marital problem
V15.81	Noncompliance with medical treatment
V62.20	Occupational problem
V61.20	Parent-child problem
V62.81	Other interperesonal problem
V61.80	Other specified family circumstances
V62.89	Phase of life problem or other life circumstance problem
V62.82	Uncomplicated bereavement

ADDITIONAL CODES (363)

300.90	Unspecified mental disorder (nonpsychotic)
V71.09*	No diagnosis or condition on Axis I

799.90*	Diagnosis or condition deferred on Axis I

V71.09*	No diagnosis or condition on Axis II
799.90*	Diagnosis or condition deferred on Axis II

MULTIAXIAL SYSTEM

Axis I	Clinical syndromes V codes
Axis II	Developmental disorders Personality disorders
Axis III	Physical disorders and conditions
Axis IV	Severity of psychosocial stressors
Axis V	Global assessment of functioning

Appendix B

NANDA-Accepted Diagnoses

Activity intolerance
Activity intolerance, potential
Adjustment, impaired
Airway clearance, ineffective
Anxiety
Aspiration, potential for
Body image disturbance
Body temperature, altered, potential
Breastfeeding, ineffective
Breastfeeding, impaired
Breathing pattern, ineffective
Cardiac output, decreased
Communication, impaired verbal
Constipation
Constipation, colonic
Constipation, perceived
Coping, defensive
Coping, family: potential for growth
Coping, ineffective family: compro-
  mised
Coping, ineffective family: disabling
Coping, ineffective individual
Decisional conflict (specify)
Denial, ineffective
Diarrhea
Disuse syndrome, potential for
Diversional activity deficit
Dysreflexia
Family processes, altered
Fatigue
Fear
Fluid volume deficit (1)

Fluid volume deficit (2)
Fluid volume deficit, potential
Fluid volume excess
Gas exchange, impaired
Grieving, anticipatory
Grieving, dysfunctional
Growth and development, altered
Health maintenance, altered
Health seeking behaviors (specify)
Home maintenance management,
  impaired
Hopelessness
Hyperthermia
Hypothermia
Incontinence, bowel
Incontinence, functional
Incontinence, reflex
Incontinence, stress
Incontinence, total
Incontinence, urge
Infection, potential for
Injury, potential for
Knowledge deficit (specify)
Mobility, impaired physical
Noncompliance (specify)
Nutrition, altered: less than body re-
  quirements
Nutrition, altered: more than body
  requirements
Nutrition, altered: potential for more
  than body requirements
Oral mucous membrane altered

Pain
Pain, chronic
Parental role conflict
Parenting, altered
Parenting, altered, potential
Personal identity disturbance
Poisoning, potential for
Post-trauma response
Powerlessness
Protective mechanisms, altered
Rape-trauma syndrome
Rape-trauma syndrome: compound
    reaction
Rape-trauma syndrome: silent reaction
Role performance, altered
Self care deficit, bathing/hygiene
Self care deficit/feeding
Self care deficit/toileting
Self-esteem, disturbance
Self-esteem, chronic low
Self-esteem, situational low
Sensory perceptual alterations (spec-
    ify) (visual, auditory, kinesthetic,
    gustatory, tactile, olfactory)

Sexual dysfunction
Sexuality patterns, altered
Skin integrity, impaired
Skin integrity, impaired, potential
Sleep pattern disturbance
Social interaction, impaired
Social isolation
Spiritual distress (distress of the human
    spirit)
Suffocation, potential for
Swallowing, impaired
Thermoregulation, ineffective
Thought processes, altered
Tissue integrity, impaired
Tissue perfusion, altered (specify type)
    (renal, cerebral, cardiopulmonary,
    gastrointestinal, peripheral)
Trauma, potential for
Unilateral neglect
Urinary elimination, altered patterns
Urinary retention
Violence, potential for self-directed or
    directed at other's

Index

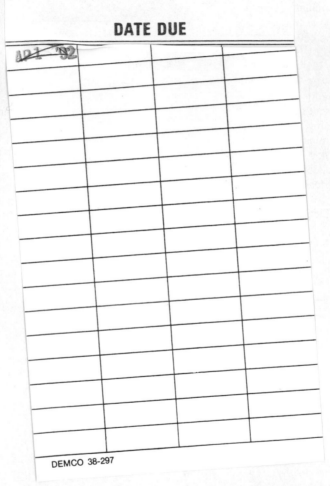

DATE DUE

APR '92

DEMCO 38-297